The
PATHOLOGY
of
DRUG ABUSE

Steven B. Karch

Trauma Office
University Medical Center
Las Vegas, Nevada

CRC Press
Boca Raton   Ann Arbor   London   Tokyo

bib: 23916   # 27800364

Library of Congress Cataloging-in-Publication Data

Catalog record is available from the Library of Congress

Direct all inquiries to CRC Press, Inc., 2000 Corporate Blvd., N. W., Boca Raton, Florida, 33431.

© 1993 by CRC Press, Inc.

International Standard Book Number 0-8493-4418-2

Printed in the United States 1 2 3 4 5 6 7 8 9 0
Printed on acid-free paper

DEDICATION

For my wife and for our friends from Kalimantan
And for Sam.

Preface

Physicians deal with the consequences of drug abuse on a daily basis, but information about the basic pathology of abused drugs is hard to come by. Hundreds of papers have been published describing the effects of drug abuse on brain neurochemistry, but practitioners are hard pressed to find out how cocaine affects blood vessels or how heroin affects the lung. I hope this book supplies the information they need. While far from encyclopedic, I think the book does provide answers to most of the questions physicians ask when they are confronted with cases of drug-related death or disability.

In the course of writing the sections on heroin, I was surprised to discover that more than twenty years have elapsed since the first papers were published by Milton Helpern, Charles Wetli, and Michael Baden. Since that time, our government has done little to foster research into the pathology of abused drugs, and knowledge has advanced very little. With the advent of the great HIV pandemic, there may be a price to pay for this lack of knowledge, and for the failure to foster meaningful research. Perhaps with changing government priorities this situation will some day be rectified.

Finally, readers of the book will notice two important omissions: alcohol and marijuana. The reason for not dealing with the former is that alcohol requires its own book. The reason for not discussing the latter is that there isn't enough good anatomic pathology to write about, although recently there have been some interesting studies dealing with marijuana toxicology. I hope that this subject can be added in future editions.

Stephen B. Karch, M.D.
Berkeley, California
November, 1992

ACKNOWLEDGMENTS

All of my teaching files were lost in the Oakland Hills Wildfire of 1991. If it were not for the generous assistance of the contributors listed below, this book would have had a lot fewer illustrations!

Dr. Margaret Billingham, Chairman, Cardiovascular Pathology, Stanford University School of Medicine
Dr. Arthur K. Cho, Department of Pharmacology, UCLA School of Medicine
Dr. Jacques Gilloteaux, Department of Anatomy, College of Medicine, Northeastern Ohio Universities
Dr. François Gray, Department of Pathology, Hôpital Henri Mondor, Creteil, France
Dr. Peter S. Hersh, Chairman, Department of Ophthalmology, Bronx-Lebanon Hospital
Dr. Robert Kloner, Hospital of the Good Samaritan, Los Angeles
Dr. Russell Kridel, University of Texas, Health Sciences Center, Houston
Dr. David A. Krendel, Section of Neurology, The Emory Clinic
Professor M. Maillet, Hôpital Lariboisère, Paris
National Library of Medicine, Bethesda, Maryland
Marilyn Masek, Laboratory of Cardiovascular Pathology, Stanford University School of Medicine
Dr. Giuseppe G. Pietra, Director, Division of Anatomic Pathology, Hospital of the University of Pennsylvania
Dr. N.G. Ryley, University of Oxford, Nuffield Department of Pathology and Bacteriology, Oxford, England
Stephen M. Roberts, University of Florida, Center for Environmental and Human Toxicology
Dr. J. M. Soares, Faculty of Sport Sciences, University of Porto, Portugal
Dr. Randall L. Tackett, Head, Department of Pharmacology and Toxicology, University of Georgia
Dr. Renu Virmani, Chairman, Department of Cardiovascular Pathology, Armed Forces Institute of Pathology
U.S. Department of Justice, Drug Enforcement Administration

I also wish to thank *Professor Henry Urich* of the London Hospital, and *Professor Margaret Billingham* of Stanford University, for their years of patient instruction. A special thanks also to Drs. *Hardwin Mead* and *Roger Winkle*. Without their help this book would not have been written. Thanks also to *William Keach* for his help in manuscript corrections, and to *Sam Karch* for his help in general.

Table of Contents

1 Cocaine

1.1 HISTORY

The word "coca" comes from the Aymara "khoka," meaning "the tree." Coca has nothing to do with the chocolate-producing nut called cocoa, and its only relation to the kola nut is phonetic. Measurable quantities of cocaine and nicotine have been detected in 3,000-year old Egyptian mummies (Balabanova, Parsche, Pirsig 1992),but both chemicals are derived from New World plants, and how they came to be used in Africa remains a mystery. Even if these plants were known to the ancient Egyptians, Europeans didn't hear about them until the Spanish colonized South America. When the Spanish took Peru in the 1500's, they encountered Indians who had been chewing coca leaf for thousands of years. The Indians' experience with coca was recounted in Nicolas B. Monardes' monograph, *Joyfulle News out of the New Founde Worlde, wherein is declared the Virtues of Herbs, Treez, Oyales, Plantes, and Stones*. Monardes' book was reprinted many times after first being published in Barcelona sometime in the early 1560's. In 1599 a translation by an English merchant was published in London. Monardes' book contained accurate descriptions of many New-World plants, including tobacco and coca. Monardes was fascinated by the fact that coca appeared to allow users to go without food, but he also was aware that coca had undesirable side effects. He observed "Surely it is a thyng of greate consideration, to see how the Indians are so desirous to bee deprived of their wittes, and be without understanding" (Guerra, 1974).

For a long time the medical community remained unimpressed with coca. Boerhave favorably mentioned coca in his textbook on medicinal plants, published in 1708 (Mortimer, 1901), however more than 100 years elapsed before the first illustration of coca appeared in an English publication. An article on coca by Sir William Hooker, then curator of the Royal Botanical Gardens at Kew, appeared in 1835. In addition to illustrations of the coca plant, the article also contained Hooker's translation of a book by the German explorer and naturalist Edward Poeppig. Poeppig thought that coca chewers were very much like opium addicts and warned against coca's immoderate use (Poeppig, 1835). Other travelers and explorers had more positive impressions, but coca's potential for toxicity was known even before it became widely available in Europe.

Johan von Tschudi was one of the early explorers of the Amazon. He was a prolific writer, and his travel books were widely read in Europe and the United States. He too was impressed with coca's apparent ability to increase endurance, but he was concerned that Europeans might develop a "habit." His book "Travels in Peru", first published in 1852, contains the first accurate description of cocaine "binging" (Tschudi, 1854). The term describes the tendency of cocaine users to consume, in one session, all the drug in their possession. According to von Tschudi, "They give themselves up for days together to the passionate enjoyment of the leaves. Then their excited imaginations conjure up the most wonderful visions...I have never yet been able to ascertain correctly the conditions the Coquero passes through on returning to his ordinary state; it however appears that it is not so much a want of sleep, or the absence of food, as the want of Coca that puts an end to the lengthened debauch."

In 1857 Von Tschudi persuaded a professor of chemistry at the University of La Paz, Enrique Pizzi, to try isolating coca's active principle. Pizzi thought he had succeeded and gave Von Tschudi a sample to take home to Europe. Returning to Göttingen, von Tschudi gave the sample to his friend Carl Wöhler, the chemist who had first synthesized urea. Wöhler gave the sample to Albert Niemann, his graduate student. Niemann found the sample contained only gypsum. Wöhler remained curious, and when he heard that Archduke Ferdinand was sending a frigate on a round the world training cruise, he approached Carl von Scherzer, chief scientist of the expedition, and asked him if he could bring back enough leaves to analyze (Scherzer, 1861). Von Scherzer returned three years later with 60 pounds of leaf and gave them to Wöhler, who again gave them to Nieman. Given an adequate supply of leaf, purification of cocaine proved relatively simple. Nieman published his Ph.D. thesis, "On a New Organic Base in the Coca Leaves" in 1860 (Niemann, 1860). Even after the purification of cocaine, interest in its therapeutic applications remained slight, and reports in journals were still mostly anecdotal. A *Lancet* editorial published in 1872, twelve years after cocaine had been purified, stated that "There is considerable difference of opinion as to its effects upon the human subject, and the published accounts are somewhat conflicting; but we think that there is a strong evidence in favor of its being a stimulant and narcotic of a peculiar kind, and of some power." (anon, 1872). The amount of cocaine contained in these products was modest. However, it is now known that when alcohol and cocaine are combined, a new metabolite called cocaethylene is formed. It has the same affinity for the dopamine receptor as cocaine itself, which means that it should be just as psychoactive. Since it has a half life that is many times longer than that of cocaine, combinations of alcohol and cocaine may be quite intoxicating.

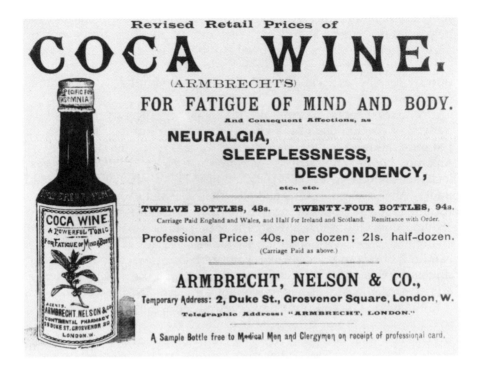

Figure 1.1 Coca containing wines
These became popular during the 1860's. The most famous was Vin Mariani, but there were many competitors. The average product contained 5 to 10 mg of cocaine per ounce. From the National Library of Medicine.

Coca-containing wines became popular in France and Italy during the late 1860's. The most famous of these was manufactured by Angelo Mariani. It contained 6 mg of cocaine per ounce and was advertised as a restorative and tonic. And that seems to have been how it was used. Satisfied customers endorsing Vin Mariani included Thomas Edison, Robert Louis Stevenson, Jules Verne, Alexandre Dumas, and even Pope Leo XIII. Within ten years of its introduction in Paris, Mariani's wines were in much demand throughout the United States (Mariani, 1872).

In the early 1880's, Parke Davis and Company began marketing a fluid extract containing 0.5 mg/mL of semipurified cocaine. At about the same time physicians began prescribing elixirs containing cocaine for a variety of ailments, including alcohol and morphine addiction. In spite of the inappropriate use of these mixtures, reports of toxicity and cocaine-related disease were rare. Concurrent with the increased dispensing by physicians, patent medicine manufacturers began adding cocaine extract to nearly all of their products. One such promoter was John Styth Pemberton. He went into competition with Mariani and began selling "French Wine Cola". His initial marketing efforts were not very successful. In what proved to be a wise marketing move, Pemberton dropped the wine from the product, and added a combination of cocaine and caffeine. The reformulated product was named "Coca-Cola."

Two events occurred in 1884 that significantly changed the pattern of cocaine use in the United States and Europe. The first was the publication of Freud's paper, Über Coca (Freud, 1884) (Andrews & Solomon, 1975). The second was Köller's discovery that cocaine was a local anesthetic (Noyes, 1884). By the time Freud sat down to write his paper, American physicians had already published over a dozen papers recommending cocaine in the treatment of morphine addiction (Bently, 1880). Freud enthusiastically accepted this American notion and even elaborated on it, recommending cocaine as a remedy for a host of conditions that are not even recognized as diseases today. Köller's discovery was probably even more important. The availability of an effective local anesthetic had tremendous impact. Cocaine was propelled into the limelight, and physicians around the world were soon experimenting with the use of cocaine in wide range of conditions. Some of the applications, such as eye and hemorrhoid surgery (anon, 1886c), were quite appropriate. Other applications, such as the treatment of hayfever, were more questionable (anon, 1886a). Still other uses were bizarre and potentially dangerous (anon, 1886b).

The first reports of cocaine toxicity appeared less than one year after Köller's and Freud's papers were published. An article in the British Medical Journal described the toxic reactions associated with cocaine use in ophthalmologic surgery (anon, 1885b), and at about the same time, reports of cocaine related death started appearing in the popular press (anon, 1885a). The first cocaine-related cardiac arrest was reported in 1886 (Thompson, 1886), as was the first stroke (Catlett, 1886). In 1887, Mattison reviewed 50 cases of cocaine toxicity, four of them fatal. Each of the fatalities had the characteristics associated with cardiac arrhythmias (Mattison, 1887b) (Mattison, 1887a). The following year Mattison published data on an additional 40 cases, including two more fatalities (Mattison, 1888).

None of these negative reports appeared to have much impact. Patent-medicine manufacturers continued to cash in on the popularity of coca by replacing low-concentration cocaine extracts with high concentrations of refined cocaine hydrochloride. Thousands of cocaine-containing patent medicines flooded the market, some with truly enormous amounts of cocaine. Dr.Tucker's Asthma Specific, for instance, contained 420 mg of cocaine per ounce and was applied directly to the nasal mucosa. Absorption was nearly total. As the cocaine content of the products increased, so did the number of reported

THE OPHTHALMOLOGICAL CONGRESS IN HEIDELBERG.

(From our Special Correspondent.)

MURIATE OF COCAINE AS A LOCAL ANÆSTHETIC TO THE CORNEA—NO RADIATING MUSCULAR FIBRES IN THE IRIS—ACTUAL CAUTERY IN SUPERFICIAL CORNEAL ULCERATIONS—OPTICO-CILIARY NEURECTOMY—IS CATARACT THE RESULT OF CHRONIC BRIGHT'S DISEASE?—PROFESSOR ARLT AND HIS RECENT WORK IN GLAUCOMA.

KREUZNACH, GERMANY, September 19, 1884.

SIR : The usual Ophthalmological Congress in Heidelberg has just closed its session, and a few cursory notes at this early date may interest some readers. At this meeting elaborate papers are not read, but condensed statements are presented of the subjects introduced. The notable feature of this Society is that only new things or new phases of old topics are presented. This is not from any expressed rule, but is from the tacit understanding which controls men who are so diligently investigating the unknown in science as are these eager workers. These men have no patience with mere reiterations. Perhaps the most notable thing which was presented was the exhibition to the Congress upon one of the patients of the Heidelberg Eye Clinic, of the extraordinary anæsthetic power which a two per cent. solution of muriate of cocaine has upon the cornea and conjunctiva when it is dropped into the eye. Two drops of the solution were dropped into the eye of the patient at the first experiment, and after an interval of ten minutes it was evident that the sensitiveness of the surface was below the normal, then two drops more were instilled and after waiting ten minutes longer there was entire absence of sensibility, a probe was pressed upon the cornea until its surface was indented, it was rubbed lightly over the surface of the cornea, it was rubbed over the surface of the conjunctiva bulbi, and of the conjunctiva palpebrarum ; a speculum was introduced to separate the lids and they were stretched apart to the uttermost ; the conjunctiva bulbi was seized by fixation forceps and the globe moved in various directions. In all this handling the patient declared that he felt no unpleasant sensation, except that the speculum stretched the lids so widely asunder as to give a little discomfort at the outer canthus. Before the experiment his eye was shown to possess the normal sensitiveness, and the other eye, which was not experimented on, was in this respect perfectly normal. The solution caused no irritation of any kind, nor did it at all influence the pupil. The anæsthetic influence seemed to be complete on the surface of the eye, and it lasted for about fifteen minutes and the parts then resumed their usual condition. This first experiment was done in the presence of Professor Arlt, of Professor Becker, of the clinical staff, of Dr. Ferrer of San Francisco, of some other physicians, and of the writer. The next day the same experiment was performed on the same patient in the presence of the Congress and with the same results. This application of the muriate of cocaine is a discovery by a very young physician, or he is perhaps not yet a physician, but is pursuing his studies in Vienna, where he also lives. His name is Dr. Koller, and he gave to Dr. Brettauer, of Trieste, a vial of it, to be used in the presence of the Congress by Dr. Brettauer. Dr. Koller had but very recently become aware of this notable effect of cocaine, and had made but very few trials with it. These he had been led to make from his knowledge of the entirely similar effect which it has for some year or more been shown to have over the sensibility of the vocal cords, and because of which laryngologists pencil it upon their surface to facilitate examinations.

The future which this discovery opens up in ophthalmic surgery and in ophthalmic medication is obvious. The momentous value of the discovery seems likely to prove to be in eye practice of more significance than has been the discovery of anæsthesia by chloroform and ether in general surgery and medicine, because it will have therapeutic uses as well as surgical uses. It remains, however, to investigate all the characteristics of this substance, and we may yet find that there is a shadow side as well as a brilliant side in the discovery. Professor Kühne, who in the Heidelberg Physiological Laboratory worked out the details of Boll's discovery of the visual purple of the retina, received the news of this new discovery with the liveliest interest. We may, perhaps, get from him a further investigation into its properties. The substance makes a clear solution, and is found in Merck's catalogue.

Another notable statement came from Dr. Eversburch, of Munich, as the result of very exact and elaborate studies, to the effect that there are no radiating muscular fibres in the iris ; in other words, that the dilator iridis has no existence in man. It is found, he says, in some animals, and especially in those which have oblong pupils, whether vertical or horizontal, and in the form of fasciculi at the extremities of the slit. He absolutely denies the existence of such fibres in the human eye, and asserts that the fibres hitherto described under this name are nerve-fibres. These revolutionary assertions were received with respect and attention, because the investigator was known to be a careful and competent anatomist. If his declarations should be confirmed, and they will not be lightly accepted, we must find out a new theory for the active dilatation of the pupil. A good deal of physiology will have to be cast into a new form. It is true that the anatomical discussion has not been closed on this point, but in favor of the existence of the dilator stand the names of Merkel, Henle, and Iwanoff among recent investigators. Eversburch has in his possession the preparations of Iwanoff, who died a few years ago, and he knows the nature of the contest into which he enters.

The uses of the actual cautery in superficial forms of corneal ulceration and in some other superficial processes, especially in those of micrococcic origin, were discussed both here and in Copenhagen. There seems to be a general consensus as to the usefulness of this treatment in selected cases of superficial corneal disease, viz., in ulcus rodens, in superficial suppurative processes, in atonic ulcers, and by Nieden in xerophthalmus. Nieden will shortly announce his views in full in an article in the *Archives for Ophthalmology*. He presented a most delicate and elegant form of galvano-cautery which he had devised, and to which he had applied a very delicate and promptly acting key invented by Professor Sattler. Another form of cautery is in use in the Heidelberg Eye Clinic, which has been devised by Professor Becker, and is a very small and utilizable Paquelin cautery. Both these instruments can be handled with nicety and delicacy, and without frightening the patient, and also in most cases without giving him any pain. This treatment, as well as the scraping of such ulcers by a sharp spoon, as does Meyer, of Paris, is founded on the micrococcic theory of the pathology of these processes, and marks another forward step in ophthalmic therapeutics.

Optico-ciliary neurectomy as a preventive of sympathetic ophthalmia has not passed out of practice, as to a considerable degree has become the case among us. So able an observer and logical a reasoner as Professor Schweigger, of Berlin, recommends its performance and holds it in higher esteem than enucleation. He divides the internal rectus muscle to gain easy approach to the nerve, and he lifts it from its bed by a sharp double hook and excises 10 mm. of it. He is said to be extremely skilful in this proceeding, and the very small disturbance which he causes in the structures of the orbit may perhaps explain the success which he has had and the confidence which he expresses in its prophylactic virtue. Among over a hundred cases which furnished the material for his conclusions, in two cases he saw occur in the opposite eye an acute neuro-retinitis, with opalescent infiltration, etc. There was no reduction of vision either central or peripheral. In two weeks the appearance

Fig. 1.1.3 Cocaine as a local anesthetic
The discovery that cocaine was a potent local anesthetic revolutionized surgery. It was first reported at an ophthalmology congress in Heidelberg and shortly thereafter an account appeared in the *Medical Record* of October 11, 1884. From the Medical Library at the University of California, San Francisco.

medical complications. The situation rapidly deteriorated when users learned they could "snort" cocaine. Until the early 1900's, cocaine had been taken mainly by mouth or by injection. The fact that the first cases of septal perforation and collapse (saddle nose deformity) were not reported until 1904 suggests that "snorting" had only became popular a year or so earlier (Maier, 1926).

The first histologic studies of cocaine toxicity were published in 1888. Vasili Zanchevski of St. Petersburg studied the acute and chronic effects of cocaine in dogs. After a single lethal dose (24 mg/kg) the animals had changes typical of acute asphyxia. Smaller daily doses given for several weeks caused a "marked hyperemic condition of the central nervous system, in contrast to the rest of the organs, which were anemic." There were focal degenerative changes in the spinal ganglia, heart and liver. In some cases the myocytes had "lost their striae and (were) intensely granular" (Zanchevski, 1888). Though illustrations are lacking, Zanchevski descriptions suggest that he was the first to observe a form of contraction band necrosis occurring as a result of cocaine toxicity.

French researchers were the first to systematically study cocaine's psychological effects, largely because cocaine and morphine addiction were such a major problem in Paris. In 1889, at a meeting of the Biological Society of Paris, Magnon presented three cases illustrating that cocaine users were subject to tactile hallucinations. The symptom complex became known as "Magnon's symptom". In 1914, Georges Guillain contrasted the differences between cocaine and alcoholic hallucinations, commenting on how variable the effects of a given dose of cocaine could be (Maier, 1926).

One psychiatric disorder that has only recently been rediscovered is cocaine-associated agitated delirium. It was first described by an American, Edward Williams, in 1914 (Williams, 1914). The syndrome consists of multiple components, including wildly irrational behavior and feats of near superhuman strength that culminate in sudden death.

Because William's writings were patently racist, and because he observed the syndrome only in blacks, later historians wrote off his observations as racist hysteria (Kennedy, 1985). New reports of the syndrome began to appear again at the start of the current pandemic. The disorder has nothing to do with race, but is quite real (Wetli & Fishbain, 1985).

The first human autopsy study was published in 1922. Bravetta and Invernizzi described a 28-year old man who had been sniffing cocaine regularly for some months before his death. He neither drank nor used other drugs (Bravetta & Invernizzi, 1922). Hyperemia of the brain, lungs, and adrenals was noted and the heart was described as "flaccid" (cardiomyopathy?). The accompanying illustrations show lesions similar to those described by Zanchevski. Animal studies by the same authors confirmed the autopsy findings and also demonstrated

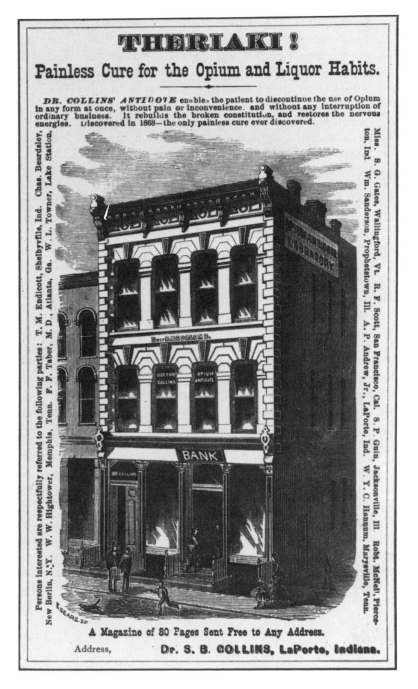

Fig. 1.1.4 Cocaine as a treatment for morphine addiction
Opiate addiction was a major problem during the 1870's. The principal ingredient in Theriaki, like most proprietary cures for addiction, was cocaine. From the National Library of Medicine.

wide-spread endothelial injuries. These studies were reprinted in Maier's classic text on cocaine abuse, published in 1926 (Maier, 1926).

Cocaine's tissue disposition was studied at an even earlier date. In 1887 a German chemist, Helmsing, published his technique for the detection of cocaine in urine and tissues. The technique was fairly sensitive, and Helmsing was able to detect cocaine in urine from a cat that had been given 8 mg of cocaine (anon, 1887). In 1951 Woods et al. developed a calorimetric technique capable of detecting levels of cocaine as low as 500 ng/mL (Woods, Cochin, Fornefeld et al., 1951). A quarter of century later Jatlow and Bailey used gas chromatography to lower the limits of detection down to 5 ng/mL (Jatlow & Bailey, 1975).

Shortly after Maier's text was published, case reports simply stopped appearing. Between 1924 and 1973 there was only one reported fatality, and it involved a surgical misadventure. In 1977 Suarez first described the "body packer" syndrome, where death results from the rupture of cocaine-filled condoms in the smuggler's intestines (Suarez, Arango & Lester, 1977). The absence of case reports no doubt reflected a decline in use, but the decline itself is difficult to explain. Certainly the outlawing of cocaine (The Pure Food and Drug Act of 1906 and the Harrison Narcotic Act of 1914) had a great deal to do with it, but other factors were involved (McLaughlin, 1973). Perhaps the most important factor may have been the introduction of the amphetamines. Although amphetamines share important mechanisms of toxicity with cocaine, the former appear to have a higher therapeutic index. In addition to being less toxic than cocaine, amphetamines are also cheaper, easier to obtain, and more socially acceptable.

Significant toxicity from the use of coca leaf and coca extract was never a problem in Europe or the United States. Toxicity only emerged when purified cocaine became readily available and individuals could increase their dosage by an order of magnitude. The small amounts of cocaine in Vin Mariani were apparently harmless, but the huge amounts in Dr. Tucker's formula were occasionally lethal. With the appearance of crack cocaine in 1986, another order of magnitude increase in dosage occurred (Jekel, Allen & Podlewski, 1986). That cocaine-related illness is now a significant cause of morbidity and mortality should not be surprising. It isn't just that more people are using the drug. They are using more of it and using it more effectively.

References
Andrews, G. & Solomon, D. (Ed.). (1975). The coca leaf and cocaine papers (1st ed.). New York and London:Harcourt Brace Jovanovich.

anon (1872). Coca. Lancet (May 25), 746.

anon (1885a). Cocaine's terrible effect. The New York Times, Vol 35 (10)684

anon (1885b). Toxic action of cucaine. Br Med J(November 21),p. 983

anon (1886a). Cucaine in hay-fever. Br Med J(May 8, 1886), 893.

anon (1886b). Cucaine in nymphomania. Br Med J(March 20), 564.

anon (1886c). Cucaine in painful defecation. Br Med J(March 27), 614.

anon (1887). The detection of cocaine in the animal body. Therapeutic Gazette, p 185.

Balabanova, S., Parsche. F., Pirsig, W. (1992). First identification of drugs in Egyptian mummies. Naturwissenschaften, 79:358

Bently, W. (1880). Erythroxylon Coca in the opium and alcohol habits. Therapeutic Gazette, i:253

Bravetta, E. & Invernizzi, G (1922).Il Cocainismo. Osservazione cliniche. Ricerche sperimentali e anatomo-patoligiche. Note Riv Psichiatr, 10, 543.

Catlett, G. (1886). Cocaine: what was its influence in the following case. Medical Gazette(February 6), 166.

Freud, S. (1884). Über coca. Wien Centralblatt für die ges Therapie, 2, 289–314.

Guerra, F. (1974). Sex and drugs in the 16th century. Br J Addict Alcohol, 69(3), 269–290.

Jatlow, P. & Bailey, D. (1975). Gas-chromatographic analysis for cocaine in human plasma, with use of a nitrogen detector. Clin Chem, 21, 918–1921.

Jekel, J.,Allen, D., Podlewski, H. et al. (1986). Epidemic freebase cocaine abuse: case study from the Bahamas. Lancet, 1, 459–462.

Kennedy, J. (1985). Coca Exotica: The illustrated story of cocaine (1st ed.). New York: Fairleigh Dickinson University Press and Cornwall Books.

Maier, H. W. (1926). Der Kokainismus (O.J. Kalant from the German 1926 edition, Trans.). Toronto: Addiction Research Foundation.

Mariani, A. (1872). La coca du Pérou. Rev de thérap méd chir Paris, 148–152.

Mattison, J. (1887a). Cocaine dosage and cocaine addiction. Pacific Med and Surg J and Western Lancet, XXX(4), 193–213; also Listed in the Index Medicus as Med Reg Phil, 1887, i:125–133

Mattison, J. (1887b). Cocaine habit. Lancet, 1, 1024.

Mattison, J. (1888). Cocaine toxemia. Am Pract and News, Louisville, 1888, n.s.v. 10–15

McLaughlin, G. (1973). Cocaine: The history and regulation of a dangerous drug. Cornell Law Rev, 58, 537–573.

Mortimer, W. G. (1901). Peru:history of coca, the "divine plant" of the Incas: with an introductory account of the Incas and of the Andean Indians of today (reprint ed.). New York: JH Vail, reprinted by AMS press in 1978.

Niemann, A. (1860). Über eine neue organische Base in den Cocablättern. Göttingen: E.A. Huth, Inaug.-diss.

Niemann, A. (1861). On the alkaloid and other constituents of coca leaves. Am J Pharmacy, 33(Third series, 9 (reprinted in), 123–127.

Noyes, H. (1884). Murate of cocaine as a local anaesthetic to the cornea; The ophthalmological Congress in Heidelberg. Med Record (October 11), 17–418.

Poeppig, E. (1835). Reise in Chile, Peru, und auf dem Amazonen Ströme während der Jahre 1827–1832 (republished in Stuttgart, Brockhaus in 1960 ed.). Leipzig: F. Fleischer.

Scherzer, K. (1861). Narrative of the circumnavigation of the globe by the Austrian Frigate Novara. London: Saunders, Otley, and Company.

Suarez, C.,Arango, A. & Lester, J. (1977). Cocaine-condom ingestion. JAMA, 238, 1391–1392.

Thompson, A. (1886). Toxic action of cucaine. Br Med J (January 9), 67.

Tschudi, J. J. (1854). Travels in Peru (Thomasina Ross, Trans.). New York: A.S. Barnes & Co.

Wetli, C. & Fishbain, D. (1985). Cocaine-induced psychosis and sudden death in recreational cocaine users. J Forensic Sci, 30(3), 873–888.

Williams, E. (1914, February 8). Negro cocaine "fiends" are a new southern menace. New York Times, p. 1.

Woods, L.,Cochin, J.,Fornefeld, E. et al. (1951). The estimation of amines in biological materials with critical data for cocaine and mescaline. J. Pharmacol Exp Ther, 101(2):188–199.

Zanchevski, V. (1888). Effects of acute and chronic cocaine-poisoning. Lancet,i (May 26), 1041.

1.2 CULTIVATION AND MANUFACTURE

1.2.1 CULTIVATION AND CROP YIELDS

Coca leaf has grown in the Andean sub-region for thousands of years. Early explorers found it all along the eastern curve of the Andes, from the Straits of Magellan to the borders of the Caribbean. Coca grows best on the moist, warm, slopes of mountains ranging from 1,500 to 5,000 feet. Coca shrubs grow to heights of 6–8 feet. The trunk of the plant is covered by rough, somewhat glossy bark that has a reddish tint. Its flowers are small, and usually white or greenish yellow. Leaves are elliptical, pointed at the apex, and dark green in color. All cultivated coca is derived from two closely related species that grow naturally only in South America, *Erythroxylum coca Lam* and *Erythroxylum novogranatense Hieron*. Each species has one distinct variety designated as *E. coca var. ipadu Plowman* and *E. Coca novogranatense var. truxillense* (Rusby) Plowman (Plowman, 1985). All four types are cultivated, though the alkaloid content of the different plants varies considerably (Plowman & River, 1983b). E. coca ipadu is cultivated only in the Amazon valley of Brazil, Colombia and Peru. Of all the cultivated varieties, ipadu contains the least alkaloid, less than 0.5%, and very little of that is cocaine. E. novogranatense is cultivated more widely and is better adapted to growth in hotter, drier climates. Although there is some controversy, it seems likely that novogranatense was the variety was cultivated in Java, Ceylon, India, and Taiwan. This variety may contain anywhere from 1 to 3% total alkaloid, with cocaine constituting as much as half of the total alkaloid present (Lee, 1981) (Bohm, Ganders & Plowman, 1982) (Plowman & River, 1983a) (Plowman, 1985) (Schlesinger, 1985). A strain of novogranatense cultivated in the desert coast region of Peru, near Trujillo, is the plant that is used to flavor Coca Cola and other cola beverages.

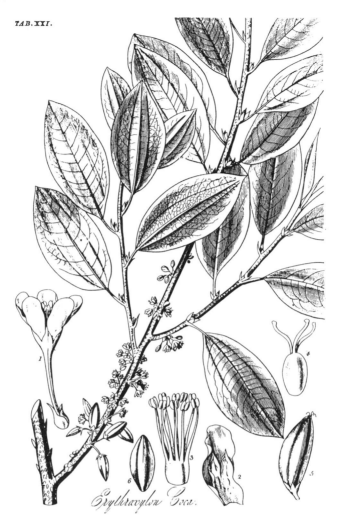

TAB.XXI.

Erythroxylon Coca.

Figure 1.2.1 The first illustrations of cocaine
The first illustration of coca to appear in an English magazine was published in
1836. It was drawn by Sir William Hooker, then director of the Royal Botanical
Gardens at Kew, and appeared in the *Companion to the Botanical Magazine*. From
the library at the Royal Botanical Gardens at Kew, England.

Major growing areas in Bolivia share many characteristics.
Yungas, which is close to La Paz, has an average annual rainfall of 45.7
inches and Chapare, which is close to Cochabamba, has an annual rainfall of 102 inches. The plantations in Yungas can be harvested three
times a year. Each harvest yields from 1 to 1.5 tons per hectare (890 to
1,336 pounds per acre) per year. The Chapare plantations, possibly
because of the higher rainfall, are harvested four times a year with a
yield of 2 to 3 tons per hectare (1,789 to 2,672 pounds per acre per year).

The average coca plantation will produce for about 20 years, but after about the tenth year, its yield steadily declines. Yields throughout South America are comparable. Both the yield per acre, and the alkaloid content of leaf, were much higher in the SE Asian plantations (at one time Indonesia exported more leaf than Peru). More than 60% of all coca leaf is grown in Peru, with another 22% coming from Bolivia and 15% from Colombia. Minor amounts come from Ecuador. When processed, 400 pounds of leaf will yield between 1 to 2 kg of coca paste, depending on the quality of the leaf and how efficiently the coca is extracted (Abruzzese, 1989).

1.2.2 COCAINE PASTE PRODUCTION

Cocaine extraction is a two or three step process, carried out in a series of laboratories. The first steps occur on site. Immediately after harvesting, leaves are placed in a shallow pit lined with heavy plastic and then soaked in a dilute solution of water and strong alkali, like lime, for 3 or 4 days. An organic solvent, which could be gasoline, kerosene, or even acetone, depending on availability, is then added to the mixture. In this way the nitrogenous alkaloids are extracted.

The extracted coca leaf is discarded and sulfuric acid is added to the extract, dissolving a complex mixture of alkaloids in the aqueous layer. If the alkaloid content of the leaves is very high (as in Bolivia), hydrochloric acid may be used instead of sulfuric. The organic solvent, usually kerosene, is then removed and the remaining aqueous solution is made alkaline by the addition of lime, ammonia, or the equivalent, causing the more basic alkaloids to precipitate out. This crude form of cocaine, called coca paste, is allowed to dry in the sun. The site where the initial steps occur is referred to as a pasta lab.   Laborers, called pisacocas, keep the alkali-coca leaf mulch mixed by stirring it with their hands and walking through it with their bare feet. The fluid is quite corrosive and the workers quickly develop large extremity ulcers. The pisacocas tolerate the ulcers only because they are given a constant supply of coca paste to smoke (Weatherford, 1988).

The dried product is a mixture of cocaine, cis - and trans- cinnamoylcocaine, tropine, tropacocaine, hygrine, cuscohygrine, ecgonine, benzoylecgonine, methylecgonine and isomers of truxillines. The mixture also contains a host of soluble organic plant waxes and benzoic acid. Depending on the alkaloid content of the leaves and on how the leaves were processed, it takes between 100 and 150 kilograms of dry leaf to produce 1 kilogram of pasta (Montesinos, 1965) (Brewer & Allen, 1991).

Once the pasta is prepared, the clandestine manufacturer has two options. The pasta may be further purified at a base lab, or the producer may go directly to a crystal lab. At base labs pasta is dissolved in dilute sulfuric acid. Potassium permanganate is added until the

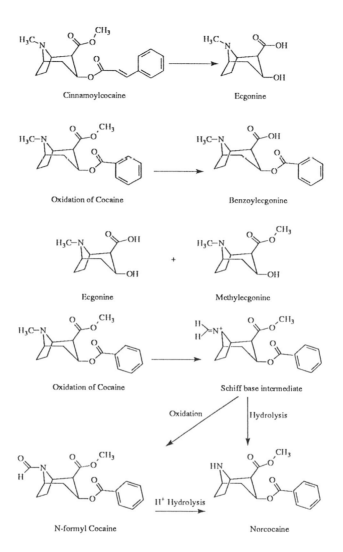

Figure 1.2.2.1 Cocaine refining
Cocaine refiners often add potassium permanganate to remove impurities. Cinnamoylcocaine is converted to ecgonine which is water soluble and easy to separate from cocaine. If the process is allowed to continue for too long, the cocaine itself is degraded and the yield drops. Norcocaine, which may be hepatotoxic, is formed at the same time.

solution turns pink, thereby destroying the cinnamoyl-cocaine isomers present as impurities in the pasta. The isomers of cinnamolycocaine are converted to ecgonine, and since ecgonine is very water soluble it is easy to separate from the cocaine. The job of the clandestine chemist is to stop the oxidation process (usually by adding ammonia or some other alkali) before the cocaine starts to oxidize, and the yield drops. Analysis

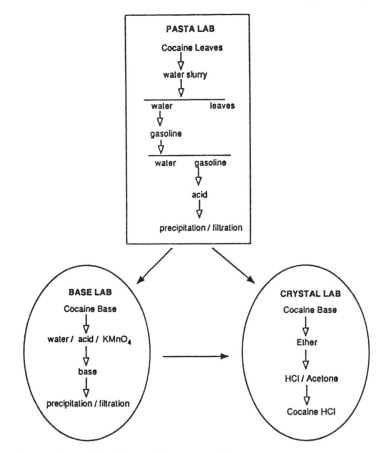

1.2.2.2 Flow chart of illicit cocaine processing
The preparation of purified cocaine from leaf, adapted from WHO bulletin

of impounded samples suggests that permanganate oxidation is used only about 60% of the time.

The reddish-pink solution is allowed to stand, then it is filtered and the filtrate is made basic with ammonia. Cocaine base precipitates out. The precipitate is filtered, washed with water, then dried. Finally it is dissolved in diethyl ether or acetone. After filtering, concentrated hydrochloric acid and acetone are added, causing purified cocaine hydrochloride to precipitate out (United Nations, 1986). This final step may be done on site, or the semipurified cocaine may be transported to a "crystal lab", usually located in one of the larger Colombian cities, although some drug producers have begun to set up labs in the United States. As much as 50 kg may be processed at one time (Lee, 1981). The semipurified cocaine is dissolved in a solvent, often ether. Hydrochloric acid is then added, along with a bridging solvent such as acetone, and white crystals precipitate out. The crystals are collected by filtration. Traces of the solvent remain and their presence can sometimes be used to identify the origin of cocaine samples. In producing countries there is a significant market for the semi-purified paste itself. Paste is smoked rolled up in pieces of newspaper or packed into cigarettes. Many of the ingredients introduced during manufacture are still present in the paste and are inhaled as pyrolysis products. Coca paste smoking is a major cause of morbidity in coca producing countries, but there is a paucity of scientific data about it (Paly, Van Dyke, Jatlow & Byck, 1980).

When permanganate is added during the refining process, cocaine's N-methyl group is oxidized, leading to the formation of N-formyl cocaine. Hydrolysis of N-formyl cocaine leads to the formation of norcocaine. The presence of the last two compounds can have forensic and clinical significance. Since N-formyl cocaine is a product of permanganate oxidation, it is not present in pasta. Accordingly, the presence of this compound may yield valuable information about how, and possibly where the cocaine sample was produced (Brewer & Allen, 1991). Norcocaine is potentially hepatotoxic. Analysis has shown norcocaine concentrations in illicit samples ranging from 0.01% to 3.70% (Kumar, 1991).

As might be expected, chemical analysis of paste has disclosed the presence of all the elements used during its manufacture, including benzoic acid, methanol, kerosene, sulfuric acid, cocaine sulfate and other coca alkaloids (Jeri, 1984; Jeri, Sanchez, del Pozo et al., 1978). Impurities may constitute anywhere from 1 to 40% of a given paste sample. Paste can be broken down into neutral, acidic and basic fractions. Gasoline residues are particularly common in the neutral fraction (ElSohly, Brenneisen & Jones, 1991). Unlike amphetamines, which may be contaminated with lead during the course of manufacture, analysis of paste samples shows them to be lead free. However, paste can contain large amounts of manganese, and the amount of manganese present is a marker for where the paste was produced. Colombian paste is manganese rich while Peruvian is not (ElSohly et al., 1991). Limited studies of blood levels suggest that the results of paste smoking are not much different than "crack" smoking (Paly, Jatlow, Van Dyke et al., 1980; Paly, Jatlow, Van Dyke et al., 1982; Paly et al., 1980).

The total synthesis of cocaine is possible, and clandestine cocaine laboratories have been confiscated. The process is, however, a great deal more demanding than the synthesis of amphetamine, and has never really been attempted on a large scale. The synthetic origin of the cocaine will be evident from the contaminants found along with the cocaine. Diastomers of cocaine, such as pseudococaine, allococaine, and the dl- form (which does not occur in nature) of cocaine are not found in cocaine refined from leaf (Soine, 1989).

The purity of confiscated cocaine is considered to be a good general indicator of availability. At wholesale levels, kilogram quantities that had been averaging 80 percent purity during 1990, increased to 87% purity during 1991. There is no recent sign that these purity levels are declining. At the retail level, ounce-sized specimens, which had been only 58% pure in 1990, had increased to 70% purity by 1991. The purity of the gram-sized samples sold on the street has increased by only 2% during the same period. From 1990 through the first nine months of 1991, the price in the U.S. for kilogram quantities ranged from $11,000 to $40,000.

References

Abruzzese, R. (1989). Coca-leaf production in the countries of the Andean subregion. Bull Narc, 41(1&2), 95–98.

Bohm, B.,Ganders, F. & Plowman, T. (1982). Biosystematics and evolution of cultivated coca (Erythroxylaceae). Systematic Botany, 7(2), 121–133.

Brewer, L. & Allen, A. (1991). N-formyl cocaine: a study of cocaine comparison parameters. J Forensic Sci, 36(3), 697–707.

Drug Enforcement Administration. (1992). Illegal drug price/purity report. United States, calendar year 1988 through September 1991. U.S. Department of Justice, DEA-92015, Washington, D.C.

ElSohly, M.,Brenneisen, R. & Jones, A. (1991). Coca paste: chemical analysis and smoking experiments. J Forensic Sci, 36(1), 93–103.

Jeri, F. (1984). Coca-paste smoking in some Latin American countries: a severe and unabated form of addiction. Bull Narc, 36(2), 15–31.

Jeri, F., Sanchez, C., del Pozo, T. et al. (1978). Further experience with the syndromes produced by coca paste smoking. Bull Narc, 30, 1–11.

Kumar, A. (1991). Identification and quantitation of norcocaine in illicit cocaine samples. In Annual Meeting of the American Academy of Forensic Sciences., (p. 73). Anaheim: AAFS.

Lee, D. (1981). Cocaine handbook. Berkeley: And/Or press.

Montesinos, F. (1965). Metabolism of cocaine. Bull Narc, 17(2), 11–17.

Paly, D., Jatlow, P., Van Dyke, C. et al. (1980). Plasma levels of cocaine in native Peruvian coca chewers. In F. Juri (Eds.), Cocaine 1980, Proceedings of the Interamerican Seminar on Coca and Cocaine (pp. 86–89). Lima: Pacific Press.

Paly, D.,Jatlow, P.,Van Dyke, C. et al. (1982). Plasma cocaine concentrations during cocaine paste smoking. Life Sci, 30 (9), 731–738.

Paly, D., Van Dyke, C., Jatlow, F. & Byck, R. (1980). Cocaine: plasma levels after cocaine paste smoking. In F. Jeri (Eds.), Cocaine: Proceedings of the Interamerican seminar on medical and sociological aspects of coca and cocaine (pp. 106–110). Lima, Peru:

Plowman, T. (1985). Coca and cocaine: effects on people and policy in Latin America. In D. Pacinie & C. Franquemont (Ed.), The coca leaf and its derivatives - biology, society and policy. Ithaca, New York: Cultural Survival, Inc.

Plowman, T. & Rivier, L. (1983b). Cocaine and cinnamoylcocaine of Erythroxylum species. Ann Botany, 51, 641–659.

Schlesinger, H. (1985). Topics in the chemistry of cocaine. Bull Narc, 37(1), 63–78.

Soine, W.H. (1989). Contamination of clandestinely prepared drugs with synthetic by-products. Proceedings of the 50th Annual Scientific Meeting, The Committee on Problems of Drug Dependence, published as NIDA Research Monograph 95:44–50.

Weatherford, J. (1988). Indian Givers. In The Drug Connection (p. 198). New York: Crown.

1.3 DRUG CONSTANTS

The free base has the formula $C_{17}H_{21}NO_4$ with a molecular weight of 303.4. It contains 67.31% carbon, 6.98% hydrogen, 4.62% nitrogen, and 21.10% oxygen. Pure cocaine forms colorless crystals or white crystalline powder. It is odorless and has a bitter taste. Its melting point is 98°C. However, it becomes volatile at temperatures over 90°C. Aqueous solutions are alkaline to litmus. The pKa at 15°C = 5.59. One gram dissolves in 600 mL of water, 6.5 mL of alcohol, 0.7mL of chloroform, 3.5 mL of ether or 12 mL of olive oil. It is also soluble in acetone and ethyl acetate.

Cocaine hydrochloride, referred to in the older literature as cocaine muriate, has the formula $C_{17}H_{22}ClNO_4$. Its composition is 60.08% carbon, 6.53% hydrogen, 4.12% nitrogen and 10.43 % chloride. Its molecular weight is 339.81. Either powdery, crystalline, or granular, it is water soluble and has a slightly bitter taste. The pKa is 8.6 and the melting point of pharmaceutical grade material is 195°C. One gram dissolves in 0.4 mL of water or 3.2 mL of cold alcohol. It is also soluble in chloroform (one gram in 12.5 mL), glycerol, and acetone. It is insoluble in ether or oils. When heated in solution it will decompose. Cocaine hydrochloride, stored in a tightly closed container at room temperature, will not decompose for at least five years. Solutions are stable for at least 21 days provided the temperature is below 24°C and the pH is below 4.0. Above that pH hydrolysis rapidly occurs (Muthadi & Al-Badr, 1986).

Reference
Muthadi, F. & Al-Badr, A. (1986). Cocaine Hydrochloride. Analyt Profiles of Drug Substances, 15, 151–230.

1.4 ROUTES OF ADMINISTRATION

1.4.1 LEAF CHEWING

Coca has been chewed for over 3,000 years, but the pharmacodynamics of the process have only been partially characterized. Habitual users chew an average of 12 to 15 grams of leaf three or four times a day. Depending on the quality of the leaf, the alkaloid content is usually less than 0.5%. Thus the total amount consumed at any one time is unlikely to amount to more than 75 mg. In one experiment, novice chewers who spit out their saliva, had average peak blood levels of 38 ng/mL at one hour. Experienced users, who swallow their saliva had mean values of 249 ng/mL, however the range was from 130 to 859 ng/mL (Paly,

Jatlow, Van Dyke, Cabieses & Byck, 1980) (Holmstedt, Lindgren, Rivier & Plowman, 1979). These levels probably lie towards the lower end of the spectrum of levels attained when the drug is snorted.

1.4.2 SNORTING

Variable levels result when cocaine is used in this fashion. In general, peak plasma concentrations are proportional to the amount of cocaine ingested (Wilkinson, Van Dyke, Jatlow, P & Byck, 1980). Because cocaine is a vasoconstrictor, it inhibits its own absorption and the time it takes to reach peak concentration gets longer as the dose gets larger. One hundred milligrams, which is approximately the equivalent of two to three "lines," will produce a blood level of 50–100 ng/mL, sufficient to cause transient increases in pulse and blood pressure (Javid, Fischman, Schuster et al., 1978) (Javid, Musa, Fischman et al., 1983) (Fischman, 1983) (Foltin, Fischman, Pedroso & Pearlson, 1988). Scanty data suggests that the "average" cocaine snorter will have blood levels not that much different from experienced leaf chewers. In one study intranasal application of 1.5 mg/kg (which would be 90 mg in a 60-kilo man, or roughly the amount of cocaine found in 15 grams of leaf) produced peak levels of 120–474 ng/mL 30 to 60 minutes afterward (Van Dyke, Barash, Jatlow & Byck, 1976). In a more recent study, a dose of 2 mg/kg (which amounted to between 100 and 255 mg total) produced peak levels ranging from 131 ng/mL up to 1,012 ng/mL, with an average of 370 ng/mL at 30 minutes. The average level fell to 295 ng/mL at 60 minutes, and 223 ng/mL at 90 minutes (Brogan, Lange, Glamann and Hillis 1992). Actual levels in abusers have not been quantitated. Clinical experience suggests that the use of a gram or more at one time is not uncommon, but ethical and safety considerations generally prohibit administration of such large doses in a laboratory setting.

1.4.3 SURGICAL APPLICATION

Blood levels after intranasal application in recreational users are generally much lower than those seen in patients undergoing surgical procedures. Otorhinolaryngologists and plastic surgeons still use combinations of epinephrine and cocaine to maintain a dry operative field. Different mixtures have been employed. The surgical application of even small amounts of cocaine will cause patients to have positive urine tests for as long as three days. In one study patients undergoing lacrimal duct surgery were anesthetized with less than 3 mL of topical 4% cocaine hydrochloride. In almost every instance, urine specimens obtained 24 hours later exceeded the 300-ng NIDA cut off, and some still exceeded it at 48 hours. In some patients cocaine was still detectable, though at levels less than 300 ng/mL, 72 hours later (Cruz, Patrinely, Reyna & King, 1991).

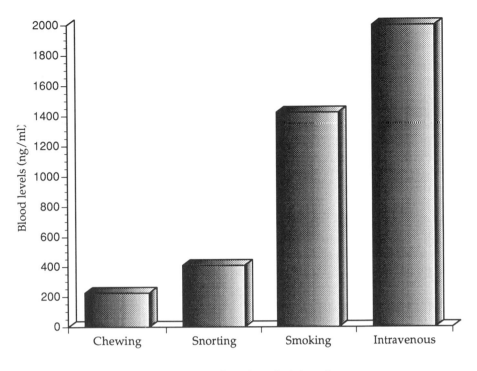

Figure 1.4.1 Blood levels and routes of administration
The route of ingestion determines cocaine blood levels. Crack smokers may have blood levels three or four times as high as leaf chewing Indians. Levels after snorting are intermediate.

Topical cocaine may be combined with submucous injections of lidocaine/epinephrine. Because pH has a significant effect on local anesthetic activity, bicarbonate is occasionally mixed with the cocaine to increase its efficacy (Sollman, 1918). Cocaine mixed with an epinephrine solution is referred to as "paste". When a mixture of cocaine and epinephrine is used, with or without the addition of bicarbonate, the resultant plasma levels can be quite high, concentrations of over 2,000 ng/mL having been observed (Lips, O'Reilly, Close et al., 1987) (Bromley & Hayward, 1988).

Injected epinephrine is, of course, absorbed along with the cocaine, and this may lead to toxicity (Taylor, Achola & Smith, 1984). Cocaine's toxic effects on the heart are at least partly mediated by catechol excess, and the potential for the occurrence of an untoward event is quite real when cocaine is combined with epinephrine. Myocardial infarction (Chiu, Brecht, Das Gupta et al., 1986) (Meyers, 1980) (Littlewood & Tabb, 1987) (Ross & Bell, 1992) and cardiac arrest have both been described as complications of cocaine and cocaine/epinephrine anesthesia. Such complications were much more common in older literature, presumably because much larger amounts of cocaine were used (Mayer, 1924). When infarction occurs in this setting, it is nearly impossible to determine the etiology. Malpractice suits have alleged that either too much epinephrine or too much cocaine had been given, but the probability is that both agents combine to cause coronary artery spasm (Karch, 1989) (Flores, Lange, Cigarroa & Hillis, 1990) (Wilkerson, Franker et al, 1990) (Ascher, Stauffer & Gaash, 1988) (Flores, 1990) (Wilkerson, 1990). Both cocaine and epinephrine can also induce lethal cardiac arrhythmias (Kabas, Blanchard, Matsuyama et al, 1990) (Laster, Johnson, Eger & Taheri, 1990) (Schwartz, Boyle, Janzen & Jones, 1988). Catechol measurements at autopsy aren't possible, and even measurements made during life, especially in the post arrest state, are impossible to interpret. Some individuals with uncomplicated infarction will have higher catechol levels than others with cardiac arrest who have been given exogenous epinephrine (Worstman, Frank & Cryer, 1984). Similarly, cocaine levels, in and of themselves, do not appear to correlate with the probability of developing coronary artery spasm, and infarction can occur when there is only metabolite present (Del Aguila & Rosman, 1990) (Levine & Nishikawa, 1991). If preexisting lesions can be demonstrated, then the at least there is a plausible mechanism for infarction. Cocaine and epinephrine increase oxygen consumption. Previously asymptomatic lesions can suddenly become symptomatic if the demand for increased blood supply becomes too great.

1.4.4 INTRAVENOUS USE

Significantly higher levels than chewing or snorting occur after intravenous use. Cone et al. found that a 40-mg intravenous bolus given to a human volunteer resulted in blood levels of between 204 and 523 ng/mL at 10 minutes (Kumor, Sherer, Thompson, et al., 1988). Chow et al. gave a 32–mg dose to volunteers and observed peak levels of approximately 250 ng/mL with a maximum increase in heart rate at 7.3 minutes (Chow, Ambre,Ruo et al, 1985). Barnett observed levels of 700–1,000 ng/mL 5 minutes after injecting 100 mg. The levels exceeded 2,500 ng/mL after 200 mg were injected (Barnett, Hawks & Resnick, 1981). One important aspect of intravenous cocaine use is that it requires multiple frequent injections to get "high". Narcotic users, by comparison, inject infrequently. The increased number of injections places the cocaine user at greater risk for HIV infection and for all the other infectious complications of intravenous drug use.

1.4.5 GENITAL APPLICATION

Genital and rectal application serves two purposes. Absorption is prompt and relatively complete, so that high blood levels are reached very quickly. In addition, cocaine used in this manner also acts as local anesthetic. For obvious reasons, rectal application has become popular among homosexual abusers. Fatalities have been reported after both rectal and vaginal application. Clinical histories in these patients suggest that death was due to arrhythmia but, interestingly, reported blood levels have not been high (Doss & Gowitt, 1988) (Ettinger & Stine, 1989) (Burkett, Bandstra, Cohen et al., 1990).

1.4.6 DERMAL ABSORPTION

Even very small amounts of cocaine applied to the skin can cause positive urine screening tests for cocaine. Resulting levels are far too low to produce symptoms, but the fact that measurable levels appear in the blood at all is troublesome. In one study, cocaine dissolved in alcohol was painted on the forearm skin of a volunteer and then the urine tested intermittently over a 96-hour period. Absorption of both free base and cocaine hydrochloride occurs when applied in this fashion. Maximal urinary benzoylecgonine concentration after the application of 5 mg of free base was 55 ng/mL at 48 hours. Much less of the cocaine hydrochloride was absorbed, with a peak urine level of only 15 ng/mL at 48 hours (Baselt, Chang & Yoshikawa, 1990). The more complete absorption of the free base can probably be accounted for by the fact that weak bases, such as cocaine, are not very lipid soluble. Free base, on the other hand, is lipophilic and is readily absorbed. Unpublished data, cited in the first study, showed a similar pattern. Five laboratory workers had 2 mg of cocaine hydrochloride, dissolved in water, placed on the palms. Urine collected three hours later was tested with the EMIT™ d.a.u. assay, and was positive in all five. In one case, the resultant blood level was above the 300 ng/mL cut off (case described by Baselt in the study cited above). A third study, done with cocaine paste, yielded much the same result (Elsohly, 1991). The risk that medical personnel might test positive because of innocent contact was assessed in still another study. Neither the placing of 2 drops of 4% cocaine on the skin, nor breathing deeply when spraying a patient with 4% cocaine aerosol, nor squeezing cocaine-soaked cotton pledgets between the fingers, caused any of 11 volunteers to test positive (Zieske, 1992). Given that skin contact can, in some situations, result in significant urinary benzoylecgonine concentrations that persist for some time, extreme caution is warranted when interpreting low-level urine drug-testing results. That is especially true when those results fall below the commonly accepted immunoassay and GC/MS limit for benzoylecgonine of 300 and 150 ng/mL respectively.

1.4.7 INHALATION

The extraction of cocaine free base with volatile solvents, popular in the early 1980s", and referred to as "free basing", gave way entirely to "crack" smoking by 1986 (Washton, Gold 1986). The origins of this practice are not entirely clear. It was first observed in Jamaica in 1983 (Jekel, Allen & Podlewski, 1986). The first mention of usage in the U.S. came from New York City in 1985 (Gross, 1985). When freebase cocaine is smoked, peak blood levels comparable to those achieved with intravenous use are rapidly attained.

There have been limited clinical studies accessing plasma levels in intoxicated "crack" smokers. "Crack" prepared on the streets contains very large amounts of bicarbonate and other contaminants. For clinical experiments, "crack" is prepared by mixing cocaine hydrochloride with an equal weight of sodium bicarbonate in sterile water and heating in a boiling waterbath. Cocaine base precipitates out and forms small pellets or "rocks" when the water is cooled. When prepared in this manner, smoking 50 mg of base delivers between 16 and 32 mg of cocaine to the subject (Perez-Reyes, Guiseppi, Ondrusek et al., 1982) (Foltin, 1991) (Paly, Van Dyke, Jatlow & Byck, 1980) (Paly, Jatlow, Van Dyke et al., 1982) (Jeffcoat, Perez-Reyes, Hill et al., 1989). The potency of smoked cocaine is about 60% of intravenous cocaine, at least in regard to the production of cardiovascular effects (Foltin, 1991).

In one study, plasma levels 6–12 minutes after smoking one 50-mg dose ranged from 250–350 ng/mL. In a second study, from the same laboratory, 2 fifty-milligram doses of free base, smoked 14 minutes apart, produced a peak level of 425 ng/mL four minutes after the last dose (Foltin, 1991). Smoking a 50-mg dose every 14 minutes, for a total of 4 doses, produced a level of over 1,200 ng/mL in one subject. To closely simulate the actual smoking patterns of crack users, volunteers smoked two 35-mg doses at intervals of 15, 30, and 45 minutes. When the doses were 15 minutes apart, plasma levels were on the order of 800 ng/mL. When the doses were 30 minutes apart, peak levels were only half as high, approximately 400 ng/mL. When 45 minutes elapsed between doses, the level rose to only 200 ng/mL (Hatsukami, Pentel, Nelson & Glass, 1991). There is, however, a great deal of variation between experimental subjects. After smoking a 50-mg dose, peak effects on blood pressure occur 2–6 minutes after inhalation and return to baseline within 30 minutes after a single dose (Foltin & Fischman, 1991) (Jeffcoat et al., 1989). In the most recent study, smoking 50 mg results in blood levels ranging anywhere from 80 to 460 ng/mL. If a second 50-mg dose was smoked 14 minutes after the first, then resultant blood levels range from 200 to 600 ng/mL (Isenschmid, Fischman, Foltin and Caplan, 1992). In both man and experimental animals, changes in heart rate and blood pressure are dose dependent and correlate temporally with peak cocaine plasma concentrations (Boni, Barr & Martin, 1991).

Side stream exposure to cocaine can cause measurable quantities of cocaine metabolite to appear in the urine. In one experiment a 73-kg adult male was exposed to 200 mg of free base that was volatilized in a confined space about the size of a closet. Serial urine specimens collected over 24 hours contained 10 to 50 ng/mL of urine (Baselt et al. 1991). Environmental exposure to cocaine is a real hazard for inner city children. Nearly 2.5% of children attending a metropolitan emergency department tested positive for cocaine or cocaine metabolite. The number would probably have been higher, but children with signs of cocaine toxicity, or history of cocaine exposure, were specifically excluded from the survey (Kharasch, Glotzer, Vinci et al., 1991). When attempting to interpret the significance of low cocaine and benzoyl-ecgonine levels, especially in children, it is important to remember that cocaine smoke, just like cigarette smoke, can be passively absorbed. The process has been described in children and can produce transient neurologic syndromes (Bateman & Heagaraty, 1989). Whether or not such exposure can lead to serious consequences is not clear.

A study of pediatric fatalities from Philadelphia identified 16 children over a two-year period who had cocaine or metabolite in their blood. The authors suggested that the presence of the cocaine may have contributed to the deaths. Scene investigations document that shortly before death these infants had been exposed to to "crack" smoke. Most of the infants were under 3 months of age, none had revealing autopsy findings, and their average cocaine blood level was 76 ng/mL, just barely over the level required to produce any measurable physiologic effects (Mirchandani, Mirchandani, Hellman et al., 1991). On the basis of this evidence alone, and in the absence of any plausible mechanism, sudden infant death syndrome would appear to be the more likely diagnosis in these particular cases (Sudden infant death syndrome has been alleged to be a complication of maternal cocaine use, but proof is lacking). In fact, the low levels of cocaine could have had their origin from other sources in the child's environment. Side stream intake of volatilized cocaine could also occur in innocent mothers. Cocaine and its metabolite would then appear in the infant, even though the mother herself was not a cocaine user. The identification of cocaine in the infant is not, necessarily, proof of abuse by the mother.

1.4.8 GASTROINTESTINAL ABSORPTION

A significant proportion of the cocaine in the blood of leaf chewers comes from gastrointestinal absorption. Chewers who swallow their saliva have higher cocaine levels than those who do not. While it is widely believed by casual users that cocaine is not absorbed from the gastrointestinal tract, in fact absorption is quite good (Wilkinson et al.,

1980). This route assumes particular importance in two special instances: in the "body packer" syndrome, and in attempts to hide evidence. It is not uncommon for a "crack" dealer facing eminent arrest to swallow his entire inventory. This may amount to ingesting several grams of cocaine. Surprisingly little happens. There are few reports of fatalities or even serious medical complications occurring secondary to the practice, and the situation has never been studied, either in animals or human volunteers. Since dealers are often users as well, tolerance may afford a degree of protection.

"Body packing", on the other hand, can be lethal (Bednarczyk, Gressmann & Wymer, 1980) (Fishbain & Wetli, 1981). The practice was first described in 1972 (Suarez, Arango & Lester, 1972). Low level smugglers ("mules") swallow packets containing hundreds of grams of cocaine. The drug to be smuggled is wrapped either in a condom, plastic bag, or aluminum foil. Packets generally contain 3 to 6 grams of drug. The radiodensity of cocaine is very close to that of stool, and that can make smugglers difficult to detect (Wetli & Mittleman, 1981) (Karhunen, Suoranta, Penttilä & Pitkäranta, 1991). If a packet should rupture the smuggler will quickly absorb a very large amount of drug. Seizures appear to be the mechanism of lethality in experimental animals given huge amounts of cocaine (Catravas, Waters, Waiz et al., 1978) (Catravas & Waters, 1981), but humans may develop pulmonary edema and heart failure, and even massive overdose is not necessarily fatal (Bettinger, 1980). Blood levels in these cases have ranged from 3 to 11 mg/L. Such levels are well in excess of levels normally seen after even intravenous abuse. Tolerance occurs and levels as high as 30 mg/L or more may be recorded as incidental findings (Howell & Ezell, 1990).

Even if the packets don't rupture, small amounts of cocaine may still appear in the urine and urine testing may be diagnostic for the syndrome (Gherardi, Baud, Leporc & Marc, 1988). Other diagnostic techniques that have been advocated included plain x-ray films, barium contrast studies, and CT scanning. As the smugglers have become more sophisticated they have improved their packing techniques to prevent leakage. They have also attempted to avoid x-ray detection by ingesting mixtures of oil which will reduce the contrast difference between the packets and surrounding bowel contents (Gherardi, Marc, Alberti et al, 1990) (Pinsky, Ducas & Ruggene, 1978) (Sinner, 1981).

1.4.9 MATERNAL / FETAL CONSIDERATIONS

In the pregnant ewe, fetal blood concentrations 5 minutes after a maternal infusion are only 12% of the values seen in the mother (Moore, Sorg, Miller & Key, 1986). In near-term Macaque monkeys 1 mg/kg injected intramuscularly in the mother yielded peak plasma concentrations of 132–312 ng/mL 10–20 minutes after injection. Fetal levels lagged behind, peaking at from 30 minutes to two hours later, but peak levels were the same (18–329 ng/mL) (Paule, Bailey, Fogle et al., 1991).

Cocaine pharmacokinetics have been studied in pregnant and lactating rats (Wiggins, Rolstein, Ruiz & Davis, 1990). From 30 minutes to three hours after injection cocaine levels are 3–4x higher in the brain and 3–5x higher in the liver than in the blood. During the period from 30 minutes to 90 minutes after injection, fetal brain concentrations were 50% to 90% of the mothers and 1.5 times as high as the blood concentration of either. Injected cocaine also appeared in the milk of lactating mothers in fairly high concentrations.

The human placenta has high affinity binding sites for cocaine (Ahmed et al. 1990), but for obvious reasons human kinetics have not been studied. What little data there is suggests that high maternal/fetal cocaine ratios occur in humans as well. In a case described by Mittleman, the ratio was 9:1 (13,700 ng/mL to 1,500 ng/mL) (Mittleman, Cofino & Hearn, 1989). The high ratio may reflect cocaine-induced vasospasm and reduced flow to the uterus, or it may simply mean that woman and child were not in equilibrium when the mother expired.

Because cocaine is a weak base and a small molecule, it diffuses freely across the placenta. That is not the case for benzoylecgonine which is highly ionized at physiological pH ranges, and which crosses the placenta hardly at all. The situation is very similar to cocaine metabolism in the brain. Benzoylecgonine does not cross the blood-brain barrier, so all the BEG found in the brain is produced by the metabolism of cocaine in the brain. All the BEG in the fetus is derived from cocaine metabolized in the fetus. Because the fetus cannot clear BEG nearly as quickly as the mother, maternal/fetal ratios are just the opposite of the case with cocaine, the parent metabolite. In Meeker's autopsy study the ratio in 6 cases was 2.44, with a range of 1.17 to 6.80 (Meeker & Reynolds, 1990). Neonates that have been exposed to drug in utero, including cocaine, marijuana, and opiates, will have measurable amounts of drugs detectable in their stools, where levels can be determined using minimally modified standard immunoassays (Maynard, Amoruso & Oh, 1991) (Ostrea, Brady et al. 1992). These same drugs can also be detected in the neonates' hair (Graham, Kren et al. 1989) (Forman, Schneiderman, Klein et al. 1992).

References

Ahmed, M., Zhou, D., Maulik, D., Elderfrawi, M. (1990). Characterization of cocaine binding site in human placenta. Life Sci, 46:553–561.

Ascher, E., Stauffer, J. & Gaash, W. (1988). Coronary artery spasm, cardiac arrest, transient electrocardiographic Q waves and stunned myocardium in cocaine-associated acute myocardial infarction. Am J Cardiol, 11, 939–941.

Barnett, G., Hawks, R. & Resbick, R. (1981). Cocaine pharmacokinetics in humans. J Ethnopharm, 3, 353–366.

Baselt, R. C., Chang, J. Y. & Yoshikawa, D. M. (1990). On the dermal absorption of cocaine. J Anal Toxicol, 14(6), 383–384.

Baselt, R. C., Yoshikawa, D. M. and Y Chang, (1991). Passive inhalation of cocaine. Clin Chem, 37(12):2160–2161.

Bateman, D. & Heagarty, M. (1989). Passive freebase cocaine ("Crack") inhalation by infants and toddlers. Am JDis Child, 143, 25–27.

Bednarczyk, L., Gressman, E. & Wymer, R. (1980). Two cocaine-induced fatalities. J Anal Tox, 4(September/October), 263–265.

Bettinger, J. (1980). Cocaine intoxication: massive oral overdose. Ann Emerg Med, 8:429–430.

Boni, J. P., Barr, W. H. & Martin, B. R. (1991). Cocaine inhalation in the rat - pharmacokinetics and cardiovascular response. J Pharmacol Exp Ther, 257(1), 307–315.

Brogan, W., Lange, R., Glamann, B and Hillis, D. (1992). Recurrent coronary vasoconstriction caused by intranasal cocaine: possible role for metabolites. Ann Intern Med, 116(7):556–561.

Bromley, L. & Hayward, A. (1988). Cocaine absorption from the nasal mucosa. Anesthesia, 43, 356–358.

Burkett, G., Bandstra, E. S., Cohen et al. (1990). Cocaine-related maternal death. Am J Obstet Gynecol, 163(1), 40–41.

Catravas, J. & Waters, I. (1981). Acute cocaine intoxication in the conscious dog: studies on the mechanism of lethality. J Pharm and Exp Ther, 217, 350–356.

Catravas, J., Waters, I., Waiz, M. et al. (1978). Acute cocaine intoxication in the conscious dog: pathophysiologic profile of acute lethality. Arch Int Pharmacodyn Ther, 235:328–340.

Chiu, Y.C., Brecht, K., Das Gupta, M. D. et al. (1986). Myocardial infarction with topical cocaine anesthesia for nasal surgery. Arch Otolaryngol Head Neck Surg, 112, 988–990.

Chow, M., Ambre, J., Ruo, T. et al. (1985). Kinetics of cocaine distribution, elimination, and chronotropic effects. Clin Pharmacol Ther, 38, 318–324.

Cruz, O. A., Patrinely, J. R., Reyna, G. S. & King, J. W. (1991). Urine drug screening for cocaine after lacrimal surgery. Am J Ophthalmol, 111(6), 703–705.

Del Aguila, C. & Rosman, H. (1990). Myocardial infarction during cocaine withdrawal. Ann Intern Med, 112(9), 712.

Doss, P. & Gowitt, G. (1988). Investigation of a death caused by rectal insertion of cocaine. Am J Forensic Med & Pathol, 9(4), 336–338.

Elsohly, M. A. (1991). Urinalysis and casual handling of marijuana and cocaine. J Anal Toxicol, 15(1), 46.

Ettinger, T. & Stine, R. (1989). Sudden death temporally related to vaginal cocaine abuse. Am J Emerg Med, 7(1), 129–130.

Fischman, M.W., Schuster, C.R. & Rajfer, S. (1983). A comparison of the subjective and cardiovascular effects of cocaine and procaine in humans. Pharmacol, Biochem, Behav, 18, 711–716.

Fishbain, D. & Wetli, C. (1981). Cocaine intoxication, delirium, and death in a body packer. Ann Emerg Med, 10(10), 531–532.

Flores, E. D., Lange, R. A., Cigarroa, R. G. & Hillis, L. D. (1990). Effect of cocaine on coronary artery dimensions in atherosclerotic coronary artery disease - enhanced vasoconstriction at sites of significant stenoses. J Am Coll Cardiol, 16(1), 74–79.

Foltin, J.F., Fischman, M., Pedroso, J. & Pearlson, G. (1988). Repeated intranasal cocaine administration: lack of tolerance to pressor effects. Drug and Alcohol Dependence, 22, 169–177.

Foltin, R. W. & Fischman, M. W. (1991). Smoked and intravenous cocaine in humans - acute tolerance, cardiovascular and subjective effects. J Pharmacol Exp Ther, 257(1), 247–261.

Forman, R., Schneiderman, J., Klein, J. et al. (1992). Accumulation of cocaine in maternal and fetal hair - the dose response curve. Life Sci, 50(18):1333–1341.

Gherardi, RK., Baud, F., Leporc, P. & Marc, B. (1988). Detection of drugs in the urine of body-packers. Lancet, 1(May 14), 1076–1078.

Gherardi, R., Marc, B., Alberti, X. et al. (1990). A cocaine body packer with normal abdominal plain radiograms. Am J Forensic Med & Pathol, 11(2), 154–157.

Graham, K., Koren, G., Klein, J. et al. (1989). Determination of gestational cocaine exposure by hair analysis. JAMA, 262(23):3328–3330.

Gross, J. (1985, November 29). New purified form of cocaine causes alarm as abuse increases. New York Times, p. 1.

Hatsukami, D., Pentel, P., Nelson, R. & Glass, J. (1991). Effects of multiple doses of smoked cocaine base in humans. In Problems of drug dependence 1991: Proceedings of the 53rd Annual Scientific Meeting of the Committee on Problems of Drug Dependence, Inc. National Institute on Drug Abuse Monograph Series, Rockville, MD. In press.

Holmstedt, B., Lindgren, J., Rivier, L. & Plowman, T. (1979). Cocaine in blood of coca chewers. J Ethnopharm, 1, 69–78.

Howell, S. & Ezell, A. (1990). An example of cocaine tolerance in a gunshot wound fatality. J Analyt Toxicol, 14, 60–61.

Isenschmid, D., Fishman, M., Foltin, R., Caplan, Y. (1992). Concentration of cocaine and metabolites in plasma of humans following intravenous administration and smoking cocaine. J Analyt Toxicol, 16:311–314.

Javaid, J., Fischman, M., Schuster, C. et al. (1978). Cocaine plasma concentrations: relation to physiological and subjective effects in humans. Science, 202, 227–228.

Javaid, J., Musa, M., Fischman, M. et al. (1983). Kinetics of cocaine in humans after intravenous and intranasal administration. Biopharm Drug Dispos, 4, 9–18.

Jeffcoat, A., Perez-Reyes, M., Hill, J. et al. (1989). Cocaine disposition in humans after intravenous injection, nasal insufflation (snorting) or smoking. Drug Metab. Dispos, 17(2), 153–159.

Jekel, J., Allen, D., Podlewski, H. et al (1986). Epidemic free base cocaine abuse: case study from the Bahamas. Lancet, 1, 459–462.

Kabas, J.,Blanchard, S.,Matsuyama, Y. et al. (1990). Cocaine-mediated impairment of cardiac conduction in the dog: a potential mechanism for sudden death after cocaine. J Pharmacol and Exp Ther, 252(1), 185–191.

Karch, S. (1989). Coronary artery spasm induced by intravenous epinephrine overdose. Am J Emerg Med, 7(5), 485–488.

Karhunen, P.J., Suoranta, P.J., Penttilä, A. and Pitkäranta, P. (1991). Pitfalls in the diagnosis of drug smuggler's abdomen. J Forensic Sci, 36(2):397–402.

Kharasch, S. J., Glotzer, D., Vinci et al. (1991). Unsuspected cocaine exposure in young children. Am J Dis Child, 145(2):204–206.

Kumor, K., Sherer, M., Thompson, L. et al. (1988). Lack of cardiovascular tolerance during intravenous cocaine infusions in human volunteers. Life Sciences, 42:2063–2071.

Laster, M., Johnson, B., Eger, E. & Taheri, S. (1990). A method for testing for epinephrine-induced arrhythmias in rats. Anesth Analg, 70, 654–657.

Levine, M. A. H. & Nishikawa, J. (1991). Acute myocardial infarction associated with cocaine withdrawal. Can Med Assoc J, 144(9):1139–1140.

Lips, F., O'Reilly, J., Close, D. et al. (1987). The effects of formulation and addition of adrenaline to cocaine for haemostasis in intranasal surgery. Anesth Intensive Care, 15, 141–146.

Littlewood, S. & Tabb, H. (1987). Myocardial ischemia with epinephrine and cocaine during septoplasty. J LA State Med Soc, 139 (5), 15–18.

Mayer, E. (1924). The toxic effects following the use of local anesthetics. An analysis of the reports of forty-three deaths submitted to the Committee for the Study of Toxic Effects of Local Anesthetics of the American Medical Association. JAMA, 82(11), 876-885.

Maynard, E., Amoruso, L.P., Oh, W. (1991). Meconium for drug testing. Am J Dis Child, 145(6) 650–652.

Meeker, J. E. & Reynolds, P. C. (1990). Fetal and newborn death associated with maternal cocaine use. J Anal Toxicol, 14(6), 379–382.

Meyers, E. (1980). Cocaine toxicity during dacryocystorhinostomy. Arch Opthalmol, 98, 842–843.

Mirchandani, H. G.,Mirchandani, I. H.,Hellman, F. et al. (1991). Passive inhalation of free-base cocaine ('Crack') smoke by infants. Arch Pathol Lab Med, 115(5), 494–498.

Mittleman, R., Cofino, J. & Hearn, W. (1989). Tissue distribution of cocaine in a pregnant woman. J Forensic Sci, 34(2), 481–486.

Moore, T., Sorg, J., Miller, L. & Key, T. (1986). Hemodynamic effects of intravenous cocaine on the pregnant ewe and fetus. Am J Obstet Gynecol, 155, 883–888.

Ostrea, E., Brady, M., Gause, S. et al. (1992). Drug screening of newborns by meconium analysis: a large scale, prospective, epidemiologic study.

Paly, D., Jatlow, P., Van Dyke, C. et al.(1980). Plasma levels of cocaine in native Peruvian coca chewers. In F. Juri (Ed.), Cocaine 1980, Proceedings of the Interamerican Seminar on Coca and Cocaine (pp. 86–89). Lima: Pacific Press.

Paly, D., Jatlow, P., Van Dyke, C. et al. (1982). Plasma cocaine concentrations during cocaine paste smoking. Life Sci, 30, 731–738.

Paly, D., Van Dyke, C., Jatlow, F. & Byck, R. (1980). Cocaine: plasma levels after cocaine paste smoking. In F. Jeri (Eds.), Cocaine: Proceedings of the Interamerican seminar on medical and sociological aspects of coca and cocaine (pp. 106–110). Lima, Peru:

Paule, M., Bailey, J., Fogle, C. et al. (1991). Maternal and fetal plasma disposition of cocaine in near-term Macaque monkeys. In Problems of drug dependence 1991: Proceedings of the 53rd Annual Scientific Meeting of the Committee on Problems of Drug Dependence, Inc. National Institute on Drug Abuse Monograph Series, Rockville, MD. In press.

Perez-Reyes, M., Guiseppi, S., Ondrusek, G. et al. (1982). Free-base cocaine smoking. Clin Pharmacol Ther, 32, 459–465.

Pinsky, M., Ducas, J. & Ruggere, M. (1978). Narcotic smuggling: the double condom sign. J Can Assoc Radiol, 29 (2), 78–81.

Schwartz, A., Boyle, W., Janzen, D. & Jones, R. (1988). Acute effects of cocaine on catecholamines and cardiac electrophysiology in the conscious dog. Can J Cardiol, 4(4), 188–192.

Sinner, W. (1981). The gastrointestinal tract as a vehicle for drug smuggling. Gastrointest Radiol, 198(6), 319–323.

Sollmann, T. (1918). Comparative activity of local anesthetics. II Paralysis of sensory nerve fibers. J Pharm and Exp Ther, 11(1), 1–7.

Suarez, C., Arango, A. & Lester, L. (1972). Cocaine-condom ingestion. Surgical treatment. JAMA, 238(13), 1391–1392.

Taylor, S., Achola, K. & Smith, G. (1984). Plasma catecholamine concentrations. The effect of infiltration with local analgesics and vasoconstrictors during nasal operations. Anesthesia, 39, 520–523.

Van Dyke, C., Barash, P., Jatlow, P. & Byck, R. (1976). Cocaine: plasma concentrations after intranasal application in man. Science, 191:859–861.

Washton, A., Gold, M. & Pottash, A. (1986). "Crack": early report on a new drug epidemic. Postgrad Med, 89(5), 52–58.

Wetli, C.V. & Mittleman, R.E. (1981). The "body packer" syndrome - toxicity following ingestion of illicit drugs packaged for transportation. J Forensic Sci,26(3):492–500.

Wiggins, R., Rolsten, C., Ruiz, B. & Davis, C. (1989). Pharmacokinetics of cocaine: basic studies of route, dosage, pregnancy and lactation. Neurotoxicology, 10(3), 367–381.

Wilkerson, R., Franker, T. et al. (1990). Cocaine-induced coronary-artery spasm. N Engl J Med, 322(17), 1235.

Wilkinson, P., Van Dyke, C., Jatlow et al. (1980). Intranasal and oral cocaine kinetics. Clin Pharmacol Ther, 27, 386–394.

Worstman, J., Frank, S. & Cryer, P. (1984). Adrenomedullary response to maximal stress in humans. Am J Med, 77, 779–784.

Zieske, LA. (1992). Passive exposure of cocaine in medical personnel and its relationship to drug screening tests. Arch Otolaryngol Head Neck Surg, 118:364

1.5 METABOLISM

1.5.1 COCAINE DISPOSITION IN MAN

1.5.1.1 General Considerations

Cocaine is rapidly cleared from the blood stream. In humans, cocaine's half-life is on the order of 40 minutes (Inaba, Stewart & Kalow, 1978) (Chow, Ambre, Ruo et al,1985) (Javid, Musa, Fischman et al., 1983) (Kumor, Sherer, Thompson et al., 1988) (Barnett,Hawks & Resnick, 1981). Cocaine has a steady-state volume of distribution of 132 liter

Cocaine blood levels after nasal administration

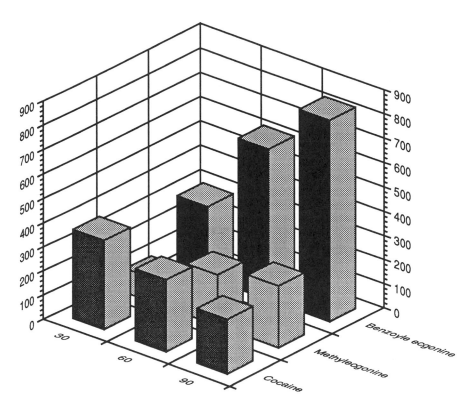

Figure 1.5.1.1 Clearance rates for cocaine and its metabolites
Blood levels of cocaine, benzoylecgonine and methylecgonine ester, measured at 30, 60 and 90 minutes after application of 2mg/kg cocaine hydrochloride solution to nasal mucosa. Adapted from Brogan et al. 1992.

or 2 L/kg. Elimination clearance is 2.0 liters per minute. Although the half-life of the drug in humans is variously reported as being between 0.5 and 1.5 hours (Jatlow, 1987) (Chow, Ambre,Ruo et al, 1985) (Kumor, Sherer, Thompson et al., 1988), more recent studies suggest it may be as short as 35 minutes. The difficulty with all of the physiological measurements is that they have been made in volunteers, chronic cocaine users admitted to detoxification programs. Whether the results from individuals can be extrapolated to the population at large has never been determined. Extrapolation from animal experiments is equally difficult, since half-life and elimination clearance differ markedly from species to species. In the rat, for instance, the plasma half life is only 18 minutes. The half-life of inhaled cocaine in ewes, which are often used as an experimental model for maternal/fetal distribution studies, is only 1.6 ± 0.5 minutes and 3.4 ± 0.9 minutes when injected intravenously (Burchfield, Abrams, Miller & Devane, 1991). Only a very small percentage of cocaine is excreted unchanged in the urine and then only for three to six hours (Jatlow, 1988). More than a dozen different breakdown products have been identified, but in humans there appear to be only two important principal metabolites: benzoylecgonine and ecgonine methyl ester. There is little evidence that either exerts toxicity in its own right.

1.5.1.2 Benzoylecgonine and ecgonine methyl ester

In the absence of alcohol, benzoylecgonine (BEG) and ecgonine methyl ester (EME) are cocaine's principal breakdown products. Both hepatic esterases and plasma pseudocholinesterases convert cocaine to benzoylecgonine. Ecgonine methyl ester forms spontaneously. The half-lives of both of these metabolites are much longer than the half-life of the parent compound. Ecgonine methyl ester has a half-life of four hours, while benzoylecgonine, with a half-life closer to six hours, can still be detected in plasma more than 24 hours after ingestion (Javid, Musa et al. 1983) (Jatlow 1987).

The role of ecgonine methyl ester is open to some debate. In one study of chronic cocaine abusers, smoked and intravenously administered cocaine resulted in very low blood levels of EME (less than 5% of benzoylecgonine levels) (Isenschmid, Fischman, Foltin and Caplan, 1992). However, when 2 mg/kg doses of cocaine were given intranasally to non-cocaine users, during angiographic evaluation of chest pain, substantial EME levels were observed. At 60 minutes, when the whole blood concentration of cocaine averaged 295 ng/mL, the EME level was 209 ng/mL, while the benzoylecgonine level was 621 ng/mL (Brogan, Lange, Glamann and Hillis, 1992). Thus it appears that EME concentrations may reach quite substantial levels in vivo.

Because plasma pseudocholinesterase and hepatic esterases play such a major role in cocaine's metabolism (Inaba et al., 1978) (Stewart, Inaba, Tang & Kalow, 1977) (Stewart, Inaba, Lucassen & Kalow, 1979), individuals with genetic defects and atypical forms of cholinesterase, as indicated by low dibucaine numbers, will metabolize cocaine more slowly than normal individuals. It has been suggested that cholinesterase deficiency may be an important mechanism contributing to cocaine's toxicity (Jatlow, Barash, Van Dyke et al., 1979). One clinical study measured plasma cholinesterase activity in cocaine-intoxicated patients presenting to the emergency department with signs and symptoms of toxicity. The results were compared with values obtained from 24 seriously ill patients who had negative drug screens. The critically ill, but cocaine-negative, patients had significantly higher cholinesterase activities than the cocaine using group (Hoffman, Henry, Weisman et al.,

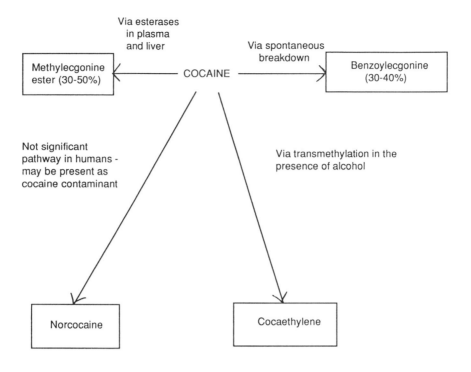

Figure 1.5.1.2 Metabolic fate of cocaine
In the absence of alcohol, benzoylecgonine (BEG) and ecgonine methyl ester
(EME) are cocaine's principal breakdown products. Cocaine is converted to BEG
by hepatic esterases and plasma pseudocholinesterase. EME forms spontaneously. In cases of cholinesterase deficiency, more cocaine is shunted via the EME
mode.

1990). Knowledge of this possible relationship has even prompted an
occasional user to take organophosphate insecticides along with their
cocaine in hope of prolonging the "high" (Herschman & Aaron, 1991).
Nonetheless, the relationship between cholinesterase activity and toxicity
is far from proven. In one interesting experiment, rats treated with
cholinesterase inhibitors were actually more resistant to cocaine toxicity
than untreated control rats (Kambam, Naukam, Paris et al., 1990).
       The argument that decreased cholinesterase activity can result
in prolonged elevation of cocaine levels and increased toxicity is based
on two questionable assumptions. The first is that blood levels can be
related to toxicity. Given the high degree of tolerance that occurs with

chronic cocaine use, inferring toxicity or impairment from isolated blood levels simply is not possible. The second problem is that other enzymes besides cholinesterase can metabolize cocaine. Hepatic microsomal enzymes and nonspecific hepatic esterases also have this ability. When pigs treated with a plasma cholinesterase inhibitor were given intravenous cocaine, the amount of ecgonine methyl ester formed did decrease, but there was a compensatory rise in the amount of benzoylecgonine formed and only very modest changes in plasma clearance of cocaine (Kambam, Mets, Hickman et al, 1992).

1.5.1.3 Cocaethylene

Other cocaine metabolites are potentially toxic. One of them, cocaethylene, is unique in that it is produced only in the presence of ethyl alcohol (Camí, de la Torre, Farré et al.,1990) (Hearn, Flynn, Hime et al., 1991) (Jatlow, Elsworth, Bradberry et al., 1991). Cocaethylene is synthesized in the liver by a transesterification reaction which adds an extra methyl group to cocaine. The reaction occurs in the microsomal fraction, but the enzymes involved are not known. Because cocaethylene is a nonpolar molecule, it crosses the blood-brain barrier easily and its concentration in the brain equals that of cocaine. In 1979 traces of cocaethylene were first detected in the urine of an individual using both alcohol and cocaine. The observation was repeated again five years later, but the possibility that cocaethylene itself might be metabolically active was not considered. Newer studies suggest that not only does cocaethylene contribute to the psychological effects produced by cocaine, it may also contribute to the toxicity (Foltin & Fischman, 1989) (Lynn, Higgins, Bickel et al, 1991) (Farré, Llorente, Uagena et al., 1990) (Woodward, Mansbach, Carroll & Balster, 1991). Animal studies have shown that cocaethylene is just as effective at blocking dopamine reuptake as cocaine in rats, and that it produces the same behavioral alterations as cocaine (Jatlow et al., 1991) (Hearn et al., 1991).

In one autopsy study, 231 cases of cocaine-associated death were retrospectively analyzed, and 124 were found to have both alcohol and cocaine in their blood. More than half (62%) of those with alcohol and cocaine present also had easily detectable levels of cocaethylene in their blood, livers and brains. Those without alcohol, or with very low alcohol levels, had no cocaethylene present (Hearn et al., 1991). In a second autopsy study postmortem blood measurements were made in a series of 7 patients whose blood alcohols ranged from 20 to 190 mg/dL. Blood cocaine levels were between 34 to 4,370 ng/mL, while cocaethylene levels were between 73 and 1,447 ng/mL. In half the cases the cocaethylene level was higher than the cocaine level (Jatlow et al., 1991). The relationship between cocaine and alcohol has been investigated in healthy volunteers. Individuals with a history of recreational drug use were given cocaine alone or a drink containing 1 gm/kg of vodka followed by 100-mg dose of cocaine hydrochloride (snorted). Coca-ethylene was detected only in the samples from the alcohol-pretreated group. The peak cocaethylene concentration was 55 ± 8 ng/mL, and serial blood measurements were consistent with a half-life of 109 minutes. Norcocaine levels were also much higher in the group that had been pretreated with alcohol. A difficult to explain observation was that the alcohol group had higher peak cocaine levels than those who had used cocaine alone (352 ±111 ng/mL vs. 258 ±115 ng/mL). It may be that spontaneous conversion to benzoylecgonine, the normal route by which 40% of a given dose of cocaine would be metabolized, is slightly inhibited by alcohol induced shifts in pH. With less of a given dose being metabolized to benzoylecgonine, more is available for hepatic metabolism, leading to increased norcocaine formation (Camí et al., 1991). In a group of patients with clinical signs of cocaine intoxication and positive alcohol screening tests, cocaine concentrations ranged from 50 ng/mL to 4,360 ng/mL, and blood alcohol levels ranged from 0.09 to 0.84 g/dL. The mean CE level was 710 ng/mL ± 0.100 (Mash, Ciarleglio, Tanis et al., 1991). Cocaethylene takes some time to form, so the time of specimen collection may make some difference. In studies using tracer quantities of C^{11} labelled cocaine, no cocaethylene could be detected until 10 minutes after the simultaneous administration of alcohol and intravenous cocaine (Fowler, Volkow, Logan et al., 1992).

1.5.1.4 Anhydroecgonine

Another metabolite of forensic interest, anhydroecgonine methyl ester (AEME) is a pyrolysis product of cocaine. It is excreted only in the urine of crack smokers. Its identification may be of some forensic significance (Jacob, Lewis, Eliasbaker & Jones, 1990), but its pharmacology has never been studied. Structurally, AEME shares features with other chemicals, such as anatoxin and arecoline that have cholinergic properties, raising the possibility that this compound may be toxic in its own right.

1.5.1.5 Norcocaine

In animals, cytochrome P450 and flavin adenine dinucleotide containing monooxygenase metabolize cocaine to norcocaine. Further enzymatic breakdown yields N-hydroxynorcocaine and norcocaine nitroxide (Shuster, Casey & Welankiwar, 1983). Norcocaine nitroxide, once thought to be a highly reactive free radical, is now known to be stable. However, further oxidation to the norcocaine nitrosodium ion produces a compound that is highly reactive with glutathione. If glutathione stores fall below a certain level, lipid peroxidation is unopposed and cocaine metabolites bind to hepatic proteins, eventually leading to cell death (Evans, 1983) (Kloss, Rosen & Rauckman, 1984). In humans only minute amounts of cocaine undergo oxidative metabolism, which may explain why liver lesions have only rarely been reported in cocaine

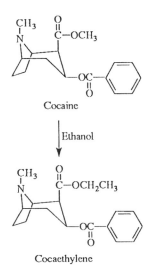

Cocaine

Ethanol

Cocaethylene

Figure 1.5.1.3 Cocaethylene formation
Cocaethylene is formed in the liver by a transesterification reaction which adds
an extra methyl group to cocaine. Cocaethylene has a much longer half-life than
cocaine, but cocaethylene binds to the dopamine receptor with the same affinity
as cocaine.

users. The higher levels of norcocaine seen when alcohol use is
combined with cocaine are yet to be explained.

1.5.2 FETAL METABOLISM

The human placenta has cholinesterase activity and metabolizes
cocaine, possibly affording the fetus a degree of protection (Roe, Little,
Bawdon & Gilstrap, 1990). Nonetheless, in animal studies, newborns develop higher blood levels than adults receiving the same dose, and their
plasma and tissue levels decline more slowly than adults (Morishima,
Khan, Hara et al., 1990). Infants born to cocaine-using mothers may
have persistently elevated cocaine levels for days (Chasnoff, Bussey,
Savich & Stack, 1986). However, a causal relationship between persistently elevated levels and the occasional case reports of perinatal stroke
and intraventricular hemorrhage in the new born has not been demonstrated.

The fetus handles BEG differently than the mother. Since BEG
is excreted primarily in the urine, and since both renal blood flow and
glomerular filtration rate double in pregnant women, mothers clear
metabolite much more quickly than their fetus, but there have been too

few studies to make any further generalizations. In one study where BEG concentrations were measured in mother and child shortly after birth, the mother's BEG concentration was nearly 20 - 30 times that of the fetus (12.2 µg/mL vs. 240 µg/mL and 10.8µg/mL vs. 378 µg/mL) (Meeker & Reynolds, 1990). Though unproven, the possibility also exists that the enzymatic pathway for conversion of cocaine to methylecgonine may not be fully developed in the newborn.

References

Barnett, G.,Hawks, R. & Resbick, R. (1981). Cocaine pharmacokinetics in humans. J Ethnopharm, 3, 353–366.

Burchfield, D. J.,Abrams, R. M.,Miller, R. L. & DeVane, C. L. (1991). Inhalational administration of cocaine in sheep. Life Sci, 48(22), 2129–2136.

Brogan, W.C. Lange, R.A. Glamann, D.B. Hillis, L.D. (1992). Recurrent coronary vasoconstriction caused by intranasal cocaine - possible role for metabolites. Ann Intern Med, 116:556–561

Camí, J.,de la Torre, R.,Farré, M. et al. (1991). Cocaine-alcohol interaction in healthy volunteers: plasma metabolic profile including cocaethylene. In Problems of drug dependency 1991: Proceedings of the 53rd Annual Scientific Meeting of the Committee on Problems of Drug Dependence, Inc. National Institute on Drug Abuse Monograph Series, Rockville, Md. in press.

Chasnoff, I.,Bussey, M.,Savich, R. & Stack, C. (1986). Perinatal cerebral infarction and maternal cocaine use. J Pediatrics, 108, 456–459.

Chow, M.,Ambre, J.,Ruo, T. et al. (1985). Kinetics of cocaine distribution, elimination, and chronotropic effects. Clin Pharmacol Ther, 38, 318–324.

Evans, M.A. (1983). Role of protein binding in cocaine-induced hepatic necrosis. J Pharmacol Exp Ther, 224 (1), 73–79.

Farré, M.,Llorente, M.,Ugena, X. et al. (1990). Interaction of cocaine with ethanol. In Problems of drug dependence 1990: Proceedings of the 52nd Annual Scientific Meeting of the Committee on Problems of Drug Dependence, Inc., Harris, L. (ed), National Institute on Drug Abuse, Rockville, MD, pg 570–571.

Foltin, R. & Fischman, M. (1989). Ethanol and cocaine interactions in humans: cardiovascular consequences. Pharmacol, Biochem, Behavior, 31 (4), 877–883.

Fowler, J., Volkow, N., Logan, J. et al. (1992). Alcohol intoxication does not change (^{11}C)Cocaine pharmacokinetics in human brain and heart. Synapse, 12:228–235.

Hearn, W. L., Flynn, D. D., Hime et al (1991). Cocaethylene - a unique cocaine metabolite displays high affinity for the dopamine transporter. J Neurochem, 56(2), 698–701.

Herschman, Z. & Aaron, C. (1991). Prolongation of cocaine effect. Anesthesiology, 74(3), 631–632.

Hoffman, R.,Henry, G.,Weisman, R. et al. (1990). Association between plasma cholinesterase activity and cocaine toxicity. Ann Emerg Med, 19(4), 467.

Inaba, T.,Stewart, D. & Kalow, W. (1978). Metabolism of cocaine in man. Clin Pharmacol Ther 23:547–552.

Isenschmid, D., Fischman, M., Foltin, R., and Caplan H. (1992). Concentration of cocaine and metabolites in plasma of humans following intravenous administration and smoking of cocaine. J Analyt Toxicol, 16:311–314.

Jacob, P.,Lewis, E. R.,Elias-Baker, B. A. & Jones, R. T. (1990). A Pyrolysis product, anhydroecgonine methyl ester (Methylecgonidine), is in the urine of cocaine smokers. J Anal Toxic, 14(6), 353–357.

Jatlow, P. (1987). Drug abuse profile: Cocaine. Clin Chem, 33(11B), 66B–71B.

Jatlow, P. (1988). Cocaine: analysis, pharmacokinetics, and metabolic disposition. Yale J Biol and Med, 61, 105–113.

Jatlow, P.,Barash, P.,Van Dyke et al. (1979). Cocaine and succinylcholine sensitivity: a new caution. Anesth Analg, 58, 235–238.

Jatlow, P.,Elsworth, J. D.,Bradberry et al. (1991). Cocaethylene - A neuropharmacologically active metabolite associated with concurrent cocaine--ethanol ingestion. Life Sci, 48(18), 1787–1794.

Javid, J.,Musa, M.,Fischman, M. et al. (1983). Kinetics of cocaine in humans after intravenous and intranasal administration. Biopharm Drug Dispos, 4, 9–18.

Kambam, J.,Naukam, B.,Paris, W. et al. (1990). Inhibition of pseudocholinesterase (PCHE) activity protects from cocaine induced cardiorespiratory toxicity (CICT) in rats. Anesthesiology, 73(3A), A581.

Kambam, J., Mets, B., Hickman, R. et al (1992). The effects of inhibition of plasma cholinesterase and hepatic microsomal enzyme activity on cocaine, benzoylecgonine, ecgonine methyl ester, and norcocaine blood levels in pigs. J. Lab Clin Med, 120 (2), 323–328.

Kloss, M.,Rosen, G. & Rauckman, E. (1984). Cocaine-mediated hepatotoxicity: a critical review. Biochem Pharmacol, 33, 169–173.

Kumor, K.,Sherer, M.,Thompson, L. et al. (1988). Lack of cardiovascular tolerance during intravenous cocaine infusions in human volunteers. Life Sciences, 42, 2063–2071.

Lynn, M.,Higgins, S.,Bickel, W. et al. (1991). In Problems of drug dependence 1991: Proceedings of the 53rd Annual Scientific Meeting of the Committee on Problems of Drug Dependence, Inc. National Institute on Drug Abuse Monograph Series, Rockland, MD. In press.

Mash, D.,Ciarleglio, A.,Tanis, D. et al. (1991). Toxicology screens for cocaethylene in emergency department and trauma admissions associated with cocaine intoxication. In Problems of drug dependence 1991: Proceedings of the 53rd Annual Scientific Meeting of the Committee on Problems of Drug Dependence, Inc. National Institute on Drug Abuse Monograph Series, Rockland, MD. In press.

Meeker, J. E. & Reynolds, P. C. (1990). Fetal and newborn death associated with maternal cocaine use. J Anal Toxicol, 14(6), 379–382.

Morishima, H.,Khan, K.,Hara, T. et al. (1990). Age-related cocaine uptake in rats. Anesthesiology, 73(3A), A929.

Roe, D. A.,Little, B. B.,Bawdon, R. E. & Gilstrap, L. C. (1990). Metabolism of cocaine by human placentas - implications for fetal exposure. Am J Obstet Gyneco, 163(3), 715–718.

Shuster, L.,Casey, E. & Welankiwar, S. (1983). Metabolism of cocaine and norcocaine to N-hydroxynorcocaine. Biochem Pharmacol, 32, 3045–3051.

Stewart, D.,Inaba, T.,Lucassen, M. & Kaklow, W. (1979). Cocaine metabolism: cocaine and norcocaine hydrolysis by liver and serum esterases. Clin Pharm Ther, 25, 464–468.

Stewart, D.,Inaba, T.,Tang, B. & Kalow, W. (1977). Hydrolysis of cocaine in human plasma by cholinesterase. Life Sci, 20, 1557–1564.

Woodward, J., Mansbach, R., Carroll, F. & Balster, R. (1991). Cocaethylene inhibits dopamine uptake and produces cocaine-like actions in drug discrimination studies. Eur J Pharm, 197(2-3), 235–236.

1.6 INTERPRETING COCAINE BLOOD LEVELS

In cases of alcohol intoxication, relatively accurate correlations can be drawn between specific blood levels and corresponding physiological and psychological states. That is not the case with cocaine. Euphoria and mood elevation do correlate well with peak blood level, but the situation is complicated by the fact that the same level can be associated with either a euphoric or a dysphoric reaction, depending on whether or not blood levels are rising or falling. Both cardiovascular effects and feelings of euphoria decline more rapidly than do cocaine blood levels (Javid, Fischman, Schuster et al., 1978), but the rush experienced by cocaine users follows a different time course than the cardiovascular changes (Kumor, 1988).

It had been thought that blood levels over 5,000 ng/mL would predictably cause seizures, respiratory depression and death (Wetli & Fishbain, 1985). In fact, that is the case only for novice and intermittent users. Tolerance on a massive scale can occur. One case report described a man who was shot while drinking in a bar. Except for being belligerent enough to warrant shooting, his behavior was normal in all other respects. After minimal attempted resuscitation he was pronounced dead. When he was autopsied several hours later, multiple specimens showed a plasma cocaine of 30 mg per liter (Howell & Ezell, 1990). In another case a young woman with a history of chronic cocaine abuse was found dead at home. Though there was no indication that the woman was a body packer attempting to smuggle drugs, or that she had attempted to overdose, she had a blood level of over 300 mg/L (Peretti, Isenschmid, Levine et al., 1990). If there is no upper limit for lethal blood concentrations, neither is there a lower limit that is safe. Death and toxicity can occur after the ingestion of trivial amounts of drug and be associated with very low plasma levels (Smart & Anglin, 1986). In a recent autopsy study of 59 cocaine-associated deaths, postmortem blood cocaine levels ranged from 0 to 12.2 mg/L with a mean of 1.2 mg/L. Benzoylecgonine concentrations were from 0.09 to 30.6 mg/L (Goggins, Roe & Apple, 1990). A second study had similar results with levels ranging from 0 to 27.6 mg/dL for cocaine and 0.2 to 30.6 mg/dL for benzoylecgonine (Mckelway, Vieweg & Westerman, 1990). There are several reasons why such a wide range of values has been reported. Tolerance is certainly a factor, since chronic users may consume massive amounts of cocaine without apparent ill effects. Another factor is the unreliability of postmortem blood levels. Changes in postmortem cocaine levels begin immediately after death, occur in an unpredictable fashion, and vary depending on what site the sample is collected from. Cocaine accumulates in some tissues and redistributes after death. One study showed that samples from the subclavian vein were generally lower at autopsy than immediately after death, while samples from the heart and femoral vein were higher. In some instances the increases were over 200% (Hearn, Keran, Wei & Hime, 1991). Apparently the release of cocaine from tissue stores more than compensates for the breakdown due to hydrolysis. Unfortunately, the change is inconsistent. In Hearn's study, half the samples of heart blood had higher levels immediately after death and half the samples had lower levels.

Perhaps the most important reason why cocaine levels can't be used to explain the cause of death is that cocaine-associated sudden death is not dose related. Chronic cocaine users may have alterations in their hearts (Karch & Stephens, 1991) and possibly their brains (Murray, 1986), that make arrhythmias more likely (see section 1.10.2 on cardiovascular effects). Given the presence of appropriate morphologic changes in the heart, in conjunction with a positive history of cocaine abuse, there is nothing unreasonable about declaring cocaine the cause of death even when no cocaine or metabolite is detectable in the blood stream.

In clinical practice, the experience has generally been that patients with myocardial infarct and stroke have low cocaine blood levels at the time of admission. Infarction may occur hours after the drug was last used (Del Aguila & Rosman, 1990). Why that should be the case has never been entirely clear. In patients with stroke the delay may be accounted for by the fact that benzoylecgonine can act as potent vasoconstrictor, at least in vitro (Madden & Powers, 1990). It takes some time for the metabolites to accumulate, and that could account for the delayed onset of vasospasm. The recent discovery of cocaethylene may have solved the riddle. Cocaethylene possesses the same ability to prevent catechol reuptake as cocaine, and it has a much longer half life. In one small study of human volunteers, the half life of cocaethylene was found to be 110 minutes, nearly 4 times as long as cocaine's (Camí, de la Torre, Farré et al.,1991)

The probability that agitated delirium will occur is not dose related either. Affected individuals are initially psychotic and ultimately die of respiratory arrest. Victims are invariably found to have only modest plasma levels (Wetli & Fishbain, 1985). The observed low levels are probably explained by the fact that they are measured late in the course of the illness. Cocaine levels are never obtained when the patient is agitated and psychotic (see discussion of agitated delirium in Section 1.10.2.6.5, below).

Other than proving that cocaine has been used, the only useful information to be derived from plasma cocaine and benzoylecgonine levels concerns the time the drug was taken. The ratio of cocaine to benzoylecgonine (BEG) offers a very useful index. Given that cocaine is rapidly converted to benzoylecgonine, and that benzoylecgonine is relatively stable (half life of 5 to 6 hours), if there is more cocaine than BEG in the plasma, then that is very strong indication of very recent ingestion. This relationship can be expressed mathematically. Using the known half life of cocaine, it is possible to estimate the time when the drug was taken. The utility of this approach is somewhat limited by the fact that the amount taken is almost never known. However, the half life of BEG is so much longer than the half life of cocaine, that inferences about time of ingestion can be drawn. Even very high levels of cocaine will be below limits of detection after 6 or 7 half lives (certainly less than 8 hours), but if a significant amount of cocaine was taken, BEG will still be detectable in the plasma more than 24 hours later. At this point, measurements of cocaethylene are problematic. The factors governing its conversion from cocaine are unknown and its presence can't be relied upon.

Very low cocaine levels are also difficult to interpret. Chronic cocaine users sequester cocaine in deep body stores. Small amounts of this sequestered cocaine can leach back into the bloodstream and saliva for days after the drug was last used (Cone & Weddington, 1989). Failing to take account of this situation can have important forensic consequences. The National Transportation Safety Board's analysis of the only commercial airline crash ever blamed on drug intoxication is a good example. In 1988, Continental Express Flight #2286 crashed on approach to the Durango, Colorado, airport; the crew and several of the passengers were killed. The Board ruled that the probable cause of the accident was error on the part of the first officer flying the approach, in conjunction with "ineffective monitoring" by the Captain due to his use of cocaine before the accident. Published reports do not mention the time elapsed between death and autopsy, but specimens obtained at autopsy, analyzed at two different laboratories, showed benzoylecgonine levels of 22 and 26 nanograms per milliliter respectively (Anon, 1989). Assuming that at one time the captain had a plasma cocaine level of 1,000 ng/mL, most of which was converted to BEG (Griesemer, 1983), then more than 30 hours must have elapsed between initial ingestion and the time samples were taken at autopsy. Even if the initial level had been several thousand (consistent with intravenous use or "crack" smoking, which seems not to have been the case in this instance), at least 24 hours would have passed between the time he used the drug and the time of the accident. Since it is now known that cocaine blood levels can actually increase after death, the captain's levels may have been even lower (Hearn et al., 1991). The amount of cocaine actually detected was not enough to have produced measurable physiological effects.

On the basis of what is known about cocaine metabolism, it could be argued that a much longer period between the time of coaine use and death had elapsed. Since unmetabolized cocaine, in addition to BEG, can be detected in the blood, saliva, and urine of chronic users for days after the last dose, attributing significance to very low cocaine levels is not a good idea.

The National Institute on Drug Abuse has promulgated regulations for drug testing which include "cut offs". For benzoylecgonine the cut off is 150 ng/mL (anon, 1988); levels below that are reported as negative. Of course these "cut-offs" were formulated with living patients in mind, but the reasoning is still valid. In the absence of any other information, cocaine or cocaine metabolite levels of less than 50 ng/mL are of only historic interest and should not be take as proof of recent ingestion. Even when levels are higher than 50 ng/mL, postmortem blood cocaine measurements must be interpreted with great care. In more than half the cases cocaine blood levels measured at autopsy are likely to be higher than they were at the time of death (Hearn et al., 1991). In the long run, measurements of cocaine and benzoylecgonine in the brain are likely to be of much more value than blood or urine determinations. Brain levels appear to be more stable after death, and measurement of brain cocaine and benzoylecgonine concentration can also yield valuable historical information about prior use of the drug.

References

Anon (1988). Mandatory guidelines for Federal workplace drug testing programs. Issued by the Department of Health and Human Services. Federal Register, p. 11970 –11989.

Anon (1989, July 17). Safety board cites captain's failure to monitor approach as key in crash. Aviation Week and Space Technology, p. 103–105.

Cami, J., de la Torre, R., Farré, M. et al. (1991). Cocaine-alcohol interaction in healthy volunteers: plasma profile including cocaethylene. In Problems of drug dependence 1991: Proceedings of the 53rd Annual Scientific Meeting of the Committee on Problems of Drug Dependence, Inc. National Institute on Drug Abuse Monograph Series, Rockland, MD. In press.

Cone, E. & Weddington, W., Jr (1989). Prolonged occurrence of cocaine in human saliva and urine after chronic use. J Analyt Toxicol, 13(2), 65–68.

Del Aguila, C. & Rosman, H. (1990). Myocardial infarction during cocaine withdrawal. Ann Intern Med, 112(9), 712.

Goggins, M.,Roe, S. & Apple, F. (1990). Cocaine and benzoylecgonine concentrations in postmortem blood and liver. Clin Chem, 36(6), 1023.

Griesmer, EC, Liu, Y, Budd, RD et al. (1983). The determination of cocaine and its major metabolite, benzoylecgonine, in postmortem fluids and tissues by computerized gas chromatography/mass spectrometry. J Forensic Sci, 28(4):894–900.

Hearn, W.,Keran, E.,Wei, H. & Hime, G. (1991). Site-dependent postmortem changes in blood cocaine concentrations. J Forensic Sci, 36(3), 673–684.

Howell, S. & Ezell, A. (1990). An example of cocaine tolerance in a gunshot wound fatality. J Analyt Toxicol, 14, 60–61.

Javid, J.,Fischman, M.,Schuster, C. et al. (1978). Cocaine plasma concentrations: relation to physiological and subjective effects in humans. Science, 202, 227–228.

Karch, S. & Stephens, B. (1991). When is cocaine the cause of death? Am J Forensic Med & Pathol, 12(1), 1–2.

Kumor, K.,Sherer, M.,Muntaner, C. et al. (1988). Pharmacologic aspects of cocaine rush. National Institute on Drug Abuse Monograph #90, ed. Harris, LS, pg 32.

Madden, J. & Powers, R. (1990). Effect of cocaine and cocaine metabolites on cerebral arteries in vitro. Life Sciences, 47(13), 1109–1114.

Mckelway, R., Vieweg, V. & Westerman, P. (1990). Sudden death from acute cocaine intoxication in Virginia in 1988. Am J Psychiatr, 147(12), 1667–1669.

Murray, G. (1986). Cocaine kindling. JAMA, 256(22), 3094–3095.

Peretti, F.,Isenschmid, S.,Levine, B. et al. (1990). Cocaine fatality: an unexplained blood concentration in a fatal overdose. Forensic Sci Int, 48, 135–138.

Smart, R. & Anglin, R. (1986). Do we know the lethal dose of cocaine? J Forensic Sci, 32(2), 303–312.

Wetli, C. & Fishbain, D. (1985). Cocaine-induced psychosis and sudden death in recreational cocaine users. J Forensic Sci, 30(3), 873–888.

1.7 COCAINE TISSUE DISPOSITION

Experimental studies have identified low-affinity cocaine receptors in the heart, lungs, gut and kidney (Calligaro & Elderfrawi, 1987) and testes (Yazigi & Polakoski, 1992). Distribution of carbon-11-cocaine has been studied in humans using PET scanning (Volkow et al. 1992), and the results generally parallel the results seen in isotopic studies done in animals (Som et al. 1989). Of course the distribution of drug immediately after it has been taken may not necessarily be the same as its distribution some hours later at autopsy. Some cocaine is metabolized by the placenta, but both cocaine and benzoylecgonine appear in the amniotic fluid and fetus (Critchley, Woods, Barson et al., 1988). Samples of brain and liver can be expected to give the highest yield at autopsy.

1.7.1 BRAIN

Cocaine is lipophilic and freely crosses the blood-brain barrier (Misra, Nayak, Bloch & Mule, 1975; Nayak, Misra & Mule, 1976) (Mule, Casella & Misra, 1976), as does cocaethylene (Hearn, Flynn, Hime, Rose et al., 1991b). Receptors with varying affinities for cocaine are found throughout the brain. The region with the highest density of cocaine receptors, which is also the region containing the receptors with the greatest affinity for cocaine, is the striatum. Lower levels of activity are found in the frontal and occipital cortices (Calligaro & Elderfrawi, 1987). In experimental animals, and in autopsied cases of cocaine-related death, the concentration of cocaine found in the brain is 4 to 10 times higher than in the plasma when measured from 0.5 to 2 hours after the drug was taken (Benuck, Reith, Sershen et al., 1988) (Spiehler & Reed, 1985). Cocaine's principal metabolite, BEG, crosses the blood brain barrier only with great difficulty (Misra et al., 1975).

In animal studies, peak cocaine concentrations in the brain were also four times higher then in the blood (Nayak et al., 1976), and that is the case in humans as well. In an autopsy study of 37 patients dying of cocaine toxicity, the mean blood cocaine concentration was 4.6 mg/L (range 0.04 to 31 mg/L) while the mean BEG level was 0.88 mg/L (range 0 to 7.4 mg/L). The mean concentration of cocaine found in the brain was 13.3 mg/kg (range 0.17 to 31 mg/kg), and that of benzoylecgonine was 2.9 mg/kg (range 0.1 to 22 mg/kg). In most cases the blood/brain ratio was close to 4. In a second study of 14 deaths, where cocaine was only an incidental finding (instances of murder, accidental death, etc.), the average blood/brain ratio was only 2.5 (Spiehler & Reed, 1985). Unmetabolized cocaine can be detected in the CSF for at least 24 hours after use (Rowbotham, Kaku, Mueller et al., 1990).

Because BEG does not cross the blood brain barrier, levels of benzoylecgonine in the brain are lower than in the blood for up to two hours after ingestion. Essentially all of the benzoylecgonine found in the brain is produced there. Not only does postmortem analysis of brain tissue give a good indication of levels at the time of death, brain levels can also be an indicator of chronic abuse, because extensive prior use is the only way to explain why a deceased person would have more BEG in the brain than in the blood. Testing brain tissue has other advantages as well, because cocaine is stable in frozen brain for months (Spiehler, 1985). There are now methods that allow the rapid extraction of cocaine from homogenized brain that make the HPLC determination of cocaine and benzoylecgonine rapid and practical (Scheurer et al., 1991).

Brain concentrations in the fetus appear to be lower than in the mother. In the case reported by Mittleman the maternal:fetal brain cocaine ratio was 6.5:1 (Mittleman, Cofino & Hearn, 1989). A study of fetal demise, including 47 cocaine related cases where both blood and brain cocaine levels were measured, found that mean blood concentrations of cocaine were 800 ng/mL, while the mean brain concentration of cocaine was 1,100 ng/mg (Morild & Stajic, 1990) (Critchley et al., 1988). At present there is too little data to be sure, but preliminary investigations suggest that cocaethylene levels in the brain are generally equal to cocaine levels (Hearn et al., 1991b).

1.7.2 HEART

PET scanning studies show that there is high uptake in the heart. Within 2 to 3 minutes after injection, 2.5% of the administered dose appears in the heart and is then cleared rapidly over the next 10 minutes. In spite of the relatively high uptake by the heart, the rapid rate at which the cocaine is cleared makes it unlikely that high levels will be detected at autopsy. This is borne out by the few measurements that have been reported. In the case described by Poklis et al., where the deceased died after an intravenous dose of undetermined size, the concentration of cocaine was 6,000 ng/mg in the heart when the cocaine concentration in the blood was only 1,800 ng/mL. Unfortunately the report does not state how many hours had elapsed between the time of death and the time of autopsy (Poklis, MacKell & Graham, 1985).

How much cocaine actually gets to the heart is a matter of some importance. Large doses of cocaine are only lethal to experimental animals when they are given via a route that guarantees that high concentrations of cocaine actually reach the heart. If the cocaine passes through the liver first, only minimal effects are observed (Jones and Tackett, 1992).

1.7.3 LIVER

Hepatic cocaine receptors are present in higher concentrations, and have greater affinity for cocaine, than those located in the brain (Calligaro & Elderfrawi, 1987). In Volkow's PET studies hepatic accumulation of drug was very high, although the rate of uptake is much slower than for most of the other organs. Peak uptake occurs 10–15 minutes after intravenous injection. More than 20% of a given dose ends up in the liver, and remains at stable levels for more than 40 minutes. The findings of these dynamic studies are generally in agreement with autopsy studies that have also shown high levels in the liver.

In Spiehler's autopsy study, the mean hepatic cocaine level in patients dying of cocaine toxicity was 6.7 mg/L and the BEG concentration was 21.3 mg/L (Spiehler & Reed, 1985). An earlier retrospective study of fifteen cases gathered from several centers yielded slightly different results. More cocaine was detected in the blood than in the liver with a blood/liver ratio of 1.4 (Finkle & McCloskey, 1977). High concentrations of BEG are hardly surprising given that the major metabolic pathways of cocaine metabolism involve plasma and hepatic esterase activity. Cocaethylene is also synthesized in the liver, and hepatic cocaethylene levels are much higher than hepatic cocaine levels (Hearn et al., 1991b).

Hepatic oxidation of the nitrogen atom in the tropane ring also occurs. The resulting products are N-hydroxynorcocaine and the free radical norcocaine nitroxide. Norcocaine also can be found as a contaminant in illicit cocaine (Kumar, 1991). Norcocaine found in illicit samples is there as a byproduct of the refining process. When potassium permanganate is added to crude cocaine mixtures, norcocaine can be formed. Norcocaine is thought to be responsible for the hepatotoxicity observed when cocaine is given to experimental animals (Thompson, Shuster & Shaw, 1979). Mice pretreated with phenobarbital, whose

P-450 microsomal systems have been activated, develop a specific type of hepatic necrosis (Kloss, 1984).

Norcocaine can be detected in man, but only in very small amounts. In addition to the norcocaine that may contaminate a sample, norcocaine can also be formed in the human body, though hepatic oxidation is not a preferred route of metabolism. Human volunteers given both cocaine and alcohol will produce more norcocaine than controls given cocaine alone. An explanation for this phenomenon is still wanting. It has been suggested that, given enough alcohol, blood pH will drop slightly and plasma cholinesterases will become less efficient, leaving more cocaine to circulate through the liver (Camí, de la Torre, Farré et al., 1991). No matter how the norcocaine gets into the body, its relationship to hepatic injury in cocaine users is unclear (Inaba, 1978). Lesions in man, histologically similar to those seen in mice, have been described, but are quite rare (Freeman & Harbison, 1981) (Marks & Chapple, 1986) (Perino, Warren & Levine, 1987) (Powell,Connolly & Charles, 1991).

1.7.4 KIDNEYS

In human radioactive uptake studies, renal uptake is higher than cardiac uptake, but still considerably less than hepatic uptake. Uptake occurs in the renal cortex only. As in the heart, peak uptake occurs at 2–3 minutes, and after 10 minutes half of the dose has been cleared (Volkow et al. 1992). Few autopsy measurements of renal cocaine levels have been reported. The values that have been observed have ranged from 1 to 28 /Kg (Poklis, Mackell & Graham, 1985) (Lundberg, Garriott, Reynolds et al. 1977) (DiMaio, Garriott, 1978) (Price, 1974), but comparing the results is difficult because, in most cases, the time elapsed from death to autopsy is not mentioned.

1.7.5 ADRENALS

In human tracer studies the adrenal glands take up is more of an intravenous tracer dose than the liver. This probably has to do with binding to noradrenergic transporters in chromaffin cells. Peak uptake occurs 10 minutes after injection. Within the adrenal, the half life of the labeled cocaine is 20 minutes (Volkow et al. 1992). There have been no reported autopsy measurements, but the relatively slow rate at which the cocaine is washed out makes it likely that significant amounts could be found at autopsy.

1.7.6 HAIR

Like most of the other abused drugs, cocaine can be detected in the hair of cocaine users (Valente, Cassini, Pigliapochi & Vansetti, 1981) (Baumgartner, Black, Jones & Blahd, 1982). Hair follicles absorb cocaine from the blood, but for reasons that are not clear, cocaine metabolites are not so readily taken up (Fritch, Groce & Rieders, 1992). A recent controlled study analyzed hair samples from patients in a detoxification program and found that cocaine and metabolites were still detectable 10 months after the last verified episode of drug use. Cocaine itself was the molecule present in the highest concentrations, but substantial amounts of benzoylecgonine, cocaethylene and norcocaine were also detected. Methylecgonine ester, one of the two principal cocaine metabolites, was present only in trace amounts (Cone et al. 1991). Given the fact that it is primarily cocaine, and not the metabolites, that accumulates in hair, antibody based screening tests that use antibody directed against metabolites are very likely to give falsely low results.

Dose-response curves have not been established and the relationship between the amount of cocaine ingested and the amount subsequently appearing in the hair is unknown. Several different analytic techniques are available that can be used to quantitate cocaine in hair (Baumgartner, Black, Jones & Blahd, 1982) (Cone, Fritch, Groce & Rieders, 1992), but specimen preparation appears to be a problem for all of them. Tests done at the Addiction Research Center have shown that when hair is externally contaminated by soaking in a cocaine solution, it is virtually impossible to wash the cocaine off (Cone, Yousefnejad, Darwin & Maguire, 1991). In the absence of established cutoffs (Fritch et al. used a cut off of 16 μg per gram of hair), such as exist for urine testing, and given the fact that external contamination may be impossible to exclude, the value of positive cocaine hair tests would seem to be somewhat limited. Only when cocaethylene is detected should a positive test be considered absolute proof of abuse (though not of impairment). Since cocaethylene is produced only when alcohol and cocaine are used at the same time, there is no circumstance where cocaethylene's presence could plausibly be explained by external contamination.

Depending on how the hair is treated, false negatives could also be a problem with this approach. Hair bleaching is done with highly alkaline solutions, and cocaine is rapidly degraded under such conditions, but the issue of environmental effects on hair testing have never been adequately evaluated.

1.7.7 BIOFLUIDS

1.7.7.1 Saliva

Saliva contains very little protein, so unbound drugs in the plasma appear in almost the same concentrations in both plasma and saliva. Because cocaine is weakly basic and saliva is normally more acidic than plasma, the concentration of ionized cocaine in saliva is frequently higher in saliva than in the blood (Thompson, 1987) (Ferko, Barabieri, Digregorio & Ruch, 1990). When human volunteers are given intravenous cocaine, saliva cocaine levels correlate well with plasma levels. Levels in both saliva and blood correlated equally well with behavioral and physiological effects. The half-life of cocaine in both fluids is the same, about 35 minutes in the case of saliva. Five hours after a 40-mg intravenous bolus of cocaine, levels in both saliva and blood are near the limits of detection (29 ng/mL for saliva and 8 ng/mL for plasma). Accordingly, if cocaine can be detected in saliva it is a good sign of very recent use (Cone & Menchen, 1988) (Ferko et al., 1990).

The same cautions apply to the interpretation of low cocaine levels in the saliva as in the blood. Chronic users may have persistent low levels even when they have abstained for several days or more. The presence of low levels in the saliva is certainly consistent with past cocaine use, but it is not necessarily diagnostic of recent ingestion. During cocaine withdrawal, lipophilic storage sites in the brain continue to release cocaine. Small amounts can appear in saliva and urine for weeks. Rats given 20 mg/kg twice a day for two weeks have cocaine detectable in their fat for as long as 4 weeks after the drug has been discontinued (Nayak et al., 1976). The same is true in man. Chronic users monitored during withdrawal continue to excrete unmetabolized cocaine, detectable by RIA, for 10 days or more after their last dose (Cone & Weddington, 1989).

1.7.7.2 Vitreous humor

Measurement of levels within the vitreous seems an obvious approach, but there have been only limited studies. Levels in blood, vitreous and liver were measured in a 28-year old woman who died shortly after an intravenous injection. When the blood cocaine was 750 ng/mL the concentration in the vitreous was 380 ng/mL and in the liver it was 130 ng/mL (Lundberg, Garriott, Reynolds et al 1977). Di Maio and Garriott described another case where the blood level was 370 ng/mL while the vitreous was 210 ng/mL (Di Maio, Garriott, 1978). Hearn et al. measured vitreous cocaine concentrations in one eye just after death and then measured concentrations in the other eye 18 hours later. The cocaine level, which was 1.0 mg/L just after death rose to 3.5 mg/L after 18 hours. Benzoylecgonine levels also rose from 1.1 mg/L to 1.7 mg/L (Hearn, Keran, Wei & Hime, 1991a). An additional study has also demonstrated postmortem elevations of cocaine in the vitreous (Beno & Kriewall, 1989), suggesting that this is not a particularly good medium for postmortem investigations.

1.7.7.3 Spinal fluid

Measurements of spinal fluid might also prove useful, especially since cocaine crosses the blood brain barrier so readily. There have been no systematic studies, but one report suggests that unmetabolized cocaine can be detected in the CSF for at least 24 hours (Rowbotham et al., 1990).

1.7.7.4 Breast milk

Cocaine can be transferred to infants via mother's milk (Chasnoff et al. 1987), but the kinetics in humans have not been studied. Cocaine levels in the milk of lactating rats reach higher levels than in the mother's liver or brain. In one experimental study, cocaine levels in rat milk were eight times higher than blood levels. This may have to do with the high lipid content of the milk (Wiggins et al. 1989).

1.7.7.5 Urine

Cocaine is eliminated almost entirely by biotransformation. Very little cocaine is excreted unchanged in the urine, and the renal clearance is less than 30 mL/minute (Chow, Ambre, Ruo et al, 1985). Eighty per cent of a given dose is converted to benzoylecgonine and ecgonine methyl ester (Fish & Wilson, 1969) (Inaba, Stewart & Kalow, 1978) (Ambre, Ruo Ih, Nelson & Belknap, 1988), and smaller amounts of ecgonine, norcocaine and various hydroxylated products, all of which appear in the urine (Ambre et al., 1988) (Zhang & Foltz, 1990). In a study of human volunteers, Ambre found an elimination half-life of 2.3 to 4.1 hours for EME and 2.8 to 6.5 hours for BEG. Because the small amounts of cocaine that do appear in the urine are cleared very quickly, commercial screening tests are designed to detect metabolite, benzoyl-ecgonine, not cocaine itself. There may be some cross reactivity, but antibody based screening tests will not detect cocaine in the urine, even if it is present. Detection of cocaine chromatographically is sign of recent ingestion, especially in occasional users. The absence of cocaine, on the other hand, is only evidence that the drug hasn't been taken within the last few hours (Jatlow, 1988).

Compared to cocaine, the half-life of benzoylecgonine is a relatively long 6.5 hours, and metabolite may appear in the urine for days. Thus the presence of benzoylecgonine is solid proof of past use, but the timing of the past use cannot be inferred from the urinalysis alone. Hospitalized patients undergoing detoxification continue to excrete metabolite for weeks after their last dose of cocaine (Weiss & Gawin, 1988) (Burke, Ravi, Dhopesh et al, 1990) (Cone & Weddington, 1989). The same caveats which apply to saliva and blood testing also apply to urine. It should also be apparent that no conclusions can be drawn about the degree of an individual's impairment, if any, at the time of urine testing. The presence of metabolite indicates only that the drug was used in the past.

References

Ambre, J., Ruo, Ih., T., Nelson, J. & Belknap, S. (1988). Urinary excretion of cocaine, benzoylecgonine, and ecgonine methyl ester in humans. J Analyt Toxicol, 12, 301–306.

Beno, J. & Kriewall, S. (1989). Post mortem elevation of cocaine levels in vitreous humor. Cited in Hearn et al. Site-dependent postmortem changes in blood cocaine concentrations, J. Forensic Sci, 36(3):673–684 (cited on pg 681)

Benuck, M., Reith, M. E., Sershen, H. et al. (1989). Oxidative metabolism of cocaine; comparison of brain and liver (42822). Proc Soc Exp Biol and Med, 190 (1), 7–13.

Burke, W., Ravi, N., Dhopesh, V. et al. (1990). Prolonged presence of metabolite in urine after compulsive cocaine use. J Clin Psych, 51, 145–148.

Calligaro, D. & Eldefrawi, M. (1987). Central and peripheral cocaine receptors. J Pharm and Exp Ther, 243 (1), 61–68.

Camí, J., de la Torre, R., Farré, M. et al. (1991). Cocaine-alcohol interaction in healthy volunteers: plasma metabolic profile including cocaethylene. In Problems of drug dependence 1991: Proceedings of the 53rd Annual Scientific Meeting of the Committee on Problems of Drug Dependence, Inc. National Institute on Drug Abuse Monograph Series, Rockland, MD. In press.

Chasnoff, I., Lewis, D., Squires, L. (1987). Cocaine intoxication in a breast fed infant. Pediatrics, 80:836–838.

Chow, M., Ambre, J., Ruo, T. et al. (1985). Kinetics of cocaine distribution, elimination, and chronotropic effects. Clin Pharmacol Ther, 38, 318–324.

Cone, E. & Menchen, S. (1988). Stability of cocaine in saliva. Clin Chem, 34(7), 1508.

Cone, E. & Weddington, W., Jr. (1989). Prolonged occurrence of cocaine in human saliva and urine after chronic use. J Analyt Toxicol, 13 (20), 65–68.

Cone, E., Yousenfnejad, D., Darwin, W. Maguire (1991). Testing human hair for drugs of abuse. II. Identification of unique cocaine metabolites in hair of drug abusers and evaluation of decontamination procedures. J Analyt Toxic, 15 (5) 250–255.

Critchley, H., Woods, S., Barson et al (1988). Fetal death in utero and cocaine abuse. Case report. Br J Obst and Gynecol, 95 (2):195–196.

DiMaio, V. and Garriott, J.(1978). Four deaths due to intravenous injection of cocaine. Forensic Sci Int., 12:119–125.

Ferko, A., Barabieri, E., Digregorio, G. & Ruch, E. (1990). The presence of cocaine and benzoylecgonine in rat parotid saliva, plasma and urine after the intravenous administration of cocaine. Res Comm in Subst Abuse, 1–2.

Finkle, B. & McCloskey, K. (1978). The forensic toxicology of cocaine (1971--1976). J Forensic Sci, 22:173–189.

Fish, F. & Wilson, W. (1969). Excretion of cocaine and its metabolites in man. J Pharm Pharmacol, 21, Suppl, 135S–138S.

Freeman, R. & Harbison, R. (1981). Hepatic periportal necrosis induced by chronic administration of cocaine. Biochem Pharmacol, 30(7), 777–783.

Hearn, W., Keran, E., Wei, H. & Hime, G. (1991a). Site-dependent postmortem changes in blood cocaine concentrations. J Forensic Sci, 36(3), 673–684.

Hearn, W. L., Flynn, D., Hime et al.(1991b). Cocaethylene - a unique cocaine metabolite displays high affinity for the dopamine transporter. J Neurochem, 56(2), 698–701.

Inaba, T., Stewart, D. & Kalow, W. (1978). Metabolism of cocaine in man. Clin Pharmacol Ther, 23:547–552.

Jatlow, P. (1988). Cocaine: analysis, pharmacokinetics, and metabolic disposition. Yale J Biol and Med, 61 (2), 105–113.

Jones, L. and Tackett, R. (1992). Differential routes of cocaine administration indicate a peripheral cardiotoxic action. Pharmacol. Biochem. Behav., 38:601–603.

Kloss.,K.W., Rosen, G.M., Rauckman, E.K. (1984). Cocaine-mediated hepatotoxicity: a critical review. Biochem Pharmacol, 33, 169–173

Kumar, A. (1991). Identification and quantitation of norcocaine in illicit cocaine samples. Read at Annual Meeting of the American Academy of Forensic Sciences., (p. 73). Anaheim: AAFS.

Lundberg, G., Garriott, J., Reynolds et al (1977). Cocaine-related death. J Forensic Sci, 22:402–408.

Marks, V. & Chapple, P. (1967). Hepatic dysfunction in heroin and cocaine users. Br J Addict, 62, 189–195.

Misra, A., Nayak, P., Bloch, R. & Mule, S. (1975). Estimation and disposition of 3H-benzoylecgonine and pharmacological activity of some cocaine metabolites. J Pharm and Pharmacol, 27, 784–786.

Mittleman, R., Cofino, J. & Hearn, W. (1989). Tissue distribution of cocaine in a pregnant woman. J Forensic Sci, 34(2), 481–486.

Morild, I. & Stajic, M. (1990). Cocaine and fetal death. Forensic Sci Int, 47, 181–189.

Mule, S., Casella, G. & Misra, A. (1976). Intracellular disposition of 3H-cocaine, 3H norcocaine, 3H-benzoylecgonine, and 3H benzoylnorecgonine in the brain of rats. Life Sciences, 19, 1585–1596.

Nayak, P., Misra, A. & Mule, S. (1976). Physiological disposition and biotransformation of 3H-cocaine in acutely and chronically treated rats. J Pharm & Exp Ther, 196(3), 556–569.

Perino, L., Warren, G. & Levine, J. (1987). Cocaine-induced hepatotoxicity in humans. Gastroenterology, 93, 176–180.

Powell, C. J., Connolly, A. K. & Charles, S. J. (1991). Shifting necrosis - butylated hydroxytoluene (BHT) and phenobarbital move cocaine-induced hepatic necrosis across the lobule. Toxicol Lett, 55(2), 171–178.

Price, K. (1974). Fatal cocaine poisoning. J Forensic Sci Soc, 14:329–333.

Rowbotham, M., Kaku, D., Mueller, P. et al. (1990). Blood, urine, and CSF levels of cocaine and metabolites following seizures in cocaine abusers. Neurology, 40, Suppl 1, 133.

Spiehler, V. & Reed, D. (1985). Brain concentrations of cocaine and benzoylecgonine in fatal cases. J Forensic Sci, 30(4), 1003–1011.

Scheurer, J., Tebbett, I. and Logan B. (1991). A rapid method for determination of cocaine in brain tissue. J. Forensic Sci,, 36(6):1662–1665.

Som, P., Oster, Z., Volkow, N. and Sacker, D. (1989). Studies on whole-body distribution and kinetics of cocaine. J. Nuc. Med, 30:831.

Thompson, M., Shuster, L. & Shaw, K. (1979). Cocaine-induced hepatic necrosis in mice - the role of cocaine metabolism. Biochem Pharmacol, 28, 2389–2395.

Thompson, L.K., Yousenfnejad, D., Kumor, K. et al. (1987). Confirmation of cocaine in human saliva after intravenous use. J Analyt Toxicol, 11, 36–38.

Volkow, N., Fowler, J., Wolf, A. et al. (1992). Distribution and kinetics of carbon-11-cocaine in the human body measured with PET. J. Nuc Med, 33:521–525.

Weiss, R. & Gawin, F. (1988). Protracted elimination of cocaine metabolites in long-term, high-dose cocaine abusers. Am J Med, 85(6), 879–880.

Wiggins, R., Rolste, C., Ruiz, B., Davis, C. (1989). Pharmacokinetics of cocaine: basic studies of route, dosage, pregnancy, and lactation. Neurotoxicology, 10:367–382.

Yazigi, R.A. and Polakoski, K.L. (1992). Distribution of tritiated cocaine in selected genital and nongenital organs following administration to male mice. Arch Pathol Lab Med, 116:1036–1039.

Zhang, J. & Foltz, R. (1990). Cocaine metabolism in man: identification of four previously unreported cocaine metabolites in human urine. J Analyt Toxicol, 14(4), 201–205.

1.8 COCAINE'S EFFECTS ON CATECHOL METABOLISM

1.8.1 GENERAL CONSIDERATIONS

Cocaine, and all of the other abused stimulants, disrupt catechol metabolism. Cocaine abusers have elevated circulating levels of catecholamines, and this has been demonstrated both in experimental animals and in humans (Gunne & Jonsson, 1964) (Chiueh & Kopin, 1978) (Karch, 1987b) (Schwartz, Boyle, Janzen & Jones, 1988) (Dixon, Chang, Machado et al., 1988) (Nahas, Trouvé & Manger, 1991) (Kiritsyroy, Halter, Gordon et al., 1990) (Conlee, Barnett, Kelly & Han, 1991) (Trouve, Nahas & Manger, 1991). Even the offspring of substance abusing mothers have abnormal sympathetic function. (Ward, Schuetz et al., 1991). In opiate abuse, most of the medical complications are infectious or secondary to the presence of drug contaminants. Many, but not all, of the pathologic changes reported in conjunction with cocaine use appear to be catechol mediated. Blood pressure elevations associated with cocaine use are centrally mediated, and the elevation is independent of any effect that cocaine exerts on peripheral catechol uptake (Schindler, Tella, Katz & Goldberg, 1992). Nonetheless, the mechanisms of catecholamine toxicity play a major role and require consideration in some detail.

Catecholamines' effects on the cardiovascular system are mediated by specific catechol receptors. A family of subtypes has been identified, but the receptors of principal concern are the $alpha_1$-adrenergic receptors which are mainly located on blood vessels, and $beta_1$

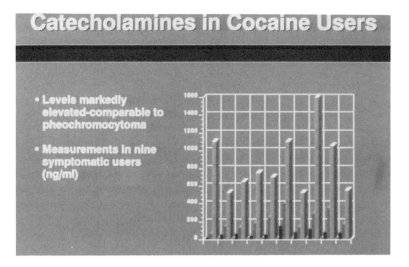

Figure 1.8.1 Elevated catecholamines in cocaine users
Catechol measurements made in crack smokers complaining of chest pain revealed substantial elevations in epinephrine and norepinephrine, but not in dopamine. Levels this high are consistent with near maximal adrenal stress and are known to be capable of producing myocardial necrosis.

receptors located in the heart. These receptors are coupled to phospholipase C via a G-protein. When the receptor is activated, phosphoinositol is cleaved into inositol phosphate and diacylglycerol. Separation of the two fragments releases free calcium into the cytosol and causes the blood vessel to contract. The alpha$_2$ receptors are found on blood vessels and neurons. When receptors on vessels are stimulated, adenyl cyclase is inhibited, intracellular levels of cyclic AMP drop, and vasoconstriction results. Stimulation of the alpha$_2$ receptors located on nerves inhibits the release of norepinephrine from postganglionic nerve endings, thus decreasing sympathetic flow.

Beta$_1$ receptors are found in the heart. When these receptors are stimulated, another G-protein is activated and adenyl cyclase activity is increased. The results include increases in heart rate, contractility, and conduction velocity. Beta$_2$ receptors are found on bronchi and smooth muscle, and also exert their effects by activating a G-protein and adenyl cyclase. Stimulation of the Beta$_2$ receptors causes dilation of bronchi and blood vessels.

The principal catecholamine of the heart is norepinephrine. Within the heart's local circulation, norepinephrine functions as a neurotransmitter. Norepinephrine is released into the synaptic cleft each time an impulse is transmitted. Impulse transmission stops when norepinephrine is pumped back into the presynaptic nerve ending. In the heart, only 30% of norepinephrine is metabolized by catechol-o-methyl transferase (Goldstein, Brush, Eisenhofer et al. 1988), the rest is actively pumped back into the presynaptic terminal. Cocaine prevents the reuptake of norepinephrine, and unmetabolized norepinephrine overflows into the systemic circulation. Once it enters the systemic circulation, norepinephrine acts as a circulating hormone (α 1,2 and ß1), not as a neurotransmitter. Epinephrine and norepinephrine bind to both alpha and beta receptors but differ in their relative affinities. Thus both are full agonists for alpha and beta$_1$ receptors, but epinephrine elicits a much greater response at beta$_2$ receptors.

Cocaine is avidly taken up by, and has a direct effect on, the adrenals (Volkow et al. 1992). In rats, cocaine causes the increased release of both epinephrine and norepinephrine (Chiueh & Kopin, 1978) (Gunne & Jonsson, 1964) (Dixon, 1989). The same is true of squirrel monkeys (Trouve, Nahas, Manger et al. 1990b). For unknown reasons, this increase in circulating catecholamines does not lead to CNS catechol depletion. Rats given repeated doses of cocaine show constant brain levels of catecholamines in the face of increased urinary excretion (Chiueh & Kopin, 1978). In a prospective study of "crack" users with chest pain, elevations in both epinephrine and norepinephrine levels were noted, but not elevations of dopamine. In ten such patients, norepinephrine levels ranged from 345 ng/L to 1,200 ng/L (normal range 0–90 ng/L) and epinephrine ranged from 135 to 300 ng/L (normal range 0–55 ng/L) (Karch, 1987b). Catechol measurements in dogs given intravenous cocaine were comparable (Schwartz, 1989), as were elevations in exercising rats (Conlee et al., 1991). Elevated plasma norepinephrine levels have even been observed in infants born to cocaine-using mothers. When catechol levels were measured in the otherwise healthy children of cocaine-using mothers, venous norepinephrine levels were 1.8x those of controls, while there were no differences in epinephrine or dopamine levels (Ward et al., 1991).

Very limited data suggests that cocaine users respond abnormally to elevated catecholamine levels. Chronic catechol excess is usually associated with down regulation of ß receptors, but cocaine users don't down regulate. Several groups have made lymphocyte receptor measurements, and found no change in binding sites or receptor affinity for either α or ß-adrenoreceptors, in spite of elevated circulating levels of catecholamines (Conlee et al., 1991) (CostardJackle, Kates & Fowler, 1989) (Trouve, Nahas & Manger, 1990a). This failure to down-regulate has also been observed in infants born to substance-abusing mothers, in spite of the fact that they too have increased circulating levels of norepinephrine.

Stimulation of both alpha and beta receptors promotes elevation of intracellular calcium. When norepinephrine and epinephrine bind to ß receptors, adenylate cyclase is activated, causing increased levels of 3'-5' cyclic AMP. The latter compound activates an AMP-dependent protein kinase capable of phosphorylating a family of regulatory

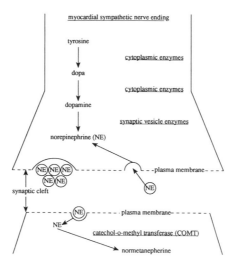

Figure 1.8.2.1
Synthesis and fate of norepinephrine produced in sympathetic nerves that supply the heart. In the heart, but not elsewhere in the body, the action of norepinephrine is terminated mainly by the reuptake of norepinephrine.

proteins, including those that control calcium movement, both on the cell surface and in the endoplasmic reticulum (Evans, 1986). As a direct consequence of catechol stimulation, calcium enters the cell and additional calcium is released from sequestered stores within the endoplasmic reticulum. Once intracytosolic calcium has risen to about 100 times resting concentrations, the myofilaments contract. The cycle terminates when the calcium is pumped back out of the cytosol. Alpha stimulation also elevates intracytosolic calcium. When alpha receptors are activated, phosphatidyl-inositol is hydrolyzed into diacylglycerol and inositol triphosphate. These two compounds are classified as "second messengers". Inositol triphosphate facilitates the release of calcium from the endoplasmic reticulum, and diacylglycerol enhances production of protein kinase C which interacts with calcium channels and beta receptors. This combination of activities further increases the amount of free calcium in the cytoplasm. If too much calcium accumulates within the cell, toxic effects can occur. These effects may be manifested as altered membrane potentials and abnormal impulse conduction, or even by the presence of visible lesions.

1.8.2 MECHANISMS OF CATECHOLAMINE TOXICITY

Elevated levels of circulating catecholamines are associated with a number of undesirable effects. Increased α adrenergic stimulation of coronary vascular smooth muscle causes vasoconstriction and ischemia

(Mathias, 1986) (Ascher, Stauffer & Gaash, 1988). The combination of simultaneous α and β stimulation means that cocaine-induced vasoconstriction is accompanied by increased oxygen demand. In individuals with preexisting lesions, myocardial infarction can probably be explained by this combination of α and β effects.

CONDITIONS ASSOCIATED WITH CONTRACTION BAND NECROSIS *

Reperfusion
Steroid therapy
Electrocution
Defibrillation
Drowning
Cocaine
Amphetamine
Epinephrine
Isoproterenol
Norepinephrine
Cobalt poisoning
Starvation
Myocardial infarction
Free-radical injuries
Brain death
Phenylpropanolamine
Intracerebral hemorrhage

*from Karch & Billingham, Contraction bands revisited. Hum Pathol 1987

At the cellular level, acutely elevated levels of epinephrine and norepinephrine can alter membrane potentials so that the occurrence of malignant ventricular arrhythmias is favored. This process was first suggested nearly fifty years ago (Bozler, 1943). Chronic exposure to high levels of catecholamines, on the other hand, can induce morphologic changes which are also associated with arrhythmias and sudden death. The specific morphologic changes induced by catechol excess are essentially the same as those associated with cocaine toxicity (Karch & Billingham,1988) (Tazelaar, Karch, Billingham & Stephens, 1987). The changes associated with cocaine and catechol toxicity are, in turn, the same as the morphologic changes associated with intracellular calcium overload. And, depending on the experimental design, the morphologic changes induced by cocaine, like the changes associated with catechol toxicity, can be prevented by calcium channel blockade (Nahas, Trouve, Demus & Sitbon, 1985) (Trouve & Nahas, 1986) (Trouve et al., 1990a). It is important to remember that calcium overload is not synonymous with catechol toxicity. Anything which disrupts membrane integrity, including ischemia, can result in calcium overload (Rona, 1985).

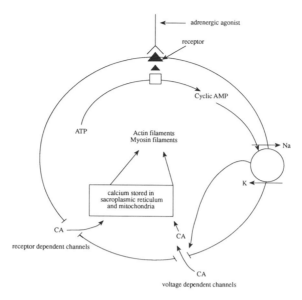

Figure 1.8.2.2 Sequence of events leading to cardiac myocyte contraction
Norepinephrine binds at both alpha and beta receptor sites but has much greater affinity for the alpha receptor. Calcium enters via voltage dependent channels (known as "slow channels") and through other calcium channels that open when norepinephrine binds to an alpha receptor. Calcium is also released from storage sites within the myocyte. Once the level of calcium within the cell has risen 100-fold, myofilaments are able to contract. If cytosolic calcium levels become too high, irreversible damage occurs to the myofilaments; this is known as "contraction band necrosis".

1.8.3 HISTOPATHOLOGY OF CATECHOL TOXICITY

Catecholamines cause a histologic change within the myocardium (Szakacs JE, 1958). The morphologic changes seen in the hearts of cocaine and amphetamine users are similar. The best known, and the most important, morphologic alteration is the injury known as contraction band necrosis. This lesion has both pathologic and forensic significance. Contraction band necrosis (CBN), sometimes referred to as coagulative myocytolysis and sometimes as myofibrillar degeneration, is a nonspecific finding. It can be seen in a variety of conditions which are apparently unrelated. Often seen after reperfusion, CBN also occurs in the hearts of patients who have been multiply defibrillated. Contraction bands are also prominent in the hearts of patients with intracerebral hemorrhage, drowning, pheochromocytoma and other conditions associated with catechol excess. CBN is frequently observed in cases of sudden cardiac death. Meticulous studies have confirmed the presence of these lesions in over 80% of individuals with non-drug related sudden death (Reichenbach & Moss, 1975) (Cebelin & Hirsch, 1980). The incidence in drug related deaths may be even higher (Rajis & Falconer, 1979) (Tazelaar et al., 1987).

The term "contraction band necrosis" was introduced by Caulfield and Kilonsky in 1959 (Caulfield & Kilonsky, 1959), but the lesion had actually been described in the heart of a cocaine user in 1922 by Bravetta and Invernizzi (Maier, 1926)! Szakacs was the first to systematically characterize the effects of catecholamines on myocardial structure and was the first to note the unique distribution of these lesions. Areas of contraction band necrosis tend to occur "without any apparent preferential distribution" (Szakacs & Cannon, 1958; Szakacs, Dimmette & Cowart, 1959). What Szakacs was referring to was the fact that severely damaged cells are often found nestled between totally normal cells. If the damage to the cell had been due to ischemia, then one would expect all the cells in a specific area show signs of injury. Szakacs made a second important observation. He realized that the changes seen after chronic catechol administration were identical to those seen in patients with pheochromocytoma (Karch & Billingham, 1988; Karch & Billingham, 1986).

Calcium overload can be initiated by many different processes. Calcium enters the cells when calcium channels are opened by catechol stimulation. When there is myocardial ischemia, a loss of cell membrane integrity can lead to the same result and the cell floods with calcium. Whatever the cause, a continuum of morphologic alterations can be seen; these may range from hypereosinophilia to total disruption of the cell. As Szakacs discovered, the lesions are characterized as much by their location as by their appearance. They bear no apparent relationship to blood supply. Contraction bands may be found in myocytes adjacent to normal capillaries. They can, and do, occur in the absence of significant coronary artery disease. Unlike the picture seen in infarction, where the myofibrillar apparatus remains visible and in register, in CBN the sarcomers are hypercontracted and distorted. The contractile apparatus may not even be visible. Milder forms of the lesion consist of eosinophilic transverse bands separated by areas containing fine eosinophilic granules.

With electron microscopy, it is apparent that the myofilaments are completely out of register and the mitochondria translocated. The dense bands visible with light microscopy are seen as amorphous gray material. This material is all that remains of both the thick and thin filaments. This exact change has been observed in the hearts of rats chronically treated with cocaine (Nahas, Maillet, Chiarasini & Latour, 1991). Z-band remnants, the hallmark of dilated, congestive cardiomyopathy, are generally not seen, however if the process were ongoing and particularly severe, then the presence of Z-band remnants would not be particularly surprising. In severe instances, as in open-heart defibrillation, the sarcomers look as if they have been torn apart, and dehiscence of the intercalated disks can occur (Karch & Billingham, 1986).

Initially, and probably not for at least 12 hours, there are no inflammatory cells in these lesions. Occasionally a mononuclear infiltrate may be seen. Eventually the injured cells are resorbed and replaced with fibrous tissue. The pattern is classically seen in patients (and experimental animals) with pheochromocytoma. Illustrating the progression of lesions in humans is quite difficult, but lesions corresponding to each stage in the evolution of catechol injury have been reported in man. The resultant fibrosis, which is occasionally quite prominent in the hearts of cocaine users, may supply the substrate for lethal arrhythmias (Merx, Yoon & Han, 1977) (Strain, Grose, Factor & Fisher, 1983).

The catechol levels required to produce necrosis have been determined, largely as a result of research in the field of heart transplantation. Hearts from donors that have been maintained with pressor therapy frequently fail after surgery. In the course of research designed to explain why, experimenters found that a surge of catecholamines accompanies brain death, and that this surge is associated with the presence of contraction band necrosis. In the baboon model of brain death, catechol elevations comparable to those seen in some cocaine users are observed (Novitzky, Cooper & Reichart, 1987; Novitzky, Cooper & Wicomb, 1988; Novitzky, Wicomb, Cooper et al, 1984; Novitzky, Wicomb et al, 1986) (Worstman, Frank & Cryer, 1984). In the experimental model of brain death, the cardiac lesions can be prevented by denervation or beta blockade. The occurrence of myocardial contraction bands must, in some way, be related to ß receptor number, density, and regulation. These parameters, in turn, depend on how much drug has been used and for how long. Unfortunately, the impact of cocaine and chronic catechol excess on receptor physiology remains, for the most part, unstudied. The limited number of studies that have addressed this question have all reached the same conclusion. There is no indication of beta receptor down regulation either in lymphocytes or myocardium (Conlee et al., 1991) (Costard-Jackle et al., 1989) (Trouve et al., 1990a) (Chiarasini, Dingeon, Latour et al, 1992). This failure of down regulation distinguishes cocaine abuse from all other chronic hyperadrenergic states.

The fact that the general tendency for down regulation to occur in hyperadrenergic states has not been confirmed in cocaine users is somewhat puzzling (Tsujimoto, Manger & Hoffman, 1984). Both the β and α receptors on lymphocytes and platelets downregulate in the presence of catechol excess, and one would expect the same result whatever the reason for the catechol elevation. It may well be that some alteration in signal transduction has occurred between the receptors and adenyl cyclase, though that possibility remains to be investigated. It has been shown that tyrosine hydroxylase activity is increased by cocaine administration (Taylor & Ho, 1977). That observation is consistent with the

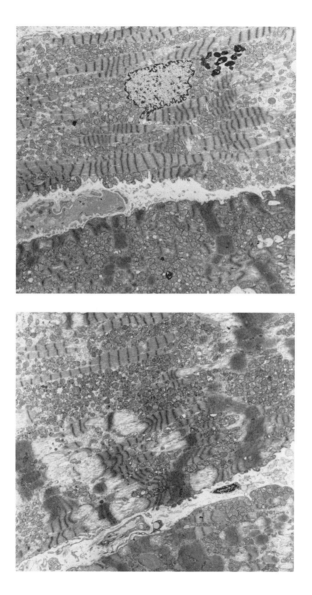

Figure 1.8.3 Effects of catecholamines on cardiac myocytes
The electron micrograph on top shows normal human myocardium. The myofilaments are in register; the mitochondria are of uniform size and are neatly packed between the filaments. The bottom micrograph illustrates the changes seen in contraction band necrosis. The dark electron-dense material is all that remains of the myofilaments; the mitochondria are swollen and translocated. Original magnification 4,320x (both A and B). Courtesy of Dr. Margaret Billingham and Marilyn Masek, Stanford University School of Medicine.

notion that increased catecholamine synthesis is occurring in an attempt to keep up with increased catechol turnover. Evidence from other fields suggests that when this happens, post synaptic calcium channel receptors will down regulate in an attempt to prevent calcium overload (Lefkowitz, Caron & Stiles, 1984).

1.8.4 CONTRACTION BAND NECROSIS AND SUDDEN DEATH

Contraction band necrosis is a marker for sudden death, whatever the cause. This has been demonstrated in a succession of studies over the last 40 years. The incidence of this finding in various autopsy studies is over 80 percent (Baroldi & Mariano, 1979) (Reichenbach & Moss, 1975) (Cebelin & Hirsch, 1980). The incidence in drug-related deaths may be even higher (Rajis & Falconer, 1979) (Tazelaar et al., 1987). Postmortem studies of addicts in general, and stimulant users in particular, have confirmed the presence of myocardial necrosis and focal fibrosis (Rajs, Härm & Ormstad, 1984) (Oehmichen, Homann & Merten, 1990).

The role of contraction band necrosis in cocaine-associated sudden death was established in a fairly large retrospective study. Myocardium from 30 individuals with cocaine associated sudden death was compared with tissue from a group of 20 patients who had died of sedative hypnotic overdose. The latter were chosen for controls because sedatives are not known to produce catechol elevations or CBN. Since CBN is a non-specific process, lesions would be expected to occur in both groups, if for no other reason than that hypoxia and resuscitation both cause contraction band necrosis (Karch, 1987a). Contraction band necrosis would, however, be expected to occur in the cocaine group much more frequently than in the controls. That was exactly what was found. Lesions occurred in both groups but were significantly much more common ($P < 0.001$) among the cocaine users. Contraction band lesions were found in 93% of the cocaine group and the lesions were judged to be diffuse in more than half the cases. In contrast, patients in the control group had CBN present less than half the time and it was diffuse in less than 10% of the cases. Also observed was a significant increase in the degree of fibrosis for the patient age group. Over 25% of the cocaine users had fibrosis, sometimes to quite striking degrees. The finding could represent previous episodes of ischemia, but more likely is a reflection of the healing process associated with recurrent bouts of contraction band necrosis.

The findings of this first systematic study, which were consistent with earlier studies on drug abuse in general, have since been confirmed in other studies of cocaine users. Contraction band necrosis has been found in other autopsy studies (Simpson & Edwards, 1986) (Roh & Hamele-Bena, 1990), and fibrosis, though at a somewhat lower incidence than observed in the San Francisco series (Mckelway, Vieweg &

Westerman, 1990). One study failed to confirm an increased frequency of CBN in cocaine users, but since the frequency of CBN in that study's control group was so much lower than what is accepted as normal for the general population, the significance of this one study is difficult to assess (Virmani, Rabinowitz, Smialek & Smyth, 1988).

Contraction band necrosis never occurs as fixation artifact (Karch & Billingham, 1986). The presence of such lesions always indicates some underlying abnormality, usually catechol excess. By themselves contraction bands constitute only presumptive indicators for cocaine use, especially if they are seen in biopsy specimens. Biopsy studies of symptomatic users have shown the same pathology as seen in the San Francisco study (Peng, 1989), but contraction bands are normally seen in biopsy specimens anyway (Adomian, Laks & Billingham, 1967). Stronger inferences can be drawn if there are other supporting findings. For instance, if microfocal fibrosis is present, the differential diagnosis then becomes quite limited. Very few conditions produce contraction band necrosis with microfocal fibrosis. In fact, the only real alternative diagnosis is pheochromocytoma, which should not be all that difficult to rule out.

References

Adomian, G., Laks, M. & Billingham, M. (1978). The incidence and significance of contraction bands in endomyocardial biopsies from normal human hearts. Am Heart J, 95(3), 348–351.

Ascher, E., Stauffer, J. & Gaash, W. (1988). Coronary artery spasm, cardiac arrest, transient electrocardiographic Q waves and stunned myocardium in cocaine-associated acute myocardial infarction. Am J Cardiol, 61 (11), 938–941.

Baroldi, G. & Mariano, F. (1979). Sudden coronary death. A postmortem study in 208 selected cases compared to 97 "control" subjects, 98, 20–31.

Bozler, E. (1943). The initiation of impulses in cardiac muscle. Am J Physiol, 138, 273–282.

Caulfield, J. & Klionsky, B. (1959). Myocardial ischemia and early infarction: an electron microscopic study. Am J Pathol, 35(3), 489–501.

Cebelin, M. & Hirsch, C. (1980). Human stress cardiomyopathy: myocardial lesions in victims of homicidal assaults without internal injuries. Hum Pathol, 11, 123–132.

Chiarasini, D., Dingeon, P., Latour, C. et al. Cardiovascular tolerance to cocaine and its correlates. Read at the Annual Meeting of the British Pharmacological Society, London, September 9, 1992.

Chiueh, C. & Kopin, I. (1978). Centrally mediated release by cocaine of endogenous epinephrine and norepinephrine from the sympathoadrenal medullary system of unanesthetized rats. J Pharmacol Exp Ther, 205, 148–154.

Conlee, R. K., Barnett, D. W., Kelly, K. P. & Han, D. H. (1991). Effects of cocaine on plasma catecholamine and muscle glycogen concentrations during exercise in the rat. J Appl Physiol, 70 (3), 1323–1327.

Costard-Jackle, A., Jackle, S., Kates, R. & Fowler, M. (1989). Electrophysiological and biochemical effect of chronic cocaine administration. Circulation, 80(4), II 15.

Dixon, W., Chang, A., Machado, J. et al. (1988). Effect of intravenous infusion and oral self-administration of cocaine on plasma and adrenal catecholamine levels and cardiovascular parameters in the conscious rat. In L. Harris (Ed.), Committee for Problems of Drug Dependency, Annual Scientific Conference; Published in National Institute on Drug Abuse Research Monograph #95. (1989),pp. 335–336.

Evans, D. (1986). Modulation of cAMP: mechanism for positive inotropic action. J Cardiovasc Pharmacol, 8, Suppl 9, S22–S29.

Goldstein, D., Brush, J., Eisenhofer, G., Stull, R. & Esler, M. (1988). In vivo measurement of neuronal uptake of norepinephrine in the human heart. Circulation, 78, 41–48.

Gunne, L. & Jonsson, J. (1964). Effects of cocaine administration on brain, adrenal and urinary adrenaline and noradrenaline in rats. Psychopharmacologia, 6(2), 125–129.

Karch, S. (1987a). Resuscitation-induced myocardial necrosis. Am J Forensic Med and Path, 8(1), 3–8.

Karch, S. (1987b). Serum catecholamines in cocaine -intoxicated patients with cardiac symptoms. Ann Emerg Med, 16(4), 481.

Karch, S. & Billingham, M. (1988). The pathology and etiology of cocaine--induced heart disease. Arch Pathol Lab Med, 112, 225–230.

Karch, S. & Billingham ME (1986). Myocardial contraction bands revisited. Hum Pathol, 17, 9–13.

Kiritsy-Roy, J. A.,Halter, J. B., Gordon et al. (1990). Role of the central nervous system in hemodynamic and sympathoadrenal responses to cocaine in rats. J Pharmacol Exp The, 255(1), 154–160.

Lefkowitz, R., Caron, M. & Stiles, G. (1984). Mechanisms of membrane- receptor regulation. N Engl J Med, 310, 1570–1579.

Maier, H. W. (1926). Der Kokainismus (O.J. Kalant from the German 1926 edition, Trans.). Toronto: Addiction Research Foundation.

Mathias, D. (1986). Cocaine-associated myocardial ischemia: review of clinical and angiographic findings. Am J Med, 81, 675–678.

Mckelway, R., Vieweg, V. & Westerman, P. (1990). Sudden death from acute cocaine intoxication in Virginia in 1988. Am J Psych, 147(12), 1667–1669.

Merx, W., Yoon, M. & Han, J. (1977). The role of local disparity in conduction and recovery of ventricular vulnerability to fibrillation. Am Heart J, 94(5), 603–610.

Nahas, G., Maillet, M., Chiarasini, D. & Latour, C. (1991). Myocardial damage induced by cocaine administration of a week's duration in the rat. In L. Harris (Ed.), Committee for Problems of Drug Dependency, Annual Scientific Conference; National Institute on Drug Abuse Research Monograph Series, in press.

Nahas, G., Trouve, R., Demus, J. & Sitbon, M. (1985). A calcium-channel blocker as antidote to the cardiac effects of cocaine intoxication. N Engl J Med, 313(8), 519–520.

Nahas, G., Trouvé, R. & Manger, W. (1990). Cocaine, catecholamines and cardiac toxicity. Acta Anesthesiol Scand, 34(Suppl 94),77–81.

Novitzky, D., Cooper, D. & Reichart, B. (1987). Haemodynamic and metabolic responses to hormonal therapy in brain dead potential organ donors. Transplantation, 43, 852–854.

Novitzky, D., Cooper, D. & Wicomb, W. (1988). Endocrine changes and metabolic responses. Transplantation Proc (5,Suppl 7), 33–38.

Novitzky, D., Wicomb, W., Cooper, D. et al. (1984). Electrocardiographic, hemodynamic and endocrine changes occurring during experimental brain death in the Chacma baboon. J Heart Transplant, 4, 63–69.

Novitzky, D., Wicomb, W., DKC, C. et al. (1986). Prevention of myocardial injury during brain death by total cardiac sympathectomy in the Chacma baboon. Ann Thorac Surg, 41, 520–524.

Oehmichen, M., Homann, P. & Pedal, I. (1990). Diagnostic significance of myofibrillar degeneration of cardiocytes in forensic pathology. Forensic Sci Int, 48, 163–173.

Peng, S.K., French, W.J., Pelikan, P.C.D. (1989). Direct cocaine cardiotoxicity demonstrated by endomyocardial biopsy. Arch Pathol Lab Med, 113 (8), 842–845.

Rajis, J. & Falconer, B. (1979). Cardiac lesions in intravenous drug addicts. Forensic Sci Int 13, 193–209.

Rajs, J., Härm, T. & Ormstad, K. (1984). Postmortem findings of pulmonary lesions of older datum in intravenous drug addicts. Virchows Arch, 402, 405–414.

Reichenbach, D. & Moss, N. (1975). Myocardial cell necrosis and sudden death in humans. Circulation, 51,52(Suppl III), III60–62.

Roh, L. & Hamele-Bena, D. (1990). Cocaine-induced ischemic myocardial disease. Am J Forensic Med & Pathol, 11(2), 130–135.

Rona, G. (1985). Catecholamine cardiotoxicity. J Mol Cell Cardiol, 17(4), 291–306.

Schindler, C., Tella, S., Katz, J. & Goldberg, S. (1992). Effects of cocaine and its quaternary derivative cocaine methiodide on cardiovascular function in squirrel monkeys. Euro J Pharmacol, 213:99–105.

Schwartz, A., Boyle, W., Janzen, D. & Jones, R. (1988). Acute effects of cocaine on catecholamines and cardiac electrophysiology in the conscious dog. Can J Cardiol, 4(4), 188–192.

Simpson, R. & Edwards, W. (1986). Pathogenesis of cocaine-induced ischemic heart disease. Arch Patho Lab Med, 110, 479–484.

Strain, J., Grose, R., Factor, S. & Fisher, J. (1983). Results of endomyocardial biopsy in patients with spontaneous ventricular tachycardia but without apparent structural heart disease. Circulation, 68(6), 1171–1181.

Szakacs, J. & Cannon A (1958). l-Norepinephrine myocarditis. Am J Clin Pathol, 30, 425–434.

Szakacs, J., Dimmette, R. & Cowart, E. (1959). Pathologic implications of the catecholamines epinephrine and norepinephrine. US Armed Forces Med J, 10,2 908–925.

Taylor, D. & Ho, B. (1977). Neurochemical effects of cocaine following acute and repeated injection. J Neurosci Res, 32(2), 95–101.

Tazelaar, H., Karch, S., Billingham, M. & Stephens, B. (1987). Cocaine and the heart. Hum Pathol, 18:195–199.

Trouve, R. & Nahas, G. (1986). Nitrendipine: an antidote to cardiac and lethal toxicity of cocaine. Proc Soc Exp Biol and Med, 183, 392–397.

Trouve, R., Nahas, G., Manger, W. et al. (1990b). Interactions of nimodipine and cocaine on endogenous catecholamines in the squirrel monkey. Proc Soc Exp Med, 193, 171–175.

Trouve, R., Nahas, G. G. & Manger, W. M. (1991). Catecholamines, cocaine toxicity, and their antidotes in the rat. Proc Soc Exp Biol Med, 196(2), 184–187.

Tsujimoto, G., Manger, W. & Hoffman, B. (1984). Desensitization of beta-adrenergic receptors by pheochromocytoma. Endocrinology, 114, 1272–1278.

Virmani, R., Rabinowitz, M., Smialek, J. & Smyth, D. (1988). Cardiovascular effects of cocaine: an autopsy study of 40 patients. Am Heart J, 115(5), 1068–1076.

Volkow, N., Fowler, J., Wolf, A. et al. (1992). Distribution and kinetics of carbon-11-cocaine in the human body measured with PET. J. Nuc Med, 33:521–525.

Ward, S. L. D., Schuetz, S., Wachsman, L. et al. (1991). Elevated plasma norepinephrine levels in infants of substance-abusing mothers. Am J Dis Chil, 145(1), 44–48.

Worstman, J., Frank, S. & Cryer, P. (1984). Adrenomedullary response to maximal stress in humans. Am J Med, 77, 779–784.

1.9 EXTERNAL MARKERS OF COCAINE ABUSE

There are external markers for cocaine abuse that may be of clinical value. None of these changes are particularly common and they are only seen with intense and repeated use. The absence of these external signs has little, if any significance. The presence of these changes, however, is a strong confirmatory sign that the individual has been a chronic user for some time.

1.9.1 PERFORATED NASAL SEPTUM

Septal perforation is the best known external manifestation of cocaine abuse. The first cases were described in the early 1900's, shortly after the practice of snorting cocaine became popular (Hutant, 1910) (Maier, 1926). The presence of this lesion is, however, not pathognomic. It can also result from chronic abuse of nose drops containing vasoconstrictors (Vilensky, 1982) (see also section 1.10.3.1)

1.9.2 COCAINE "TRACKS"

The adulterants most commonly found in cocaine are water soluble, and their repeated injection tends not to produce the chronic inflammatory reactions and granulomas associated with narcotic abuse. Recent injection sites appear as salmon colored bruises, sometimes with a clear central zone about the needle puncture site (Wetli, 1987a; Wetli, 1987b). As lesions become older they turn blue and yellow, eventually disappearing without leaving any scar. Slowly healing cutaneous ulcers are also seen. The base of the ulcer may be red to gray and the margins of the ulcers will have a pearly white appearance consistent with epidermal overgrowth (Yaffee, 1968). In experimental animals, healing of lesions is relatively rapid and complete (Bruckner, Beng & Levy, 1982).

The histopathologic effects of subcutaneous cocaine injection have been studied on a limited scale. Subcutaneous injections of 0.1 to 2.0% cocaine solutions cause blanching and hemorrhage. Fifteen minutes post injection, blood vessels are engorged and there is hyalinization of scattered muscle bundles. Cocaine is directly toxic to vascular endothelium. Hemorrhage of the vessels in the mid and upper dermis is seen within 15 minutes of injection. The change is not due to cocaine induced vasoconstriction and ischemia, because epinephrine, which is a more powerful vasoconstrictor, doesn't produce similar lesions (Bruckner et al., 1982).

1.9.3 "CRACK KERATITIS"

Because "crack" smoke is a local anesthetic, the corneas of crack smokers may inadvertently be anesthetized. When the smoker rubs his eyes, too much pressure may be applied and a sizable piece of the cornea may be rubbed off. This sort of corneal abrasion has been referred to as "crack eye" (Ravin & Ravin, 1979). The same mechanism may lead to keratitis with corneal ulcers and infections (Strominger, Sachs & Hersh, 1990). Microbial and monilial keratitis have both been reported in crack smokers, suggesting that more than mechanical factors may be involved (Zagelbaum, Tannenbaum & Hersh, 1991). The results of some studies suggest that abnormalities of cell-mediated immunity develop in chronic cocaine users (Watzl & Watson, 1990). Chronic crack smokers may have a diminished ability to cope with normal bacterial flora.

1.9.4 DENTAL EROSIONS

Chronic intranasal cocaine users may have erosions on the enamel of the upper front teeth. Erosions result when the teeth are bathed with acid cocaine hydrochloride that has trickled down from the sinuses and the posterior oropharynx (Krutchkoff, Eisenberg, O'Brien & Ponzillo, 1990).

1.9.5 "CRACK THUMB"

This sign was first described in 1990, and is a "repetitive use" type of injury. Crack smokers often use disposable cigarette lighters to heat their pipes. They may do this many times a day, and a callus can result from repeated contact of the thumb with the serrated wheel that ignites the lighter. The callus is usually located on the ulnar aspect of the thumb (Larkin, 1990). Constant handling of a heated crack pipe can lead to superficial burns on the palmar aspect of the hands. The same

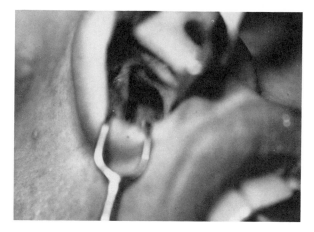

Figure 1.9.1 Perforated nasal septum
This lesion was first reported in conjunction with cocaine use in 1904. It is not absolutely diagnostic for cocaine abuse, since the same defect can be produced by the chronic use of vasoconstrictive nose drops. The first cases of cocaine-related septal perforation were reported just after the turn of the century. Courtesy of Dr. Russel Kridel, University of Texas, Health Sciences Center, Houston.

sort of thing happens in "ice" smokers.

1.9.6 "CRACK HANDS"

This finding has much in common with "crack thumb". Examination of chronic "crack" smokers may disclose blackened, hyperkeratotic lesions on the palmar aspect of the hands. The pipes used to smoke cocaine can become quite hot, and chronic users are likely to sustain multiple small burns (Feeny and Briggs, 1992).

1.9.7 EVIDENCE OF TERMINAL SEIZURES

Another occasionally observed external marker is a bite mark on the lips and tongue. A minority of cocaine users may experience seizure activity as a terminal event (Wetli, 1987a; Wetli, 1987b). However, since seizures don't always occur, even in conjunction with massive overdose, and since many other agents can cause terminal seizure activity, the usefulness of this sign is somewhat limited.

References

Bruckner, J.,Jiang, W. & Beng,T. Ho. (1982). Histopathological evaluation of cocaine induced skin lesions in the rat. J Cutaneous Pathol, 9, 83–95.

Feeny, C. and Briggs, S. (1992). Crack hands: a dermatologic effect of smoking crack cocaine. Cutis, 50:193–194.

Hautant, A. (1910). Über den chronischen Kokainismus mit nasaler Anwendung. Int Zentralbl. Laryngol Rhinol, 25, 138.

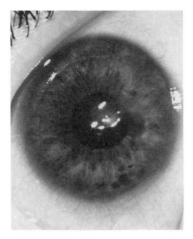

Figure 1.9.2 Crack keratitis
Volatilized cocaine anesthesizes the cornea so that abusers can't feel how hard they're rubbing their eyes. There is also evidence that crack smokers may be less able to resist corneal infection. Infected ulcers with corneal clouding may be the result. Courtesy of Dr. Peter S. Hersh, Chairman, Department of Ophthalmology, Bronx-Lebanon Hospital. Published with permission from the American Journal of Ophthalmology. Copyright 1991 by the Ophthalmic Publishing Co. Am J Opth Vol.111, No.3, p. 247-248.

Krutchkoff, D.,Eisenberg, E.,O'Brien, J. & Ponzillo, J. (1990). Cocaine-induced dental erosions. N Engl J Med, 322(6), 408.

Larkin, R. (1990). The callus of crack cocaine. N Engl J Med, 323(10), 685.

Maier, H. (1926). Der Kokainismus (O.J. Kalant from the German 1926 edition, Trans.). Toronto: Addiction Research Foundation.

Ravin , J. & Ravin, L. (1979). Blindness due to illicit use of topical cocaine. Ann Opthalmol, 11(6), 863-864.

Strominger, M.,Sachs, R. & Hersh, P. (1990). Microbial keratitis with crack cocaine. Arch Ophthalmol, 108(12), 1672.

Vilensky, W. (1982). Illicit and licit drugs causing perforation of the nasal septum: case report. J Forensic Sci, 27(4), 958-962.

Watzl, B. & Watson, R. (1990). Immunomodulation by cocaine-a neuroendocrine mediated response. Life Sci, 46 (19), 1319-1329.

Wetli, C. (1987a). Fatal reactions to cocaine. In A. Washington & M. Gold (Eds.), cocaine: a clinician's handbook New York, London: Guilford Press.

Wetli, C. (1987b). Fatal cocaine intoxication. Am J Forensic Med and Pathol, 8(1), 1-2.

Yaffee, H. (1968). Dermatologic manifestations of cocaine addiction. Cutis, 4, 286-287.

Zagelbaum, B.,Tannenbaum, M. & Hersh, P. (1991). Candida Albicans corneal ulcer associated with crack cocaine. Am J Ophthalmol, 111(2), 248-249.

1.10 TOXICITY BY ORGAN SYSTEM

1.10.1 INTUGEMENT

Scleroderma is an uncommon disease. The estimated annual incidence is between 4 and 12 new cases per million per year. Scleroderma is three times more common in females, but when it occurs in young people, it is fifteen times more common in women than men (Medsger & Masi, 1979). The median age of onset for scleroderma is between 40 and 50. Three cases of scleroderma have been reported in cocaine users, all were in males, two of whom were in their twenties. The third male was 40 years old (Kerr, 1989) (Trozak & Gould, 1984).

The principal abnormality in scleroderma is the deposition of pathologic amounts of normal collagen. In some instances, the process may be confined to the skin, but pathologic deposition may also be generalized. The etiology of scleroderma is not understood. Various theories have implicated alterations in cellular immunity, fibroblast function, and small vessel disease (Gay, Buckingham, Prince et al., 1980). The final common pathway by which the disease is manifest is thought to be small vessel disease that eventually produces fibrosis of the affected organ (Follansbee, Curtiss, Medsger et al., 1984). Cocaine abuse and scleroderma share certain common features. Vascular abnormalities are common in both, particularly in the heart. In classic scleroderma the heart becomes fibrotic and contraction band necrosis is frequently seen (Follansbee et al., 1984). The presence of myocardial fibrosis predisposes both groups to conduction defects and arrhythmias. Both groups are prone to heart failure and sudden death. The morphologic changes in the hearts of both groups are similar enough to raise the possibility that catechol toxicity is common to both.

There are other similarities. Both cocaine users and patients with scleroderma may develop isolated cerebral vasculitis. It is an uncommon complication of both disorders, but it has been observed in both, even in the absence of systemic vasculitis. In the two biopsy-proven cases of cocaine-associated vasculitis, the vessels were infiltrated with lymphocytes. In the one case of scleroderma-associated vasculitis the biopsy was non-diagnostic (Pathak & Gabor, 1991).

References

Follansbee, W.,Curtiss, E.,Medsger, T. et al. (1984). Physiologic abnormalities of cardiac function in progressive systemic sclerosis with diffuse scleroderma. N Engl J Med, 310, 142–148.

Gay, R.,Buckingham, R.,Prince, R. et al. (1980). Collagen types synthesized in dermal fibroblast cultures from patients with early progressive systemic sclerosis. Arthritis Rheum, 23 (2), 190–196.

Kerr, H. (1989). Cocaine and scleroderma. Souther Med J, 82(10), 275–276.

Medsger, T. & Masi, A. (1979). The epidemiology of systemic sclerosis. Clin
    Rheum Dis, 5, 15–25.
Pathak, R. & Gabor, A. (1991). Scleroderma and central nervous system vascu-
    litis. Stroke, 22, 410–413.
Trozak, D. & Gould, W. (1984). Cocaine abuse and connective tissue disease. J
    Am Acad Dermatol, 10, 525.

1.10.2 CARDIOVASCULAR SYSTEM

Cocaine causes vascular disease. Vessels throughout the body
can be involved, but the brunt of the injury is borne by the heart. In
general there is little to distinguish cocaine-induced disease from
naturally occurring disease, and no single abnormality is absolutely
diagnostic for cocaine-associated disease. However, in some instances
the pattern of histologic changes can be diagnostic. Specifically, the
changes associated with catechol toxicity are distinctive and are common
to stimulant abuse in general. In this section the pathology of cocaine-
-associated vascular disease will be reviewed with special emphasis on
the problem of catecholamine toxicity.

1.10.2.1 Coronary artery disease

Myocardial infarction is a relatively frequent complication of
cocaine use, but several years into the second cocaine pandemic there
still is a paucity of autopsy data. Three separate mechanisms have been
identified which could account for infarction in cocaine users. Most
infarcts are due to the presence of fixed lesions. In various reported
series, the incidence of fixed lesions, presumably atheromatous, but
possibly thrombotic, has been anywhere from 0% (Virmani, Rabinowitz
& Smialek, 1987) to well over 50% (Mathias, 1986) (Minor et al, 1991).
Only a handful of published reports have included autopsy findings
(Stenberg, Winniford, Hillis et al, 1989) (Young & Glauber, 1947) (Nanji
& Filpenko, 1984) (Kossowsky & Lyon, 1984) (Isner, Estes, Thompson
et al., 1986) (Simpson & Edwards, 1986), and occasionally angiographic
findings (Kossowsky & Lyon, 1984) (Pasternack, Colvin & Bauman,
1986) (Cregler & Mark, 1985) (Howard, Hueter & Davis, 1985) (Wilkins,
Mathur, Ty & Hall, 1985) (Weiss, 1986) (Ascher, Stauffer & Gaash, 1988)
(Isner et al., 1986) (Rollingher, Belzberg & Macdonald, 1986) (Rod &
Zucker, 1987) (Smith, Liberman, Brody et al., 1987) (Smith et al., 1987)
(Zimmerman, Gustafson & Kemp, 1987) have been described. In about
half the individual case reports, lesions have been demonstrated.

Failure to demonstrate lesions angiographically does not
necessarily mean that they are not there. Certain types of cocaine related
coronary lesions are neither thrombotic nor atherosclerotic and may
involve long segments of vessels in a concentric fashion. The lesions
may not be noticed on angiography unless earlier films are available for
comparison (Karch & Billingham, 1988) (Simpson & Edwards, 1986)

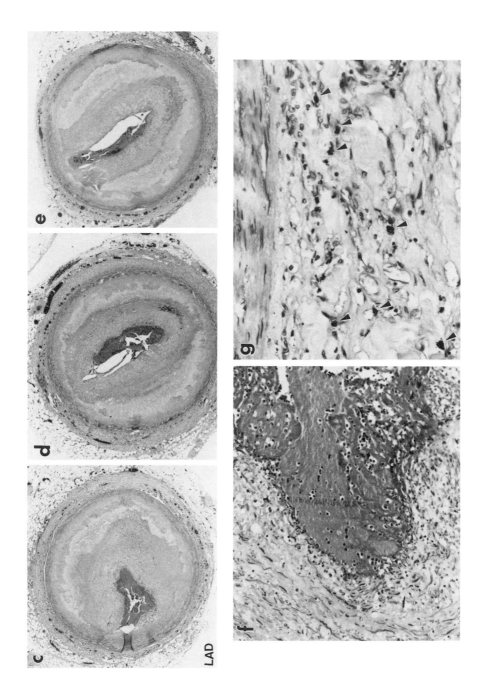

(Chow, Robertson & Stein, 1990). An arteriogram which looks normal may actually be missing serious underlying disease. It may very well be that the frequency of these lesions is significantly underestimated.

Simpson and Edwards were the first to describe intimal hyperplasia as a cause of myocardial infarction in a cocaine user (Simpson & Edwards, 1986). The patient, a 21-year old construction worker, had multivessel obstruction due entirely to intimal hyperplasia. There was no sign of collagen or elastin deposition. This sort of lesion is routinely seen in transplanted organs and also occurs in some connective tissue disorders (Dawkins, Jamieson,Hunt et al., 1985) (Bywater, 1957). It is classified as a type of "chronic rejection" and presumably occurs secondary to an immunologic abnormality. Simpson and Edwards postulated that recurrent episodes of coronary spasm might lead to endothelial injury with platelet aggregation and release of smooth muscle growth factor producing obstructive intimal hyperplasia. Whether or not their explanation is correct, similar alterations have been observed in the hearts of other cocaine users (Roh & Hamele-Bena, 1990).

Lesions nearly identical to those described by Simpson and Edwards can be produced by catechol excess. Even though modern histologic studies of cocaine induced changes are almost non-existent, the older literature contains many observations on what catecholamine treatment does to blood vessels. Thirty years ago, Szakacs found that dogs infused with norepinephrine at 1–1.5 μg/minute/kg would consistently develop coronary artery lesions. The initial response was fibrinoid necrosis, followed by intimal hyperplasia. Szakacs also observed exactly the same sorts of lesions in humans who died after receiving prolonged infusions of pressors and in patients dying of pheochromocytoma. Similar lesions were also found in the gastrointestinal tract. Occasionally these lesions completely obstructed the small arteries, resulting in bowel infarction and perforation (Szakacs, Dimmette & Cowart, 1959). Bowel infarction and perforation have also been seen in cocaine users (Endress & King, 1990) (Freudenberger, Cappell & Hutt, 1990) (Nathan & Hernandez, 1990) (Nalbandian, Sheth, Dietrich & Georgiou, 1985) (Mizrahi, Laor & Stamler, 1988). Histologically the picture is no different than the one described by Simpson and Edwards in the coronary arteries. A

Figure 1.10.2.1 1 Adventitial mast cells in cocaine users
Compared to age and sex matched controls, more mast cells are present in the adventitia of cocaine users' coronary arteries, and the degree of luminal narrowing correlates well with the number of mast cells present. On the left are three cross-sections of severely diseased LAD from a chronic cocaine user. On the right are higher-power views of the adventitia in this vessel. Toluidine blue staining demonstrates the presence of numerous mast cells; orig. magnification 150x. Courtesy of Dr. Rene Virmani, Chairman, Dept of Cardiovascular Pathology, Armed Forces Institute of Pathology.

slight variation on this theme was seen in one patient with cocaine related bowel infarction who had abnormalities of the submucosal arterioles with disruption of the internal elastic membrane that projected into and obstructed the lumen (Garfia, Valverde, Borondo et al., 1990). Endomyocardial biopsies from eleven cocaine users with symptoms of myocardial ischemia demonstrated marked medial thickening of small intramyocardial arteries (20 to 40 μM) in 7 of the 11 patients (Majid, Patel, Kim et al, 1990). In all 11 of these cases arteriography, including ergonovine challenge, was unremarkable.

Thickening of the media and intimal hyperplasia has also been seen in the nasal submucosal vessels of chronic cocaine addicts (Chow et al., 1990), suggesting that the process occurs throughout the body. Further support for this notion is lent by the fact that similar changes are also seen in patients with pheochromocytoma (Szakacs et al., 1959). More modern studies on cocaine's effects, done with scanning electron microscopy, have tended to confirm Szakacs' earlier work with catecholamines. Coronary arteries from dogs chronically treated with cocaine show signs of endothelial cell sloughing and occasional thrombus formation. Blood vessels from the same animals have also demonstrated increased responsiveness to norepinephrine and serotonin (Jones & Tackett, 1990).

Whatever the etiology of the underlying fixed lesions, cocaine use can make coronary artery lesions symptomatic. Intranasal cocaine (2 mg/kg body weight) causes increases in arterial pressure and rate-pressure product. At the same time the rate-pressure product is rising, coronary sinus blood flow significantly decreases (Lange, Cigarroa, Flores et al., 1990). As a result, cocaine increases myocardial work and oxygen demand while, at the same time, decreasing blood flow. If asymptomatic lesions are already present, the extra work load imposed by the cocaine can lead to infarction, even without coronary spasm. Increased oxygen demand in the presence of preexisting lesions can be sufficient to cause infarction. The results of earlier studies suggested that cocaine induces platelet aggregation, thereby increasing the likelihood of thrombosis and infarction (Tonga, Tempesta, Tonga et al, 1985). More recent studies have found no evidence that cocaine mediates increases in platelet aggregation or dense granule release (Kugelmass & Ware, 1992), but many other cocaine induced changes could lead to the same result. Increased thromboxane generation in the presence of underlying endothelial injuries can lead to thrombosis and infarction. (Stenberg et al., 1989) (Kolodgie, Virmani, Cornhil et al., 1990; Virmani, Kolodgie, Robinowitz et al, 1989). Clinical experience suggests that it is the combination of increased oxygen demand and decreased blood supply, with or without thrombosis, that has probably accounted for the majority of reported cases of infarction.

Autopsy studies and other epidemiologic data suggest that cocaine itself is atherogeneic (Escabedo, Ruttenber, Anda et al. 1992). In

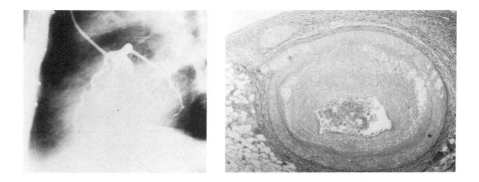

Figure 1.10.2.1 2 and 3: Coronary artery disease in cocaine users
The coronary arteries of cocaine users may undergo the same type of intimal hyperplasia as seen in transplant recipients. Because this sort of lesion concentrically involves the entire length of the involved vessel, obstructions may not be apparent unless earlier studies are available for comparison. The normal appearing study on the left was obtained just two weeks before the patient died of myocardial infarction. On the right is a cross section of the LAD from the same patient. Concentric intimal hyperplasia has almost entirely obstructed the lumen. H&E. Courtesy of Margaret Billingham, Stanford University School of Medicine.

one study, over 60% of patients with cocaine associated sudden deaths had moderate to severe coronary atherosclerosis (the patients had a mean age of 47). In such a young age group a much lower percentage of significant lesions would be expected (Dressler, Malekzadeh & Roberts, 1990). Other autopsy studies have also noted the increased incidence of significant atherosclerotic lesions (Virmani, Rabinowitz, Smialek & Smyth, 1988) (Kolodgie et al., 1990) (Dressler et al., 1990). In the most recent of these studies the coronary arteries of cocaine abusers dying of thrombosis were compared to those of cocaine users without thrombosis and cases of sudden death unassociated with cocaine use. The average age for the cocaine-thrombosis group was only 29 years and the degree of luminal narrowing was much higher than would be expected in this age group. In the patients with thrombosis, there was moderate to severe coronary atherosclerosis and increased numbers of adventitial mast cells (Kolodgie et al., 1991). One feature that distinguished the cocaine group was the fact that, even though thrombi were present in vessels that had extensive atherosclerosis, there was no plaque rupture or hemorrhage as would normally be seen in atherosclerotic lesions not associated with cocaine use.

The role of histamine in atherosclerosis is controversial (Born, 1991), but there is good evidence that histamine containing mast cells

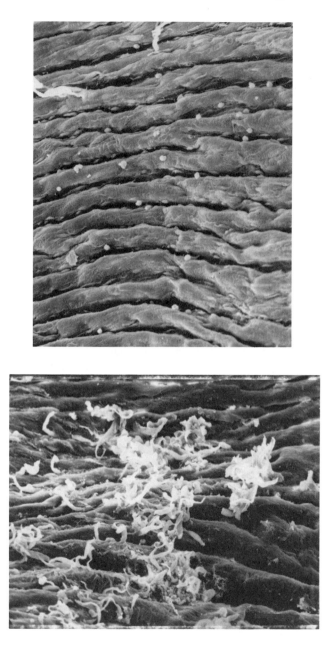

Figure 1.10.2.1 4 and 5 Effects of cocaine on endothelium
Both scanning micrographs are of a canine coronary artery. The photograph on
top is from a control animal; orig. magnification 312x. The lower photograph is
from a dog that received 1 mg/kg/day of cocaine for 4 weeks. Sloughing of
endothelial cells is evident; orig. magnification 520x. Courtesy of Dr. Randall L.
Tackett, Head, Dept. of Pharmacology and Toxicology, University of Georgia.

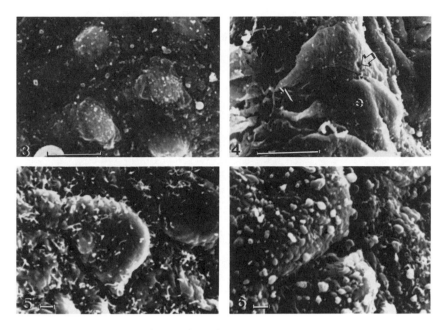

Figure 1.10.2.1 6 Transplacental cardiotoxicity
Whether or not cocaine exerts cardiotoxic effects in humans remains an open question. In animal models, toxicity is easily demonstrated. This pair of scanning micrographs shows endothelial sloughing in hamster neonatal right atrium. The photograph on the left is a scanning micrograph of control right atria. The photograph on the right is from a neonate whose mother received cocaine on the 6th, 7th and 9th day of gestation. The endothelium is abnormally flattened and no longer completely covers the underlying myocytes. Both scans are at the same magnification (scale bar = 10 μm). Courtesy of Dr. Jacques Gilloteaux, Department of Anatomy, College of Medicine, Northeastern Ohio Universities.

may be implicated in the pathogenesis of human coronary vasospasm (Ginsberg, Bristow, Kantrowitz et al., 1981). The presence of increased numbers of histamine-rich mast cells has been noted in atherosclerotic coronary vessels, even in non-drug using populations. Histamine isn't the only vasoactive compound contained in mast cells. Prostaglandin D_2, and leukotrienes C_4 and D_4 have also been demonstrated (Maseri, L'Abbate, Baroldi, et al., 1978). The potential exists for a large number of potentially harmful interactions between elevated circulating catecholamines, cytokines, and other tissue factors, and it would not be surprising if cocaine users did have accelerated atherosclerosis. Cocaine users have elevated circulating catecholamines, and it has been shown that LDL uptake by arterial walls is accelerated by both epinephrine and norepinephrine (Born, 1991). The difficulty in interpreting these studies is that the patients involved are frequently polydrug abusers and, more often than not, cigarette smokers. Singling out one causal agent on the

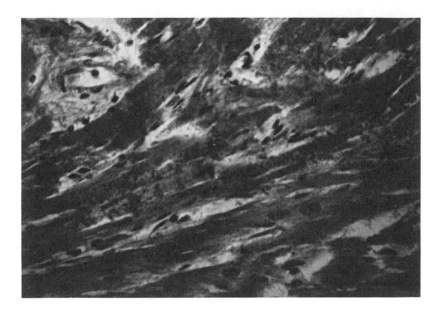

Figure 1.10.2.3.1 Contraction band necrosis in cocaine user's heart
This section of myocardium, stained with H&E, is from the heart of a cocaine
user with sudden death syndrome. The dark bands traversing the cells are
composed of clumped myofilaments that are no longer functional. Lesions are
extremely focal, with damaged myocytes surrounded by apparently normal cells.

basis of such limited retrospective will be a formidable task.

1.10.2.2 Coronary artery spasm

Cocaine induced spasm has been demonstrated angiographically,
but the mechanism remains a matter of contention. Human and animal
studies give conflicting results. Isolated rat hearts perfused with cocaine
(100 μg to 500 μg/mL) display both physiologic and morphologic evidence of spasm (Vitullo, Karam, Mekhail et al., 1989). Several morphologic alterations were apparent in the isolated rat heart model. In the
smaller vessels (10 μm–65 μm) endothelial cells were seen bulging into
the lumen of constricted vessels. Scalloping of the internal elastic lamina
and separation of the vessels from surrounding tissues was also observed. Ultrastructural studies showed vacuolization of the cytoplasm in
both endothelial and smooth muscle cells. Langendorff perfusion measurements in this same model showed decreases in myocardial flow rate,
along with decreased contractility as reflected by decreased left ventricular pressure and decreased contractility (dp/dt).

Using arteriography and microsphere tracers, Hale et al.,
working with a different experimental model, also was able to induce

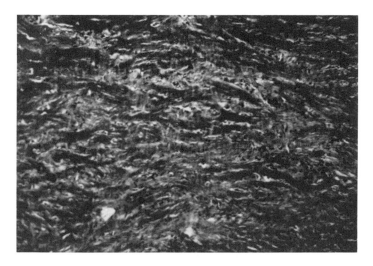

Figure 1.10.2.3.2 Contraction band necrosis results in patchy fibrosis
Section of myocardium from rat implanted with pheochromocytoma cells. Initial
lesions of contraction band necrosis have been replaced with multiple small foci
of fibrosis. Courtesy of Margaret Billingham, Stanford University Medical
Center.

significant decreases in coronary diameters. An average 15% decrease in
the cross-sectional area of the circumflex artery occurred 3–5 minutes
after cocaine administration, and decreased regional myocardial flow
was seen at 15 minutes (Hale, Alker, Rezkalla et al, 1989). As in the rat
studies, contractility was decreased. Others, however, have observed
quite different results. Bedotto et al. could find no sign of spasm or
decreased contractility, though he did note peripheral venous and arterial constriction. Coronary angiograms obtained at peak aortic pressure
(during infusions of 0.5 gm/kg) failed to demonstrate any cross sectional
narrowing (Bedotto, Lee, Lancaster et al., 1988). Even more confusing
is that fact that one well designed experiment showed that intravenous
cocaine could produce rapid, dose-dependent coronary vasodilation in
anesthetized beagles. One minute post injection, flow increased by up
to 175% (Friedrichs, Wei & Merrill, 1990).

In another experiment, segments of rabbit aorta exposed to
cocaine or norcocaine, in concentrations of 10^{-9} to 10^{-10} M, constricted,
but constriction doesn't occur when the segments were exposed to other
metabolites such as benzoylecgonine. The degree of constriction is not
affected by the presence or absence of endothelium (Chokshi, Gal &
Isner, 1989a). But another study, using similar, but not identical metho-
dology, found that cocaine neither constricted nor dilated rabbit aortic
rings, and the results were the same whether or not the endothelium
was intact (Pol, Morley, Zhang & Bove, 1991). More recently, other

workers have shown that the coronary spasm induced by intravenously administered cocaine in dogs occurs regardless of whether or not the endothelium is present (Kuhn, 1992).

Vasoconstriction in cat cerebral arteries is greater after exposure to benzoylecgonine than after treatment with either cocaine or norepinephrine. Segments of bovine coronary artery develop increased tension when exposed to cocaine, and experiments with various blocking agents suggest that serotonin or histamine may be the mediator of cocaine induced contractions (Foy, 1991). In still another model, solutions of benzoylecgonine produced a nearly 50% decrease in cross sectional area of coronary arteries (Madden & Powers, 1990). On the other hand, vasodilation of cat pial arterioles occurs when they are exposed to a broad range of cocaine concentrations (Dohi, Jones, Hudak & Traystman, 1990). Of course, all of these studies were undertaken before the existence of cocaethylene was recognized. Cocaethylene, formed only when cocaine is used with alcohol, binds to the dopamine receptor with the same affinity as cocaine, but cocaethylene has a much longer half-life (Camí, de la Torre, Farré et al., 1991) (Hearn, Flynn, Hime et al., 1991). The presence of this metabolite might explain some cases of spasm which have occurred many hours after cocaine was last used.

The obvious conclusion to be drawn from these animal studies is that not only are there considerable differences in the way various animals respond to cocaine, but there are also differences between the ways different blood vessels from the same individual respond. Such a conclusion is hardly surprising. The number and density of beta receptors can be affected by many factors, including preexisting physiologic state and age. Furthermore, the rate at which cocaine is metabolized in different species is widely disparate and could well account for the different responses that have been observed.

Even if the mechanism may be obscure, there is no question that cocaine causes coronary spasm in humans. Many reports have described myocardial infarction in cocaine users who have normal coronary arteries. Well designed clinical studies have also demonstrated cocaine mediated coronary artery constriction in man. Lange et al. showed that a dose of 2 mg per kg, given to a group of 45 patients undergoing cardiac catheterization for the evaluation of chest pain, decreased coronary sinus blood flow and decreased the diameter of the left coronary artery by at least 8 to 12 percent. In spite of the decreased flow, none of the patients developed symptoms and the spasm was reversed by treatment with phentolamine (an alpha blocking agent) (Lange, Cigarroa, Flores et al., 1989; Lange, Cigarroa & Hillis, 1989). In a related study, the same workers compared coronary artery cross-sectional areas in diseased and nondiseased segments of coronary artery before and 15 minutes after 2mg/kg of intranasal cocaine. The lumenal areas decreased in both groups, but there was more vasoconstriction in the diseased segments (Flores, Lange, Cigarroa & Hillis, 1990). This is consistent with the generally held clinical impression that coronary artery spasm tends to occur at the site of preexisting constrictions.

Coronary vasospasm is associated with alterations in adrenergic function. The first suggestion that there was a relationship came from studies of Prinzmetal's angina. In that disorder, repolarization abnormalities (QT prolongation) precede episodes of spasm (Roberts, Curry, Isner et al., 1982) (Ricci, Orlick, Cipriano et al., 1979), and it is well known that QT interval prolongation may be secondary to increased sympathetic discharge. In animal studies, unilateral stellate ganglion stimulation causes selective coronary spasm, QT prolongation, and a marked increase in coronary artery resistance. These changes can all be prevented with alpha adrenergic blockade (Randall, Armour, Geis et al., 1972). All of these changes can be produced by giving cocaine. Animals infused with cocaine develop PR and QT prolongation (Parker, Beckman, Bauman & Hariman, 1989) (Rosen, Leopold & Danilo, 1988) (Beckman, Parker, Hariman et al., 1991). Torsades-de pointes (reciprocating ventricular tachycardia associated with QT interval prolongation) has occurred in cocaine-intoxicated patients (Rosen et al., 1988), and a report describing cocaine-induced torsades in a patient with congenital idiopathic long QT syndrome lends further support to the notion that sympathetic function is altered in cocaine users (Schrem, Belsky, Schwartzman & Slater, 1990).

It has been argued that contraction band necrosis is an anatomic marker for coronary spasm. Factor has identified what he feels are contraction bands in the media of coronary arteries (Factor & Cho, 1985), and other studies have confirmed the findings in cases of brain death (Novitzky, Wicomb, Cooper et al, 1984). Lesions appear in the media as discrete zones of hypereosinophilia, usually in widened cells with rarefaction of the cytoplasm on either side of the eosinophilia area. It has been suggested that this morphologic finding is a marker both for coronary artery spasm and sudden death. Similar lesions have been produced in the coronary arteries of animals infused with catecholamines (Joris & Majno, 1981). When observed in humans, such lesions are frequently associated with the presence of nonocclusive microthrombi and, more often than not, are found adjacent to atherosclerotic plaque ruptures and mural plaque hemorrhages. Unfortunately, the lesion has yet to be identified in cocaine users.

1.10.2.3 Myocardial diseases

Both epidemiologic (Ruttenber et al. 1991) and echocardiographic (Brickner et al., 1991) studies show that cocaine users may be prone to left ventricular hypertrophy. This finding has also been confirmed at autopsy (Escobedo, Ruttenber, Anda et al., 1992). Controlled echocardiography measurements indicate that significant increases in left ventricular mass and posterior wall thickness both occur. If that is the case, it

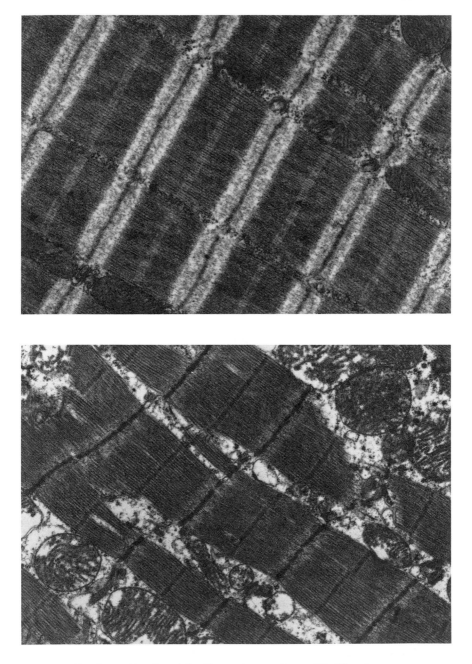

Figure 1.10.2.3.3 Mitochondria disruption and myofibrillar damage
The photograph on top is from a control rat, that below is from a rat infused
with 40 mg/kg/day for 21 days. The mitochondria are swollen and translocated,
and many of the myofilaments are degenerating. Original magnification 7,200x.
Courtesy of Prof. M. Maillet, Hôpital Lariboisière, Paris.

could explain many of the ischemic and arrhythmic events that have been described in cocaine users.

A handful of clinical reports have noted an association between dilated cardiomyopathy and long-term cocaine use. Most of these reports are not very informative, since they merely describe the occurrence of heart failure in polydrug abusers. Without angiography or biopsies, the diagnosis remains in question (Wiener, Lockhart & Schwartz, 1986) (Chokshi, Moore, Pandian & Isner, 1989b) (Duell, 1987) (Wolfson, 1990) (Mendelson & Chandler, 1992). The limited number of morphologic observations that have been published suggest that cardiomyopathy, when it occurs in cocaine and amphetamine users, is catechol mediated (Karch & Billingham, 1988) (Peng, French, Pelikan, 1989) (Henzlova, Smith, Prchal & Helmcke 1991). The myocardial response to chronic catechol toxicity has been well characterized and is the same in man and animals. Norepinephrine "myocarditis" was observed almost as soon as intravenous pressor agents were introduced (Szakacs & Cannon A, 1958). Histologically, this type of necrosis is indistinguishable from the picture seen in patients and animals with pheochromocytoma (Rosenbaum, Billingham, Ginsburg et al., 1987). Contraction band necrosis is the earliest recognizable lesion.

TABLE 1.10.2.3.1
DIFFERENCES BETWEEN ISCHEMIC AND CATECHOL NECROSIS

Ischemic Necrosis	Catechol Necrosis
Involves many cells in area supplied by a single vessel	Very focal, necrotic cell may be surrounded by normal cells
Myofilaments remain in register	Myofilaments destroyed, forming eosinophilic clumps
Mitochondria remain neatly packed and are of uniform size	Mitochondria are translocated with distorted shapes

Catechol-induced necrosis and ischemic necrosis can be distinguished by their pattern of distribution. In cases of ischemic injury, all the cells supplied by a given vessel will be affected. When the injury is due to catechol excess, individual necrotic myocytes are found interspersed between normal cells. Distribution is, in fact, one of the principal diagnostic features of catechol injury. Another feature separating the two is the arrangement of the myofilaments. When the insult is ischemic, the myofilaments remain in register. When the damage is due to catechol excess, the filaments are disrupted. There is no "zone" of injury with catechol necrosis and there is no apparent relationship to blood supply. After 12 or more hours have elapsed, a mononuclear infiltrate, predominantly lymphocytic, may be seen. The necrotic myocytes are eventually reabsorbed and replaced by non-conduction fibrous tissue.

The hallmark of both the acute and healed catechol lesions is that they are extremely focal.

One study describes the findings in three patients with histories of cocaine abuse and end-stage chronic heart failure who underwent cardiac transplantation. The morphologic changes in the native hearts were noted to be distinctly different from those seen in other patients with the same clinical diagnosis. There were fewer nuclear abnormalities and less myocyte hypertrophy. The fibrosis was much more focal in distribution and there were focal lymphocytic infiltrates (Karch & Billingham, 1988). Biopsy findings in a second group of seven patients, six with recent onset of congestion failure and one with chest pain, showed very similar changes. There was myocyte necrosis in five of the seven patients, and its distribution was identical to that seen when contraction band necrosis occurs as a result of catechol toxicity. Necrotic cells were found next to normal cells with no apparent relationship to blood supply. Focal interstitial fibrosis, of varying degrees of severity, was noted throughout. In two specimens necrosis was associated with predominantly lymphocytic infiltrates. Nor was there eosinophilia (Peng, French & Pelikan, 1989) (see below). Very much the same picture has also been seen in chronic amphetamine abusers (Smith, Roche, Jagusch & Herdson, 1976).

TABLE 1.10.2.3.2
MORPHOLOGIC DIFFERENCES BETWEEN DRUG-INDUCED TOXIC MYO-CARDITIS AND HYPERSENSITIVITY MYOCARDITIS. TOXIC MYOCARDITIS IS INVARIABLY DOSE RELATED, WHILE HYPERSENSITIVITY MYOCARDITIS IS NOT.

Toxic Myocarditis	Hypersensitivity Myocarditis
Lesions of varying ages	Lesions all the same age
Myocyte necrosis	No necrosis
Necrotizing vasculitis	Non-necrotizing vasculitis
No esosinophilic infiltrates	Eosinophilic infiltrates
Fibrosis a prominent feature	No fibrosis

Adapted from Billingham, 1985

Contraction band necrosis is a prominent feature of all myocardial biopsies, regardless of the underlying cause. For that reason, contraction bands found in biopsy material are difficult to assess (Adomian, Laks & Billingham, 1967) (Karch & Billingham, 1986). Clinical experience suggests that the presence of nuclear pyknosis may be one way to distinguish preexisting contraction band lesions from those produced by the biopsy process itself, but that has never been proven in a controlled study. In some of the biopsies, Z-band remnants can be seen with electron microscopy. This particular finding is classically associated with dilated congestion cardiomyopathy and is not generally associated with the sort of necrosis resulting from catechol toxicity. While it has not been observed in any other patients with cocaine-related heart disease, it has been seen in patients with amphetamine toxicity (Smith et al., 1976). Its presence probably signifies only that necrosis was very severe.

Bravetta and Invernezzi were the first to report finding cellular infiltrates in the heart of a cocaine user, and that was nearly seventy years ago (Bravetta & Invernizzi, 1922)! Since then, the observations have been repeated many times. However, fifty years elapsed between the publication of the Bravetta and Invernezzi paper and the appearance of a paper by Isner et al. that reported finding eosinophilic infiltrates in an endomyocardial biopsy specimen from a 29-year old man with cocaine-related cardiac symptoms (Isner et al., 1986). Others have observed both lymphocytic and eosinophilic interstitial infiltrates (Simpson & Edwards, 1986) (Virmani et al., 1987) (Virmani et al., 1988) (Talebzadeh, Chevrolet, Chatelain et al., 1990). In the San Francisco study, mononuclear infiltrates were frequently seen, but they weren't associated with myocyte necrosis (Tazelaar, Karch, Billingham & Stephens, 1987).

The presence of eosinophilic infiltrates suggests that what is being described is a hypersensitivity phenomenon. Hypersensitivity myocarditis is distinguished from toxic myocarditis by the fact that its occurrence is not dose-related. Lesions are all of the same age, hemorrhages are rare, and their is no myocyte necrosis. The list of drugs causing hypersensitivity myocarditis is increasing (Billingham 1985). Eosinophilic myocarditis is a very rare disorder. Fewer than six instances were observed in 10,000 biopsies done at Stanford. When it occurs, it's usually as the result of a hypersensitivity reaction. When eosinophils have been observed in the myocardium of cocaine users, it has often been as an incidental finding, either as surprise finding at autopsy or in biopsy specimens obtained to evaluate chest pain, heart failure or arrhythmia. Most of the time, the clinical manifestations of this disorder are so nonspecific that the diagnosis is rarely suspected during life (Taliercio, Olney & Lie, 1985).

None of the cocaine users with eosinophilic infiltrates have had signs of extracardiac involvement such as polyarteritis nodosa or eosinophilic leukemia. These patients do not match the picture classically associated with acute necrotizing myocarditis (Herzog, Snover & Staley, 1984), nor do they resemble patients with eosinophilic coronary arteritis (Churg-Strauss syndrome, also called allergic granulomatosis angiitis).

A heterogeneous group of agents can cause toxic myocarditis, and since cocaine can be adulterated with an even longer list of agents, implicating cocaine as the cause of eosinophilic myocarditis becomes very difficult. Further confounding the issue is the fact that most adult drug abusers are polydrug abusers. Virtually all the patients in the San Francisco study had other drugs present (Tazelaar et al., 1987). Benzo-diazepines were found in over half the San Francisco cases and opiates were identified nearly as often. A review paper published in 1988 listed sugars (lactose, sucrose and manitol) as the most common cocaine adul-terants, followed by stimulant drugs (caffeine, amphetamines) and local anesthetic agents (Shannon, 1988).

TYPES OF COCAINE ADULTERANTS

A. SUGARS
   dextrose
   lactose
   manitol
   sucrose

B. STIMULANTS
   caffeine
   ephedrine
   phenylpropanolamine
   phentermine

C. LOCAL ANESTHETICS
   lidocaine
   benzocaine
   procaine
   tetracaine

D. INERT AGENTS
   inositol
   corn starch

E. OTHERS
   acetaminophen
   aminopyrine
   aspirin acid
   ascorbic acid
   boric acid
   diphenhydramine
   niacinamide
   phenacitin
   quinine

Based on information supplied by the Drug Enforcement Agency, and from Shannon, 1988

After an initial flurry of reports in 1986 and 1987, recent mentions of eosinophilic infiltrates have become uncommon. One explanation might be that most cocaine users are now "crack" smokers. And "crack", while it may contain large amounts of bicarbonate, is otherwise largely free of contaminants. Finally, it must be emphasized that the mere presence of cells in the myocardium does not necessarily mean that there is active myocarditis. The lymphocytic infiltrates seen in cocaine users are gene-rally not accompanied by myocyte necrosis and, according to the Dallas criteria, infiltrates without necrosis are not myocarditis (Aretz, Billing-ham, Edwards et al., 1986). What these infiltrates represent is not clear, but similar infiltrates are also seen in experimental animals with catechol toxicity and the same process may be occurring in cocaine users. Another possibility that must be considered when infiltrates are encountered in the hearts of drug users is that they have AIDS. A variety of opportunistic infections occur. In most areas of the country the probability is that an obvious infiltrate in the heart of an HIV+ cocaine user represents an opportunistic infection and not a cocaine related injury.

The first report describing AIDS related myocardial disease was published in 1985. An assortment of opportunistic agents were found in 10 of the 41 hearts studied (Commarosano & Lewis, 1985). In a second series of 82 patients dying of AIDS, infectious agents were found in 17%. The usual pathogens associated with decreased immune function, including toxoplasmosis, mycobacteria, histoplasmosis, cryptococcus, cytomegalovirus and pneumocystitis, have all been reported (Anderson, Virmani & Macher, 1987). Several studies have noted histologic changes consistent with the diagnosis of myocarditis (inflammatory infiltrates with myocardial cell necrosis) in anywhere between one-third and one-half of autopsied cases (Anderson, Garabed, Gold et al., 1988) (Lafont, Marche, Wolff et al., 1988). There is even evidence that HIV virus itself invades the myocardium (Grody, Cheng & Lewis, 1990). Kaposi's sarcoma, most often involving the pericardium, has been reported (Anderson et al., 1987), as has lymphomatous infiltration of the heart.

1.10.2.4 Valvular Heart Disease

Intravenous drug users get endocarditis and there is no reason to suppose that the subgroup of cocaine abusers is any different. Unfortunately, there is no autopsy data to review and no animal models. One clinical study reviewed the records of 115 intravenous drug abusers who were admitted to the hospital for evaluation of fever (Chambers, Morris, Tauber et al., 1987). Endocarditis was proven in 20%. When the subgroup was further analyzed, 80% of those with endocarditis were found to be intravenous cocaine users. Logistic regression analysis of the patients' histories demonstrated that cocaine use was the single variable most strongly predictive for endocarditis. History of cocaine use was, in fact, a better predictor than even the presence of a mitral or aortic murmur, the findings classically associated with endocarditis. These retrospective findings have never been confirmed by any other clinical observations, and valvular pathology in experimental animals has not been studied. If there is a relationship between intravenous cocaine use and endocarditis, it might have to do with the fact that injected cocaine has a very short half-life. Maintaining a "high" takes repeated injections - many more injections than will be required by an opiate addict. That should increase the probability of sepsis.

1.10.2.5 Aorta and Peripheral Vessels

Fewer than a dozen cases of aortic dissection have been described. Most have been type I dissections with the process extending from the ascending aorta to the iliacs (Barth, Bray & Roberts, 1986) (Gadaleta, Hall & Nelson, 1989) (Edwards & Rubin, 1987) (Tardiff, Gross, Wu et al, 1989) (Grannis, Bryant, & Caffaratti, 1988) (Om, Porter & Mohanty, 1992). None of these individuals had Marfan's syndrome or any other significant medical history. Two recognized factors contribute to aortic dissection: aortic medial disease and hypertension. Cocaine use is certainly associated with at least one, and possibly with both disorders. Transient hypertension occurs in virtually all users, and some preliminary studies have shown damage to the media and elastic layers in the aortas of rats chronically treated with cocaine (Langner and Bement, 1991).

Aortic dissection is initiated by transverse tears in the aortic wall. For dissection to occur, tears must extend through the intima and at least halfway through the media (Crawford, 1990). The case reported by Barth is interesting because the initiating tear was so extensive. A 45-year old crack smoker, with a blood cocaine level of 9 mg/liter, suddenly collapsed and could not be resuscitated. The heart weighed 500 grams. A circumferential tear through the intima and media was found in the ascending aorta 2 cm above the sinotubular junction. There was no distal dissection but there was medial extension proximally to the level of the aortic valve cusps and there was adventitial hemorrhage around the aortic root extending into the proximal portion of right and left coronary arteries (without compression). Adventitial hemorrhage even extended down into the pulmonary arteries (Barth et al., 1986). The most plausible explanation for these changes is hypertension induced shearing injury to an aortic media that had, in some way, been weakened by chronic cocaine exposure. However, in the most recently reported case (Bacharach, Colville, Lie 1992), aneurysmal dilatation was seen in conjunction with nonspecific aortitis. A predominantly lymphoplasmacytic infiltrate in the media was interspersed with occasional scattered giant cells. Since this individual's serology was negative, and since there was nothing in the history to suggest Takayasu's disease or giant cell arteritis, it seems likely that cocaine was responsible for the process.

Superficial and deep thrombophlebitis both occur as complications of cocaine abuse. Superficial venous involvement as a consequence of intravenous cocaine abuse is no way different from the phlebitis that results from the abuse of any other drug. Much more interesting is the apparent increased risk of Paget-Schroetter syndrome, deep vein thrombosis of the upper extremity. In one retrospective study, 12 radiologically proven cases of upper extremity thrombosis were identified over a three-year period. Five of the cases were in intravenous cocaine users. Compared to non-drug related cases, the cocaine users were much younger (mean age 35.8 years versus 56.5 years) and were all males, compared to 57% females in the non-drug related group (Lisse, Davis & Thurmond-Anderle, 1989; Lisse, Davis & Thurmond-Anderle, 1990). There is no experimental model for this condition and its mechanism remains obscure. Thrombosis might be the result of cocaine-enhanced platelet aggregation and thromboxane production (Tonga et al., 1985), or it might be due to some adulterant that was injected with the cocaine.

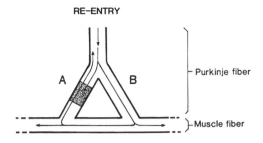

Figure 1.10.2.6 (1) Unidirectional heart block
Zones of patchy myocardial fibrosis may provide the anatomic substrate for
reentry arrythmia. This mechanism is thought to account for many cases of
cardiac sudden death. Reprinted with permission. Textbook of Advanced
Cardiac Life Support, 1987. Copyright American Heart Association.

1.10.2.6 Sudden cardiac death

Sudden death is certainly the most dramatic consequence of
cocaine abuse, and it is also the least understood. This syndrome poses
major problems for medical examiners and clinicians alike. Clearly, the
probability of a lethal outcome is unrelated to the amount of cocaine
ingested (Smart & Anglin, 1986) (Karch & Stephens, 1991). However,
the explanation of why that should be the case is far from clear.
Depending on whether or not the victim is a novice or chronic user,
different mechanisms may come into play. Federally sponsored research
efforts have been carried out mainly with rats. In that particular model,
doses of cocaine required to produce cardiovascular death are much
higher than the doses required to trigger fatal convulsions. On the basis
of such experiments it has been suggested that sudden death in humans
may be primarily a neurologic event as well (Anon, 1992). The problem
with such theories is that the rodent heart, like the hearts of other small
animals, is extremely resistant to the induction of lethal arrythmias. A
critical mass of myocardium is needed in order to sustain rhythms such
as ventricular tachycardia, and in the absence of sufficient mass
abnormal rhythms terminate spontaneously (McWilliam, 1887) (Porter,
1894) (Zipes, 1975). In 1914 Garrey found that when pieces of fibrillating
left ventricle with a surface area of less than 4 cm^2 were shaved from a
heart, they stopped fibrillating but the remaining ventricle continued to
fibrillate until three quarters of the ventricle had been removed. It isn't
very surprising that the results of the rodent experiments favor neurologic mechanisms.

More often than not, the mechanism appears to be a lethal
arrhythmia. While experimental studies have been largely unsatisfactory,
clinical observations have some bearing on the problem. Malignant
rhythm disturbances occur when the orderly progression of impulses
through the ventricle is disrupted (the process is called wave front

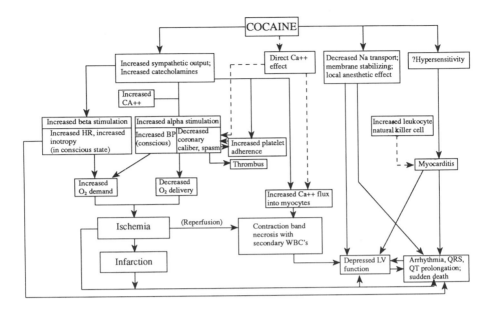

Figure 1.10.2.6 (2) Mechanisms for sudden death in cocaine users
A complex series of interrelated events may lead to sudden death in a cocaine
abuser. Some of the more important factors are indicated in this flow diagram.
The diagram is from Kloner et al., *Circulation* 1992 and is reprinted with
permission.

dispersion). Cocaine produces distinct morphologic and physiologic alterations in the heart, and each of these can result in wave front dispersion and reentry. Cardiomegally increases the distance impulses must traverse, while myocardial fibrosis may disrupt impulse transmission. Even without producing histologically identifiable changes, cocaine can cause conduction abnormalities. Cocaine is a local anesthetic and sodium channel blocker and it may induce repolarization abnormalities that disrupt impulse conduction. Both functional and morphologic alterations can occur at the same time, which is the reason that explanation of sudden death in cocaine users remains so elusive. To fully understand the complexity of the issue, each of these possible mechanisms have to be considered separately.

1.10.2.6.1 Acute Anesthetic Related Effects

Sudden death in novice users probably has more to do with cocaine's anesthetic properties than with its adrenergic effects. In addition to its effects on catechol metabolism, which ultimately result in intracytosolic calcium elevations and cellular necrosis, cocaine also blocks the fast sodium channel, thereby inhibiting action potential generation (Weidmann, 1955). It also blocks potassium efflux channels (Przywara, 1989), further inhibiting generation of the action potential generation. Conduction velocity in cardiac tissue depends on how fast depolarization occurs. If sodium influx and potassium efflux are blocked, impulse propagation is impaired and conduction is depressed. Different areas of the heart respond differently to local anesthetic agents and the refractory period in each of the different locations will lengthen by variable amounts. Orderly transmission of impulses is interrupted by cocaine use and the result is temporal dispersion of the wavefronts. Occasionally an impulse may arrive at a point where it can't be conducted. Described as a unidirectional conduction block, such blocks can be caused by any amide local anesthetics (Kasten & 1986, 1986). The process has been demonstrated in animals but clinical studies are still lacking (Schwartz, 1989). Another local anesthetic effect which might lead to sudden death is conduction block. Dogs given intravenous cocaine in quantities mimicking "recreational" doses (infusions starting at 3 mg per kg over 30 seconds) develop severe prolongation of conduction times through the His-Purkinje system into the ventricle. Slowing of conduction is dose dependent. The more cocaine given, the slower conduction (Kabas, Blanchard, Matsuyama et al, 1990). In other animal studies high dose cocaine treatment has been noted to have potent negative inotropic and type I electrophysiological effects. Blood pressure drops, while both coronary blood flow and cardiac output decrease. At the same time the PR, QRS, QT and QTc intervals all increase (Beckman et al., 1991). Rats given cocaine by inhalation develop blood levels comparable to those seen in humans. In one rat experimental model 70% of the animals demonstrated electrophysiological abnormalities, including atrial arrhythmias and incomplete heart block (Boni, Barr & Martin, 1991). Electrophysiologic measurements in a dog model of acute intoxication showed that ectopic activity and ventricular tachycardia were easily induced and that cocaine had a proarrhythmic effect due to multiple mechanisms (Gantenberg & Hageman, 1992). These experimental models may or may not be relevant to humans. Cocaine users will take ever increasing amounts to maintain their "high", and they will keep on taking the drug so long as it is available. Tolerance to the stimulant effects and some of the vascular effects may occur, but tolerance to the local anesthetic effects does not. If sufficient drug is taken, complete heart block can result. Cocaine induced asystole and complete heart block have been described clinically and experimentally (Nanji & Filpenko, 1984) (Watt & Pruitt, 1964).

1.10.2.6.2 Acute Catechol Related Effects

Electrophysiologic studies strongly suggest that acute changes occurring in the hearts of cocaine users are the result of both local anesthetic and adrenergic effects of cocaine (Temsey-Armos, Fraker, Brewster and Wilkerson 1992). Myocardial alterations are associated with chronic cocaine use, and these changes could well provide a substrate for arrhythmic sudden death. What happens acutely is less clear. Very large, non-physiologic, doses of cocaine given to rats will produce focal hemorrhages, contraction band necrosis, and ultimately death from prolonged seizure activity (Nahas, Trouve, Demus & Sitbon, 1985) (Trouve & Nahas, 1986) (Maillet, 1991) (Chiarasini, Dingeon, Latour et al 1992).

The most obvious explanation for cocaine-related sudden death is catechol induced ischemia. Enhanced alpha-adrenergic stimulation results in coronary artery contraction, decreased blood flow, and ischemia. Decreased epicardial artery diameters have been demonstrated in man, even at relatively low doses, making ischemic induction of arrhythmias a real possibility, especially in an individual who has preexisting disease (Flores et al., 1990) (Lange et al., 1990). At the same time alpha stimulation is increasing, beta adrenergic stimulation occurs and also leads to elevated intracytosolic calcium. Moderate elevations can cause the type of after-depolarizations that are associated with ventricular tachycardia (Bozler, 1943). If myocytes accumulate even more calcium, contraction band necrosis occurs and these lesions certainly can provide an adequate substrate for arrhythmic generation (Michelson, Spear & Moore, 1980). The association between contraction band necrosis and sudden death is well established (Reichenbach & Moss, 1975) (Cebelin & Hirsch, 1980). Even if contraction band necrosis isn't apparent at autopsy, catechol induced changes still may be responsible for sudden death. Calcium overload is not an all-or-nothing phenomenon. A spectrum of cellular alterations precede frank contraction band necrosis. Some of the alterations, such as mild eosinophilia, may be reversible. Similarly, changes in the cell membrane which allow the excessive entry of calcium may also be reversible. Even though there are no apparent abnormalities seen at autopsy, that doesn't necessarily mean that the changes are "functional". It may be that changes are present, but only detectable with electron microscopy. These studies are yet to be done.

1.10.2.6.3 Chronic Cocaine Effects

Many different anatomic alterations have been reported in the hearts of cocaine users with sudden death. In the San Francisco study, nearly one-third had patchy myocardial fibrosis not present in controls. Most had prominent contraction band necrosis and many had mononuclear infiltrates (Tazelaar et al., 1987). Myocardial fibrosis is a multifactorial process, but in cases of cocaine and catechol toxicity, it is probably the result of healing contraction band necrosis. If fibrosis is extreme, cardiomyopathy may result (Karch & Billingham, 1988) (Karch & Billingham, 1986). Cardiomyopathy is a major risk factor for malignant rhythm disorders and so is myocardial fibrosis. In the population of non-drug using patients with spontaneous ventricular tachycardia or fibrillation and normal arteriograms (which is a somewhat small group), nearly all patients will be found to have abnormal endomyocardial biopsies. In Strain's series over half the patients had interstitial and perivascular fibrosis associated with other cardiomyopathic changes such as myocellular hypertrophy. Nearly 20% had histologic alterations consistent with the diagnosis of subacute myocarditis (Strain, Grose, Factor & Fisher, 1983). If these changes are associated with serious ventricular arrhythmias in patients who are not drug users, there is every reason to suppose the same holds true in the drug using population. Abnormal interstitial fibrosis is found in other types of drug abusers as well (Kringsholm & Christoffersen 1987).

1.10.2.6.4 Relationship between seizures and sudden death

Cocaine-associated seizures have been recognized for over a century and can occur after relatively small doses of the drug. They are usually a benign phenomenon, and close questioning of users will often elicit a history of "small fits" that may temporarily interrupt a smoking session, but that are not severe enough to warrant seeking medical attention. Except in the case of the occasional body packers, continuous seizure activity is rarely the cause of death in humans. That is not true in some experimental models. In dogs infused with massive amounts of cocaine, continuous seizure activity is the cause of death (Catravas & Waters, 1981; Catravas, Waters, Waiz et al., 1978). That is not the case in mice and rats, where seizures and lethality appear to be mediated by different mechanisms (George, 1991).

The origin of cocaine-induced seizures is not known with certainty. Contrary to what might be expected, experiments have shown that cocaine seizures are not mediated by noradrenergic mechanisms (Jackson, Ball & Nutt, 1990), but may be due to interference with the serotonin transporter (in contrast to the behavioral effects which appear to be secondary to cocaine's effects on the dopamine transporter) (George & Ritz, 1991). Repeated use of cocaine increases susceptibility to seizures, and it has been argued that this process is a result of cocaine's local anesthetic properties. Animal studies confirm the tendency to increased seizure susceptibility, but also suggest that some other property, besides cocaine's local anesthetic effects, is responsible (Marley et. al. 1991). Whatever the cause, the important relationship in humans is that what begins as a cocaine-induced seizure discharge may end up as a cardiac arrhythmia. Epileptogenic foci can cause sudden cardiac death.

A relationship between cerebral epileptogenic foci and cardiac arrhythmias has been recognized for years. Electrocardiographic abnormalities as a consequence of central nervous system disease were first described nearly fifty years ago (Byer, Ashman & Toth, 1947). Patients with subarachnoid hemorrhage and other severe neurologic diseases exhibit a stereotyped pattern of EKG changes with peaked T waves and QT prolongation (Burch, Myers & Abildskov, 1954). Sometimes the T and QT changes are associated with ventricular ectopy (Novitzky et al., 1984) (Samuels, 1987). Ectopy and T wave elevation are both seen in case of brain death and the pattern abruptly reverts to normal when brain herniation is complete. The rapidity with which the EKG tracing returns to normal suggests strongly that neural, rather than hormonal, events are involved.

Most epileptics who die suddenly do so as a result of trauma or status epilepticus. A small percentage of young patients with infrequent seizure activity, and subtherapeutic anticonvulsant levels, will have no cause of death identifiable at autopsy (Hirsch & Martin, 1971). An emerging consensus holds that arrhythmias may be the cause of death in this subgroup (Oppenheimer, 1990) (Lip and Brodie 1992). The reverse sequence also occurs. Investigation of patients with cardiac arrhythmia occasionally discloses the presence of a seizure focus, the treatment of which abolishes the arrhythmia (Gilchrist, 1985) (Kiok, Terrence, Fromm & Lavine, 1986).

The relationship between seizures and arrhythmia has been studied in animals. Chemical induction of seizures (pentylenetetrazol) in paralyzed, ventilated cats causes measurable increases in the discharge rate from the cardiac sympathetic nerve and also the vagus. Electrocardiograms show ventricular ectopic beats, T wave changes and QT prolongation, similar to the pattern seen in humans with subarachnoid hemorrhage. Larger doses of pentylenetetrazol result in more intense seizure activity as well as ventricular fibrillation and/or asystole supervene (Lathers & Schraeder, 1982). As seizure activity becomes more intense, the normal synchronization between the branches of the cardiac nerve is lost. It has been suggested that, because these branches supply different areas of the myocardium, unbalanced activity results in temporal dispersion of the depolarizing wave front (Oppenheimer, 1990). The result would be much the same as with sodium channel blockade: malignant reentry arrhythmia (Oppenheimer, 1990).

1.10.2.6.5 Agitated Delirium & the Neuroleptic Malignant Syndrome

The first modern mention of cocaine-associated agitated delirium was in 1985 (Wetli & Fishbain, 1985). Reports of patients with similar symptoms had appeared in the early 1900's (Williams, 1914), but because these reports were deeply interwoven with elements of racist hysteria, they were never taken very seriously. The syndrome is comprised of four components which appear in sequence: hyperthermia, delirium with agitation, respiratory arrest, and death. Individuals succumbing to this disorder uniformly have low to modest cocaine blood levels and do not behave like patients with massive overdose (continuous seizures, respiratory depression and death). In the early stages of the disorder, victims are hyperthermic and grossly psychotic, with marked physical agitation. They often perform amazing feats of strength. What happens next is not entirely clear. For whatever reason (perhaps the cocaine blood level drops), agitation ceases and the patient becomes quiet. Shortly afterward he dies.

Wetli described seven cases. All had fairly stereotyped histories. Typical was the case of a 33-year old man who started pounding on the door of a house he had moved out of some time previously. *He was shouting that he wanted to see his wife and daughter. The occupants informed him that nobody by that name resided there, yet he pursued his actions. Four bystanders finally restrained him and assisted police units upon their arrival. The subject was handcuffed and put into a police car, whereupon he began to kick out the windows of the vehicle. The police subsequently restrained his ankles and attached the ankle restraints and handcuffs together. He was than transported to a local hospital. While enroute the police officers noted he became tranquil (about 45 minutes after the onset of the disturbance). Upon their arrival at the hospital a few minutes later, the subject was discovered to be in a respiratory arrest. Resuscitative attempts were futile. A postmortem examination was performed 1 hour and 45 minutes later (about 3 hours after the onset of the disturbance), and a rectal temperature of 41°C (106°F) was recorded. He had needle marks typical of intravenous drug abuse and pulmonary and cerebral edema. Abrasions and contusions of the ankles and wrist were also evident from his struggling against the restraints. Toxicologic analysis of postmortem blood disclosed 52.3 mg/L of lidocaine and 0.8 mg/L of cocaine. No lidocaine was administered to the victim during resuscitative attempts.*

Agitated delirium can be the result of other medical disorders, not just cocaine toxicity. It has been suggested that this constellation of symptoms is actually a variant of neuroleptic malignant syndrome (Kosten & Kleber, 1988; Kosten & Klever, 1987). Neuroleptic malignant syndrome (NMS) is a highly lethal disorder seen in patients taking dopamine antagonists, and in individuals who have been withdrawn from dopaminergic agents such as bromocriptine and levodopa (Levinson, 1985) (Friedman, Feinberg & Feldman, 1985). NMS is usually associated with muscle rigidity, though variants of the syndrome without rigidity are also recognized. At the cellular level the mechanism is thought to be either receptor blockade or neurotransmitter deficiency. Cocaine acutely elevates extracellular dopamine levels in experimental animals (Pettit, Pan, Parsons & Justice, 1990). With long-term use, net reductions of dopamine content occur (Karoum, Fawcett & Wyatt, 1988; Karoum, Suddath & Wyatt, 1990), and it is generally believed that cocaine users suffer from a relative dopamine deficiency (Taylor & Ho, 1977). Other factors implicated in the pathogenesis of this syndrome include altered dopaminergicserotonergic transmission, enhanced synthesis and action of prostaglandin E1 and E2, and a modification of calcium mediated signal transduction (Ebadi, Pfeiffer & Murrin, 1990).

One explanation for the syndrome holds that while a cocaine user has high cocaine blood levels, CNS dopamine levels will remain elevated, in spite of a relative central deficiency induced by chronic use. If levels are high enough, paranoid psychosis may be the result. As cocaine levels fall, so does postsynaptic dopamine availability and the syndrome is set off, much in the same fashion as a patient with Parkinsonism who has been withdrawn from levodopa. As cocaine levels drop the psychotic behavior tapers off, but is followed by hyperthermia - relative dopamine deficiency interfering with heat dissipation. The type of dopamine receptor associated with hypothermia rapidly down-regulates in the presence of high dopamine levels, but that is not the case for receptors responsible for temperature elevation. For a more thorough explanation, see Danielson, Coutts, Coutts et al., 1985. Rigidity is not apparent in the cocaine users, but akinesia involving the respiratory muscles may be the final event leading to death (Kosten & Kleber, 1988).

This symptom complex seems to be occurring with some regularity. And, because violent behavior is usually exhibited, the police are frequently involved. As a result, the affected individual dies in police custody or on his way to the hospital. Because cocaine blood levels are low at autopsy, and because there is a general misunderstanding about cocaine blood levels and the probability of death, the issue of police brutality is often raised. In some cases, death has been attributed to police use of a "choke hold" while restraining the agitated victim (Luke, Reay 1992). Unless the findings of strangulation are specifically ruled out at autopsy, considerable liability may result. In some jurisdictions "Tasers" are used to subdue violently agitated individuals. The "Taser" is a device which delivers an electrical charge sufficient to produce immobilization. Use of this device in instances of agitated delirium may result in fatalities. While the mechanism is unclear, essentially all of the fatalities associated with the use of this device have occurred in agitated cocaine or phencyclidine users (Kornblum & Reddy, 1991).

References

Adomian, G.,Laks, M. & Billingham, M. (1978). The incidence and significance of contraction bands in endomyocardial biopsies from normal human hearts. Am Heart J, 95, 348–351.

Anderson, D.Virmani, R, Reilly, J et al. (1988). Prevalence of myocarditis at necropsy in acquired immunodeficiency syndrome. J Am Coll Cardiol, 11(4), 729–799.

Anderson, D.,Virmani, R. & Macher, A. (1987). Cardiac pathology and cardio-vascular cause of death in patients dying with the Acquired Immunode-ficiency Syndrome (AIDS). In The Third International Conference on AIDS, Cited in Curr Probl in Cardiol, June 1991, 389.

Anon (1992). NIDA researchers investigate cocaine toxicity, seizures link. DAWN Briefings, September 1992. National Institute on Drug Abuse. Bethesda, MD.

Aretz, TH.,Billingham, M.,Edwards, W. et al. (1986). Myocarditis: a histopatho-logic differentiation and classification. Am J Cardiovasc Path, 1(1), 3–14.

Ascher, E.,Stauffer, J. & Gaasch, W. (1988). Coronary artery spasm, cardiac arrest, transient electrocardiographic Q waves and stunned myocardium in cocaine-associated acute myocardial infarction. Am J Cardiol, 61, 939–941.

Bacharach, J., Colville, D., Lie, J. (1992). Accelerated atherosclerosis, aneurysmal disease, and aortitis: possible pathogenetic association with cocaine abuse. Int Angiol, 11:83–86.

Barth, C. W III, Bray, M. & Roberts, W. (1986). Rupture of the ascending aorta during cocaine intoxication. Am J Cardiol, 57, 496.

Beckman, K. J., Parker, R. B., Hariman et al. (1991). Hemodynamic and electro-physiological actions of cocaine - effects of sodium bicarbonate as an antidote in dogs. Circulation, 83(5), 1799–1807.

Bedotto, J., Lee RW, Lancaster, L. et al (1988). Cocaine and cardiovascular function in dogs: effects on heart and peripheral circulation. J Am Coll Cardiol, 11(6), 1337–1342.

Billingham, M.E. (1985). Pharmacotoxic myocardial disease: an endomyocardial study. Heart Vessels, 1 (Suppl.1):386–394.

Boni, J. P.,Barr, W. H. & Martin, B. R. (1991). Cocaine inhalation in the rat -pharmacokinetics and cardiovascular response. J Pharmacol Exp Ther, 257(1), 307–315.

Born, G. (1991). Recent evidence for the involvement of catecholamines and macrophages in atherosclerotic process. Ann Med, 23:569–572.

Bozler, E. (1943). The initiation of impulses in cardiac muscle. Am J Physiol, 138, 273–282.

Bravetta, E. & Invernizzi, G (1922).Il Cocainismo. Osservazione cliniche. Ricerche sperimentali e anatomo-patoligiche. Note Riv Psichiatr, 10, 543.

Brickner, E., Willard, J., Eichhorn, E. et. al. (1991). Left ventricular hypertrophy associated with chronic cocaine abuse. Circulation, 84(3) 1130–1135.

Burch, G.,Meyers, R. & Abildskov, J. (1954). A new electrocardiographic pattern observed in cerebrovascular accidents. Circulation, 9, 719–723.

Byer, E.,Ashman, R. & Toth, L. (1947). Electrocardiogram with large upright T waves and long QT intervals. Am Heart J, 33, 796–801.

Camí, J., de la Torre, R., Farré, M. et al. (1991). Cocaine-alcohol interaction in healthy volunteers: plasma metabolic profile including cocaethylene. In Committee on Problems of Drug Dependency Annual Scientific Meeting, in press. West Palm Beach: National Institute on Drug Abuse.

Catravas, J. & Waters, I. (1981). Acute cocaine intoxication in the conscious dog: studies on the mechanism of lethality. J Pharm Exp Ther, 217, 350–356.

Catravas, J., Waters, I., Walz, M. et al. (1978). Acute cocaine intoxication in the conscious dog: pathophysiologic profile of acute lethality. Arch Int Pharmacodyn Ther, 235 (328–340).

Cebelin, J. & Hirsch, C. (1980). Human stress cardiomyopathy: myocardial lesions in victims of homicidal assaults without internal injuries. Hum Pathol, 11, 123–132.

Chambers, H., Morris, D., Tauber, M. et al. (1987). Cocaine use and the risk for endocarditis in intravenous drug users. Ann Intern Med, 106, 833–836.

Chiarasini, D., Dingeon, P., Latour, C. et al. Cardiovascular tolerance to cocaine and its correlates. Read at annual meeting of The British Pharmacological Society, London, September 1992.

Chokshi, S.,Gal, D. & Isner, J. (1989a). Vasospasm caused by cocaine metabolite: a possible explanation for delayed onset of cocaine-related cardiovascular toxicity. Circulation, 80(4), II–351.

Chokshi, S., Moore, R., Pandian, N. & Isner, J. (1989b). Reversible cardiomyopathy associated with cocaine intoxication. Ann Intern Med, 111, 1039–1040.

Chow, J., Robertson, A. & Stein, R. (1990). Vascular changes in the nasal submucosa of chronic cocaine addicts. Am J Forensic Med & Pathol, 11(2), 136–143.

Cammarosano, C. & Lewis, C. (1985). Cardiac lesions in acquired immune deficiency syndrome (AIDS). J Am Coll Cardiol, 5, 703–706.

Crawford, E. (1990). The diagnosis and management of aortic dissection. JAMA, 264(19), 2537–2541.

Cregler, L. & Mark, H. (1985). Relation of acute myocardial infarction to cocaine abuse. Am J Cardiol, 56, 794.

Danielson, T., Coutts, R., Coutts, K. et al. (1985). Reserpine induced hypothermia and its reversal by dopamine antagonists. Life Sci, 37, 31–38.

Dawkins, K., Jamieson, S., Hunt, S. et al. (1985). Long-term results, hemodynamic, and complications after combined heart and lung transplantation. Circulation, 71, 919–926.

Dohi, S., Jones, M. D., Hudak, M. L. & Traystman, R. J. (1990). Effects of cocaine on pial arterioles in cats. Stroke, 21(12), 1710–1714.

Dressler, F., Malekzadeh, S. & Roberts, W. (1990). Quantitative analysis of amounts of coronary arterial narrowing in cocaine addicts. Am J Cardiol, 65(5), 303–308.

Duell. P. (1987). Chronic cocaine abuse and dilated cardiomyopathy. Am J Med, 83, 601.

Ebadi, M., Pfeiffer, R. & Murrin, L. (1990). Pathogenesis and treatment of neuroleptic malignant syndrome. Gen Pharmac, 21(4), 367–386.

Edwards, J. & Rubin, R. (1987). Aortic dissection and cocaine abuse. Ann Intern Med, 107(5), 779–780.

Endress, C. & King, G. (1990). Cocaine-induced small-bowel perforation. Am J Radiol, 154, 1346–1347.

Escobedo, L., Ruttenber, A., Anda, R. et al (1992). Coronary artery disease, left ventricular hypertrophy, and the risk of cocaine overdose death. Coronary Artery Disease, 3:853–857.

Factor, S. & Cho, S. (1985). Smooth-muscle contraction bands in the media of coronary arteries: postmortem marker of antemortem coronary spasm? J Am Coll Cardiol, 6, 1329–1337.

Flores, E. D., Lange, R. A., Cigarroa, R. G. & Hillis, L. D. (1990). Effect of cocaine on coronary artery dimensions in atherosclerotic coronary artery disease - enhanced vasoconstriction at sites of significant stenoses. J Am Coll Cardiol, 16(1), 74–79.

Freudenberger, R. S., Cappell, M. S. & Hutt, D. A. (1990). Intestinal infarction after intravenous cocaine administration. Ann Intern Med, 113(9), 715–716.

Friedman, J., Feinberg, S. & Feldman, R. (1985). A neuroleptic malignant like syndrome due to levodopa therapy withdrawal. JAMA, 254, 2792–2795.

Friedrichs, G. S., Wei, H. M. & Merrill, G. F. (1990). Coronary vasodilation caused by intravenous cocaine in the anesthetized beagle. Can J Physiol Pharmacol, 68(7), 893–897.

Gadaleta, D., Hall, M. & Nelson (1989). Cocaine induced acute aortic dissection. Chest, 96(5), 1203–1205.

Gantenberg, N. and Hageman, G. (1992). Cocaine-enhanced arrhythmogenesis: neural and nonneural mechanisms. Can J Physiol Pharmacol, 70: 240–246.

Garfia, A., Valverde, J., Borondo, J. et al. (1990). Vascular lesions in intestinal ischemia induced by cocaine-alcohol abuse: report of a fatal case due to overdose. J Forensic Sci, 35(3), 740–745.

Garrey, W. (1914). The nature of fibrillatory contraction of the heart - its relation to tissue mass and form. Am J Physiol, 33:397–414.

George, F. & Ritz, M. (1991). Cocaine-induced seizures are inhibited by serotonergic 5HT2 and 5HT3 receptor antagonists. In L. Harris (ed.) Committee for Problems of Drug Dependence, Annual Conference, published in National Institute on Drug Abuse Monograph Series, in press.

George, F., (1991). Cocaine toxicity: genetic evidence suggests different mechanisms for cocaine-induced seizures and lethality. Psychopharmacology, 104(3):307–311.

Gilchrist, J. (1985). Arrhythmogenic seizures: diagnosis by simultaneous EEG/ECG recording. Neurology, 35, 1503–1506.

Ginsburg, R., Bristow, M., Kantrowitz, N. et al. (1981). Histamine provocation of clinical coronary artery spasm: implications concerning pathogenesis of variant angina pectoris. Am Heart J, 102, 819–822.

Grannis, F., Bryant, C.,JD, Caffaratti. & Turner, A. (1988). Acute aortic dissection associated with cocaine abuse. Clin Cardiol, 11(8), 572–574.

Grody, W., Cheng, L. & Lewis, W. (1990). Infection of the heart by the Human Immunodeficiency Virus. Am J Cardiol, 66, 203–206.

Hale, S., Alker, K., Rezkalla, S. et al. (1989). Adverse effects of cocaine on cardiovascular dynamics, myocardial blood flow, and coronary artery diameter in an experimental model. Am Heart J, 118(5, Part 1), 927–933.

Hearn, W. L., Flynn, D. D., Hime, G. W., Rose, S. et al (1991). Cocaethylene - A unique cocaine metabolite displays high affinity for the dopamine transporter. J Neurochem, 56(2), 698–701.

Henzlova, M., Smith, S., Prchal, V. & Helmcke, F. (1991). Apparent reversibility of cocaine-induced cardiomyopathy. Am Heart J, 122(2):577–579.

Herzog, C., Snover, D. & Staley, N. (1984). Acute necrotising eosinophilic myocarditis. Br Heart J, 52, 343–348.

Hirsch, C. & Martin, D. (1971). Unexpected death in young epileptics. Neurology, 21, 682–690.

Howard, R., Hueter, D. & Davis, G. (1985). Acute myocardial infarction following cocaine abuse in a young woman with normal coronary arteries. JAMA, 254(1), 95–96.

Isner, J., Estes, N., Thompson, P. et al. (1986). Acute cardiac events temporally related to cocaine abuse. N Engl J Med, 315, 1438–1443.

Jackson, H. C., Ball, D. M. & Nutt, D. J. (1990). Noradrenergic mechanisms appear not to be involved in cocaine-induced seizures and lethality. Life Sci, 47(4), 353–359.

Jones, L. F. & Tackett, R. L. (1990). Chronic cocaine treatment enhances the responsiveness of the left anterior descending coronary artery and the femoral artery to vasoactive substances. J Pharmacol Exp Ther, 255(3), 1366–1370.

Joris, I. & Majno, G. (1981). Medial changes in arterial spasm induced by L-norepinephrine. Am J Pathol, 105 (3), 212–222.

Kabas, J., Blanchard, S., Matsuyama, Y. et al. (1990). Cocaine-mediated impairment of cardiac conduction in the dog: a potential mechanism for sudden death after cocaine. J Pharmacol and Exp Ther, 252(1), 185–191.

Karch, S. & Billingham, M. (1988). The pathology and etiology of cocaine-induced heart disease. Arch Pathol Lab Med, 112, 225–230.

Karch, S. & Billingham M. (1986). Myocardial contraction bands revisited. Hum Pathol, 17, 9–13.

Karch, S. & Stephens, B. (1991). When is cocaine the cause of death? Am J Forensic Med & Pathol, 12(1), 1–2.

Karoum, F., Fawcett, R. & Wyatt, R. (1988). Chronic cocaine effects on peripheral biogenic amines: a long-term reduction in peripheral dopamine and phenylethylamine production. Euro J Pharm, 148, 381–388.

Karoum, F., Suddath, R. L. & Wyatt, R. J. (1990). Chronic cocaine and rat brain catecholamines - long-term reduction in hypothalamic and frontal cortex dopamine metabolism. Eur J Pharmacol, 186(1), 1–8.

Kasten, G. & 1986 (1986). Amide local anesthetic alterations of effective refractory period temporal dispersion: relationship to ventricular arrhythmias. Anesthesiology, 65, 61–66.

Kiok, M., Terrence, CF, Fromm, G. & Lavine, S. (1986). Sinus arrest in epilepsy. Neurology, 36, 115–116.

Kolodgie, F., Virmani, R., Cornhill, JF. et al. (1990). Cocaine: an independent risk factor of atherosclerosis. Circulation, 82, Supplement III(4), III-447.

Kolodgie, F. D., Virmani, R., Cornhill, J.F. et al. (1991) Increase in atherosclerosis and adventitial mast cells in cocaine abusers: an alternative mechanism of cocaine-associated coronary vasospasm and thrombosis. J Am Coll Cardiol, 17(7), 1553–1560.

Kornblum, R. & Reddy, S. (1991). Effects of the taser in fatalities involving police confrontation. J Forensic Sci, 36(2), 434–449.

Kossowsky, W. & Lyon, A. (1984). Cocaine and acute myocardial infarction: a probable connection. Chest, 86, 729–731.

Kosten, T. & Kleber, H. (1988). Rapid death during cocaine abuse: a variant of the neuroleptic malignant syndrome? Am J Drug Alcohol Abuse, 14(3), 335–346.

Kosten, T. & Kleber, H. (1987). Sudden death in cocaine abusers: relation to neuroleptic malignant syndrome (letter). Lancet, 1, 1198–1199.

Kringsholm, B. & Christoffersen, P. (1987). Lung and heart pathology in fatal drug addiction. A consecutive autopsy study. Forensic Sci Int, 34, 39–51.

Kugelmass, A. & Ware, J.(1992). Cocaine and coronary artery thrombosis. (letter). Ann Intern Med, 116(9):776–777.

Kuhn, F.E., Gillis, R.A., Virmani, R. et al. (1992). Cocaine produced coronary artery vasoconstriction independent of an intact endothelium. Chest, 102:581–585.

Lafont, A., Marche, C., Wolff, M. et al. (1988). Myocarditis in acquired immuno-deficiency syndrome (AIDS) . Etiology and prognosis (abstract). J Am Coll Cardiol, 11, 196A.

Lange, R., Cigarroa, R., Yancy, C. et al. (1989). Cocaine-induced coronary-artery vasoconstriction. N Engl J Med, 321(23), 1557–1562.

Lange, R., Cigarroa, R., Flores, E. et al. (1990). Potentiation of cocaine-induced coronary vasoconstriction by beta-adrenergic blockade. Ann Intern Med, 112(12), 897–903.

Lange, R., Cigarroa, R. & Hillis, L. (1989). Cocaine-induced reduction in cross--sectional area of coronary artery stenoses in man: a quantitative assessment. Circulation, 80(4), II-351.

Langner, R., Bement, C. (1991). Cocaine-induced changes in the biochemistry and morphology of rabbit aorta. NIDA Research Monograph, 108: 154–166.

Lathers, CZ. & Schraeder, P. (1982). Autonomic dysfunction in epilepsy: chara-cterization of autonomic cardiac neural discharge associated with pentylenetetrazol-induced epileptogenic activity. Epilepsia, 23 (6), 633–647.

Levinson, J. (1985). Neuroleptic malignant syndrome. Am J Psychiatry, 142: 1137–1145.

Lip, G. and Brodie, M. (1992). Sudden death in epilepsy: an avoidable outcome. J Royal Soc Med, 85:609–613.

Lisse, J., Davis, C. & Thurmond-Anderle, M. (1989). Upper extremity deep venous thrombosis: increased prevalence due to cocaine abuse. Am J Med, 87(4), 457–458.

Lisse, J., Davis, C. & Thurmond-Anderle, M. (1989). Cocaine abuse and deep venous thrombosis. Ann Intern Med, 110(7), 571–572.

Luke, J., Reay, D. (1992). The perils of investigating and certifying death in police custody. Am J Forensic Med & Pathol, 13 (2):98–100.

McWilliam, J. (1887). Fibrillar contraction of the heart. J Physiol, 8:296–310.

Madden, J. & Powers, R. (1990). Effect of cocaine and cocaine metabolites on cerebral arteries in vitro. Life Sciences, 47(13), 1109–1114.

Majid, P., Patel, B., Kim, H. et al. (1990). An angiographic and histologic study of cocaine-induced chest pain. Am J Cardiol, 65(11), 812–814.

Marley, R., Witkin, J. and S. Goldberg. (1991). A pharmacogenetic evaluation of the role of local anesthetic actions in the cocaine kindling process. Brain Res, 562:251–257.

Maseri, A., L'Abbate, A., Baroldi, G. et al. (1978) Coronary vasospasm as a possible cause of myocardial infarction: a conclusion derived from the study of "preinfarction" angina. N Engl J Med, 299 (23), 1271–1277.

Mathias, D. (1986). Cocaine-associated myocardial ischemia: review of clinical and angiographic findings. Am J Med, 81, 675–678.

Mendelson, M., and Chandler, J. (1992). Postpartum cardiomyopathy associated with maternal cocaine abuse. Am J Cardiol, 70:1092–1094.

Michelson, E.,Spear, J. & Moore, E. (1980). Electrophysiologic and anatomic correlates of sustained ventricular tachyarrhythmias in a model of chronic myocardial infarction. Am J Cardiol, 45, 583–590.

Minor, Jr. R., Scott, B., Brown, D. et al. (1991). Cocaine-induced myocardial infarction in patients with normal coronary arteries. Ann Intern Med, 115(10):797–806.

Mizrahi, S., Laor, D. & Stamler, B. (1988). Intestinal ischemia induced by cocaine abuse. Arch Surg, 123, 394.

Nahas, G., Trouve, R., Demus, J. & Sitbon, M. (1985). A calcium-channel blocker as antidote to the cardiac effects of cocaine intoxication. N Engl J Med, 313(8):519–520.

Nahas, G., Maillet, M., Chiarasini, D. & Latour, C. (1991). Myocardial damage induced by cocaine admnistration of a week's duration in the rat. In L. Harris (ed.) Committee for Problems of Drug Dependency, Annual Conference, Published in National Institute on Drug Abuse Monograph Series. In Press.

Nalbandian, H., Sheth, N., Dietrich, R. & Georgiou, J. (1985). Intestinal ischemia caused by cocaine ingestion: report of two cases. Surgery, 97(3), 374–376.

Nanji, A. & Filipenko, J. (1984). Asystole and ventricular fibrillation associated with cocaine intoxication. Chest, 85:132–133.

Nathan, L. & Hernandez, E. (1990). Intravenous substance abuse and a presacral mass. JAMA, 263(11), 1496.

Novitzky, D., Wicomb, W., Cooper, D. et al. (1984). Electrocardiographic, hemodynamic and endocrine changes occurring during experimental brain death in the Chacma baboon. J Heart Transplant, 4, 63–69.

Om, A., Porter, T., and Mohanty, P. (1992). Transeophageal echocardiographic diagnosis of acute aortic dissection complicating cocaine abuse. Am Heart J, 123(2) 532–534.

Oppenheimer, S. (1990). Cardiac dysfunction during seizures and the sudden epileptic death syndrome. J Royal Soc Med, 83(3), 134–136.

Parker, R., Beckman, K., Baumann, J. & Hariman, R. (1989). Sodium bicarbonate reverses cocaine-induced conduction defects. Circulation, 80(4), II–15.

Pasternack, P., Colvin, S. & Bauman, F. (1986). Cocaine-induced angina pectoris and acute myocardial infarction in patients younger than 40 years. Am J Cardiol, 55, 847.

Peng, S., French, W. & Pelikan, P. (1989). Direct cocaine cardiotoxicity demonstrated by endomyocardial biopsy. Arch Pathol Lab Med, 113(8), 842–845.

Pettit, H. O., Pan, H. T., Parsons, L. H. & Justice, J. B. (1990). Extracellular concentrations of cocaine and dopamine are enhanced during chronic cocaine administration. J Neurochem, 55(3), 798–804.

Pol, S., Morley, D., Zhang, X. & Bove, A. (1991). Cocaine has no direct vasoconstrictor effect. In L. Harris (ed.) Committee for Problems of Drug Dependency, Annual Conference. Published in National Institute on Drug Abuse Monograph Series. In Press.

Porter, W. (1894). On the results of ligation of the coronary arteries. J Physiol (London), 15:121–138.

Przywara, D.A. and Dambacon, G.E., (1989). Direct actions of cocaine on cardiac cellular electrical activity. Circulation Res, 65, 185–192.

Randall, W., Armour, J., Geis, W. et al. (1972). Regional cardiac distribution of the sympathetic nerves. Fed Proc, 21, 1199–1208.

Reichenbach, D. & Moss, N. (1975). Myocardial cell necrosis and sudden death in humans. Circulation, 51,52(Suppl III), III 60–62.

Ricci, D., Orlick, A., Cipriano, P. et al. (1979). Altered adrenergic activity in coronary arterial spasm: insight into mechanism based on study of coronary hemodynamics and the electrocardiogram. Am J Cardiol, 43, 1073–1079.

Roberts, W., Curry, R. Jr., Isner, J. et al. (1982). Sudden death in Prinzmetal's angina with coronary spasm documented by angiography. Am J Cardiol, 50, 203–210.

Rod, J. & Zucker, R. (1987). Acute myocardial infarction shortly after cocaine inhalation. Am J Cardiol, 59, 161.

Roh, L. & Hamele-Bena, D. (1990). Cocaine-induced ischemic myocardial disease. Am J Forensic Med & Pathol, 11(2), 130–135.

Rollingher, I., Belzberg, A. & Macdonald, I. (1986). Cocaine-induced myocardial infarction. Can Med Assoc J, 135, 45–46.

Rosen, T., Leopold, H. & Danilo, P. (1988). The effects of cocaine on the isolated fetal and adult guinea pig heart. Circulation, 78(4, Suppl-II), II–359.

Rosenbaum, J., Billingham, M., Ginsburg, R. et al. (1987). Cardiomyopathy in a rat model of pheochromocytoma: morphological and functional alterations. J Pharmacol Exp Ther, 241, 354–360.

Ruttenber, H., Sweeny, P., Mendelin, J. & Wetli, C. (1991). Preliminary findings of an epidemiologic study of cocaine related deaths in Dade County, Florida, 1978-1985, in Epidemiology of cocaine use and abuse, Schober, S and Schade, C (eds.), NIDA Research Monograph 110, U.S. Government Printing Office, Washington, D.C., 95-112

Samuels, M. (1987). Neurogenic heart disease: a unifying hypothesis. Am J Cardiol, 60, 15J–19J.

Schwartz, A.B., Janzen, D., Jones, R.T., and Boyle, W., (1989). Electrocardiographic and hemodynamic effects of intravenous cocaine in awake and anesthetized dogs. J Electrocardiol, 22(2), 159–166.

Schrem, S., Belsky, P., Schwartzman, D. & Slater, W. (1990). Cocaine-induced Torsades de Pointes in a patient with the idiopathic long QT syndrome. Am Heart J, 120(4), 980–984.

Shannon, M. (1988). Clinical toxicity of cocaine adulterants. Ann Emerg Med, 17(11), 1243–1247.

Simpson, R. & Edwards, W. (1986). Pathogenesis of cocaine-induced ischemic heart disease. Arch Patho Lab Med, 110, 479–484.

Smart, R. & Anglin, R. (1986). Do we know the lethal dose of cocaine? J Forensic Sci, 32(2), 303–312.

Smith, H., Liberman, H., Brody, S. et al. (1987). Acute myocardial infarction temporarily related to cocaine use. Ann Intern Med, 107, 13–18.

Smith, H., Roche, A., Jagusch, M. & Herdson, P. (1976). Cardiomyopathy associated with amphetamine administration. Am Heart J, 91, 792–797.

Stenberg, R., Winniford, M., Hillis, D. et al. (1989). Simultaneous acute thrombosis of two major coronary arteries following intravenous cocaine use. Arch Pathol Lab Med, 113, 521–524.

Strain, J., Grose, R., Factor, S. & Fisher, J. (1983). Results of endomyocardial biopsy in patients with spontaneous ventricular tachycardia but without apparent structural heart disease. Circulation, 68(6), 1171–1181.

Szakacs, J. & Cannon A (1958). l-Norepinephrine myocarditis. Am J Clin Pathol, 30, 425–434.

Szakacs, J., Dimmette, R. & Cowart, E. (1959). Pathologic implications of the catecholamines epinephrine and norepinephrine. US Armed Forces Med J, 10, 908–925.

Talebzadeh, V., Chevrolet, J., Chatelain, P. et al. (1990). Myocardite à éosinophiles et hypertension pulmonaire chez une toxicomane. Ann Pathol, 10(1), 40–46.

Taliercio, C., Olney, B. & Lie, J. (1985). Myocarditis related to drug hypersensitivity. Mayo Clin Proc, 60, 463–468.

Tardiff, K., Gross, E., Wu, J. et al. (1989). Analysis of cocaine-positive fatalities. J Forensic Sci, 34(1), 53–63.

Taylor, D. & Ho, B. (1977). Neurochemical effects of cocaine following acute and repeated injection. J Neurosci Res, 3, 95–101.

Tazelaar, H., Karch ,S., Billingham, M. & Stephens, B. (1987). Cocaine and the heart. Hum Pathol, 18, 195–199.

Tella, S., Korupolu, G., Schindler, C., and Goldberg, S. (1992). Pathophysiological and pharmacological mechanisms of acute cocaine toxicity in conscious rats. J Pharm Exp Ther, 262:936–946.

Temsey-Armos, P., Fraker, T., Brewster, P. and Wilkerson, D. (1992). The effects of cocaine on cardiac electrophysiology in conscious, unsedated dogs. J. Cardiovasc Pharmacol, 19:883–891.

Togna, G., Tempesta, E., Togna, A. et al. (1985). Platelet responsiveness and biosynthesis of thromboxane and prostacylin in response to in vitro cocaine treatment. Haemostasis, 15, 100–107.

Trouve, R. & Nahas, G. (1986). Nitrendipine: an antidote to cardiac and lethal toxicity of cocaine. Proc Soc Exp Biol and Med, 183, 392–397.

Virmani, R., Kolodgie, F., Rabinowitz, M. et al. (1989). Cocaine associated coronary thrombosis coexists with atherosclerosis and increased adventitial mast cells. Circulation, 80(4), II-647.

Virmani, R., Rabinowitz, M. & Smialek, J. (1987). Cocaine-associated deaths: absence of coronary thrombosis and a high incidence of myocarditis. Lab Invest, 56, 83.

Virmani, R., Rabinowitz, M.,Smialek, J. & Smyth, D. (1988). Cardiovascular effects of cocaine: an autopsy study of 40 patients. Am Heart J, 115(5), 1068–1076.

Vitullo, J., Karam, R., Mekhail, N. et al. (1989). Cocaine-induced small vessel spasm in isolated rat hearts. Am J Pathol, 135(1), 85–91.

Watt, T. & Pruitt, R. (1964). Cocaine-induced incomplete bundle branch block in dogs. Circ Res, 15, 234–239.

Weidmann, S. (1955). Effects of calcium ions and local anaesthetics on electrical properties of Purkinje fibers. J Physiol, 129, 568–582.

Weiss, R. (1986). Recurrent myocardial infarction caused by cocaine abuse. Am Heart J, 111(793).

Wetli, C. & Fishbain, D. (1985). Cocaine-induced psychosis and sudden death in recreational cocaine users. J Forensic Sci, 30(3), 873–880.

Wiener, R., Lockhart, J. & Schwartz, R. (1986). Dilated cardiomyopathy and cocaine abuse: report of two cases. Am J Med, 81, 699–701.

Wilkins, C., Mathur, V., Ty, R. & Hall, R. (1985). Myocardial infarction associated with cocaine abuse. Texas Heart Inst J, 12, 385–387.

Williams, E. (1914,). Negro cocaine "fiends" are a new Southern menace. New York Times, p. 12, Section 5. February 8

Wolfson, H. and Hoyga, PT. (1990). Chronic cocaine abuse associated with dilated cardiomyopathy. Am J Emerg Med.

Young, D. & Glauber, J. (1947). Electrocardiographic changes resulting from acute cocaine intoxication. Am Heart J, 34, 272–279.

Zimmerman, F., Gustafson, G. & Kemp, H. (1987). Recurrent myocardial infarction associated with cocaine abuse in a young man with normal coronary arteries: evidence for coronary artery spasm culminating in thrombosis. J Am Coll Cardiol, 9, 964–968.

Zipes, D., Fischer, J., King, R., et al. (1975). Termination of ventricular fibrillation in dogs by depolarizing a critical amount of myocardium. Am J Cardiol, 36:37–44.

1.10.3 PULMONARY DISEASE

Cocaine-related pulmonary disorders can be grouped into four categories: local inflammatory and infectious processes, barotrauma, parenchymal disease, and vascular adaptations. Most of the changes in the upper airway are a result of local inflammatory processes, but all four types of alterations may be seen in the lower portions of the airway. Cocaine's effects on the upper airway are primarily local. The most common cocaine induced disorder of the upper airway is perforation of the nasal septum. This disorder has been recognized for nearly 100 years (Maier, 1926). Much less common are chronic inflammatory processes involving the oropharynx. Occasionally the inflammatory process may be so intense that it mimics limited Wegner's granulomatosis (Daggett, Haghighi & Terkeltaub, 1990).

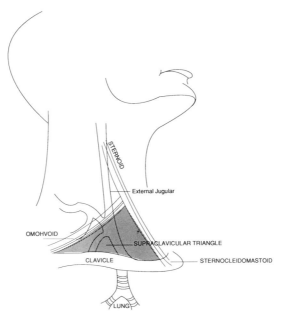

Figure 1.10.3.2 The supraclavicular fossa
As peripheral veins become sclerosed, chronic abusers resort to injecting themselves in the supraclavicular fossa and in the femoral triangle. The supraclavicular fossa overlies the great vessels and the apex of the lung. Pneumothorax and hemothorax are the predictable results.

A heterogeneous group of disorders, ranging from decreased diffusing capacity (Itkonen, Schnoll & Glassroth, 1984) and pneumomediastinum (Hunter, Loy, Markovitz & Kim, 1986) to bronchiolitis obliterans (Patel, Dutta & Schonfeld, 1987), and pulmonary edema (Allred & Ewer, 1981) have all been attributed to cocaine use. It is not known with any certainty whether intravenous cocaine abuse carries with it the same increased risks for community acquired pneumonia and septic pulmonary emboli as heroin use, and experimental studies of the effects of cocaine on the lung are non-existent. There is now a rat model for cocaine smoking (Boni, Barr & Martin, 1991), and hopefully the situation may become clearer in the next few years. For the present, however, the histologic effects of cocaine on the human lower airway remain too poorly documented to permit many generalizations.

Because intravenous cocaine abuse is less common than intravenous heroin abuse, and because the contaminants in illicit cocaine are water soluble while those in heroin are not, the complications of intravenous abuse are seen less frequently in cocaine users. Nonetheless, intravenous cocaine abuse can lead to infectious complications such as pneumonia, vascular complications such as foreign particle embolization, and mechanical complications such as pneumothorax. Perhaps the most important difference between intravenous heroin and cocaine abuse is that cocaine users inject themselves much more frequently. As a consequence they are at a greater risk of developing infectious complications, and that includes HIV infection.

1.10.3.1 Local inflammation

Chronic coca leaf chewers may develop stomatitis, glossitis and buccal mucosal leukoderma (Hammer & Villegas, 1969). The practice of "snorting" probably didn't begin until shortly before 1903, the year when the first cases of septal perforation were reported (Maier, 1926). Septal perforation is now a well known complication of drug abuse (Pearman, 1979), but little is known about the histologic changes accompanying the process. One controlled autopsy study compared histological findings in septal mucosa from 20 individuals with proven histories of chronic nasal inhalation of cocaine and 15 controls. As might be expected, chronic inflammatory disease was seen in the cocaine users. The glandular elements were in total disarray and mononuclear cells, particularly lymphocytes, were seen surrounding arterioles and glands. An unexpected finding was the presence of thickened submucosal arterioles. Intimal hyperplasia and fibrosis of these vessels was seen in the majority of cases. There was also increased perivascular deposition of collagen (Chow, Robertson & Stein, 1990). The arterial findings were similar to, but not nearly so marked, as those that have been observed in the coronary arteries of cocaine users (Simpson & Edwards, 1986) (Roh & Hamele-Bena, 1990), or in cases of catechol toxicity (Szakacs, Dimmette & Cowart, 1959). Sampling septal mucosa at autopsy might prove quite useful in confirming a suspected diagnosis of cocaine toxicity, since the finding would suggest a pattern of chronic prior use. At a minimum, the mucosa should be swabbed with saline, since cocaine may be recovered for some time, possibly days, after it was last used. Besides the changes in the septum, upper respiratory tract necrosis, sometimes on a fairly massive scale, also occurs (Becker & Hill, 1988) (Deutsch & Millard, 1989) (Daggett et al., 1990). The etiology is thought to be ischemic, secondary to chronic cocaine-induced vasoconstriction, but could also be secondary to contaminants in the inhaled cocaine. Biopsies of a posterior oropharyngeal ulcer in one patient showed only necrosis and a mixed inflammatory cell infiltrate, and there is nothing diagnostic about the tissue changes. The causative role of cocaine is generally confirmed by the resolution of the lesions with cocaine abstinence.

1.10.3.2 Barotrauma

The general classification of barotrauma includes disorders where increased intraalveolar pressure or decreased interstitial pressure lead to rupture of an alveolus with leakage of air. Whether pneumothorax or pneumomediastinum occurs depends on the location of the alveolus. Abnormalities have been recognized in cocaine users that could account for this pressure imbalance. Increased intraalveolar pressure is usually the result of coughing or performing the Valsalva maneuver, which crack smokers routinely do. There are, however, other possibilities. Pulmonary inflammation could weaken the alveolar wall and lead to leakage of air. Alternatively, vasoconstriction in the vessels adjacent to an alveoli could cause decreased interstitial pressure, leading to alveolar rupture without any great increase in intraalveolar pressure (Seaman, 1989) (Macklin & Macklin, 1944). In cocaine users, all of these possibilities need to be considered.

Another possible cause for pneumo and hemothorax is injection into central veins, although this practice is much more common in heroin abusers. Heroin tends to be adulterated with material that is not water soluble. Repeated injections of adulterated heroin can lead to sclerosis of peripheral veins. When that happens, the user is forced to inject central veins. The two most popular central sites are the great vessels in the neck ("pocket shot") (Lewis, 1980) and the vessels of the femoral triangle ("groin shot") (Pace, Doscher & Margolis, 1984). Injections are made into the general area of the supraclavicular fossa, either by the addict himself or by a hired "street doc". Since the lung apex is directly contiguous with the area, pneumothorax not uncommonly results (Kurtzman, 1970), (Lewis, 1980), (Merhar, 1981), (Douglas, 1986).

Cocaine-associated pneumomediastinum occurs with some frequency (Aroesty, Stanley & Crockett, 1986; Mir, Galvete et al., 1986; Brody, Anderson & Gutman, 1988; Bush, Rubenstein, Hoffman & Bruno, 1984; Christou, Turnbull & Cline, 1990; Hunter et al., 1986; Leitman, Greengart & Wasser, 1988; Luque, Cavallaro, Torres et al., 1987; Mir, Galvette, Plaza et al, 1986; Morris & Shuck, 1985; Poon, Ruiz, Toole & Stern, 1987; Salzman, Khan & Emory, 1987; Savader, Omori & Martinez, 1988; Schweitzer, 1986; Shesser, Davis & Edelstein, 1981) (Luque et al., 1987) (Savader et al., 1988). Since pneumomediastinum is a benign condition, and since no fatal cases of pneumothorax have been reported, there are no autopsy studies. Presumably the mechanism has to do with the performance of a Valsalva maneuver by a deeply inhaling smoker. No cases have been reported after intravenous or intranasal use. Surprisingly, barotrauma has not been proposed as the mechanism for the increasing number of cocaine-related strokes that have been reported (see section 1.10.5), but it might offer just as good an explanation as cocaine induced vasospasm. Air from ruptured alveoli may diffuse into pulmonary capillaries and veins, then pass through the left side of the heart and embolize, via the systemic arteries, to the brain. The diagnosis is particularly difficult to make. If the patient survives for more than a few hours, the air bubbles will have dissolved and typical morphologic changes (multiple small, well-circumscribed foci of cortical necrosis, sometimes associated with laminar necrosis) will not have had time to develop (Wolf, Moon, Mitchell & Burger, 1990).

1.10.3.3 Parenchymal disease

Pulmonary congestion and edema are common findings in drug related deaths. Osler first wrote about morphine-induced pulmonary edema over 100 years ago (Osler, 1880), and turn-of-the-century pathologists also recognized a connection between pulmonary congestion and opiate related deaths (Hamilton, 1905). Edema secondary to heroin abuse has been a common problem since the 1960's (Steinberg & Karliner, 1968) (Duberstein & Kaufman, 1971). Pulmonary congestion in cocaine-related deaths was also recognized at the turn of the century (Hamilton, 1905), but pulmonary edema in cocaine users also occurs in non-fatal cases (Allred & Ewer, 1981) (Hoffman & Goodman, 1989) (Efferen, Palat & Meisner, 1989) (Cucco, Yoo, Cregler & Chang, 1987) (Purdie, 1982) (Kline & Hirasuana, 1990) (Bakht, Kirshon, Baker & Cotton, 1990). The etiology of cocaine-associated pulmonary edema is obscure. It could be another manifestation of catechol toxicity (Kurachek & Rockoff, 1985) (Karch, 1990), and it might share common mechanisms with "neurogenic" pulmonary edema (Robin, Wong & Ptashne, 1989). Cocaine-induced pulmonary edema could also be explained by the fact that both cocaine and catecholamine excess can lead to decreased contractility (Perreault, Allen, Hague et al, 1989) (Strichartz, 1987) (Szakacs et al., 1959). If contractility is depressed enough to lower cardiac output, heart failure and pulmonary edema could develop. Still another possible mechanism might be a direct effect of cocaine on the lung, though, at the moment, there is nothing to support such a notion.

Hemosiderin-laden macrophages are a common finding in the lungs of drug abusers. This change was first recognized in narcotic abusers (Siegel, 1972) (Rajs, Härm & Ormstad, 1984) (Kringsholm & Christoffersen, 1987), but similar macrophages are commonly seen in the subgroup abusing cocaine. Hemosiderin laden cells are not seen in any particular relationship to recent hemorrhage and their etiology is obscure. Siegel thought that hypoxia was in some way responsible (Siegel, 1972) though that has never been established, and would not explain the presence of these cells in cocaine users who, unless they have massively overdosed, are not hypoxic. Diffuse alveolar hemorrhage has been described (Murray, Albin, Megner & Criner, 1988), and clinical reports suggest that spontaneously resolving hemoptysis is not that uncommon among cocaine smokers (Forrester, 1990) (Murray et al., 1988) (Murray, Simalek, Golle & Albin, 1989) (Bouchi, Asmar, Covetil et al., 1992). One retrospective autopsy study of cocaine users found hemosiderin-laden macrophages in 27% to 35% of the patients (Murray et al., 1988). But by comparison, the incidence of this finding is much higher in narcotic abusers (>90%) (Kringsholm & Christoffersen, 1987).

The results of other studies suggest that the change may simply be the result of alveolar deposition of particulate matter (Klinger, Bensadoun & Corrao, 1992). Accordingly, the presence of iron containing macrophages has little diagnostic value and is, in fact, more consistent with a history of narcotic abuse than with cocaine.

Prior to the advent of smokable cocaine, mentions of cocaine related pulmonary disease were rare. As smoking cocaine became more popular, reports of patients with inflammatory infiltrates, sometimes associated with fever, hypoxia, hemoptysis and even respiratory failure, began to appear (Forrester, Steele, Waldron & Parsons, 1990). Specimens from several of these patients have demonstrated diffuse alveolar damage with hyaline membrane formation and Type II cell hyperplasia as well as intraalveolar and interstitial inflammatory infiltrates with eosinophilia. Some cocaine users with x-ray demonstrated inflammatory infiltrates have had peripheral eosinophilia (Murray et al., 1988; Murray et al., 1988) while others did not (Forrester et al., 1990) (Patel et al., 1987) (Cucco et al., 1987) (Talebzadeh, Chevrolet, Chatelain et al., 1990) (Oh and Balter, 1992). As with many of the other syndromes that have been attributed to cocaine use, there is virtually no experimental data that would suggest a mechanism for these changes. Nonetheless a reasonable argument could be made that hypersensitivity is at least partially responsible. Several biopsy specimens have shown deposition of IgE in both lymphocytes and alveolar macrophages (Forrester et al., 1990), and eosinophilic infiltrates have been observed in the heart (see section 1.10.2.3 for discussion of eosinophilic infiltrates in myocardium), and the pulmonary findings could be just another manifestation of the same underlying process. The difficulty with this theory is that at least half of the reported cases have been in polydrug abusers, and it is hard to know which drug is the culprit. Finally, the high rate of HIV infection among intravenous drug users should not be forgotten. Most of the pathology encountered in cocaine users is non-infectious. But like other patients with AIDS, any number of opportunist and non-opportunistic infections can be encountered.

1.10.3.4 Vascular adaptations

Hypertrophy of the smooth muscle in the walls of pulmonary arteries, along with proliferation of the elastic fibers, is consistent with the diagnosis of pulmonary hypertension. This alteration is seen in the lungs of narcotics abusers and is the result of intravascular deposition of foreign materials that have been injected along with the narcotic. Granuloma formation results, and sets in train a series of events which eventually lead to pulmonary hypertension. The three agents most commonly responsible for granuloma formation are talc, corn starch, and microcrystalline cellulose (Radow, Nachamkin, Morrow et al., 1983). All three materials are strongly birefringent. Starch granules are particularly simple to identify because they exhibit the "Maltese cross" pattern when viewed with polarized light. Particles can also be differentiated by their staining properties. Both starch and cellulose are both PAS-positive, while microcrystalline cellulose stain black with GMS (Tomashefski, Hirsch & Jolly, 1981).

In autopsy studies of narcotic and polydrug abusers the incidence of medial hypertrophy has ranged from 8% (Hopkins, 1972) to as high as 40% (Rajs et al., 1984). The mechanism, however, remains controversial, and in at least two controlled studies, intravenous drug users with multiple talc induced granulomas had no more medial hypertrophy than controls (Tomashefski & Hirsch, 1980) (Kringsholm & Christoffersen, 1987) (see section 5.8.1.4 for a more complete discussion of talc granulomas and angiothrombosis). Medial hypertrophy and talc granulomas can be seen in the lungs of cocaine users. Murray et al. examined the lungs of 20 individuals who had died of cocaine intoxication. Individuals with histories of polydrug abuse, or with toxicology screens that were positive for drugs beside cocaine, were specifically excluded from the study. Also excluded were cases in which birefringent material was found within the lungs. Four patients (20%) were found to have medial hypertrophy involving either the small or medium sized pulmonary arteries (Murray, Simalek, Golle & Albin, 1989). The authors suggest that chronic exposure to cocaine induced high levels of catecholamines, and that catechol excess may have resulted in pulmonary hypertension. Other authors have made the same suggestion (Itkonen et al., 1984). The variable rates of medial hypertrophy found in different autopsy studies might be explained by the drug-use practices of the local populations. Narcotic abuse is not associated with catechol excess, but stimulant abuse is. The problem with the catechol thesis is that patients with pheochromocytoma are not prone to pulmonary hypertension, except as a consequence of heart failure (Rose, Novitzky & Cooper, 1988). The patients in Murray's study with medial hypertrophy had no other signs of heart disease. Without more data the significance of medial hypertrophy in cocaine users is impossible to assess. Another inconsistency with the argument is the fact that granulomatous changes can also occur in the lungs of individuals who only sniff cocaine. Cellulose granulomas were identified in a patient who denied intravenous drug use and who had no occupational exposure to cellulose products (Cooper, Bai & Heyderman, 1983), and talc granulomas have been identified in two other patients (Buchanan, Lam & Seaton, 1981) (Oubeid, Bickel, Ingram & Scott, 1990).

Finally, the great vessels of the neck are subject to mechanical injury. "Pocket shooters" may lacerate the brachial, subclavian, or jugular veins. Hemothorax, hematoma and pseudoaneurysm are all recognized complications of central venous injection. Since the material injected is far from sterile, local and distant complications may occur. Mycotic aneurysm formation, local cellulitis and abscess formation have all been described, though the incidence is much higher in heroin than in cocaine users (McCarroll and Rozler, 1991).

References

Allred, R. & Ewer, S. (1981). Fatal pulmonary edema following intravenous "freebase" cocaine use. Ann Emerg Med, 10(8), 441–442.

Aroesty, D., Stanley, R. & Crockett, D. (1986). Pneumomediastinum and cervical emphysema from the inhalation of "free based" cocaine: report of three cases. Otolaryngol Head Neck Surg, 3:372–374.

Bakht, F., Kirshon, B., Baker, T. & Cotton, D. (1990). Postpartum cardiovascular complications after bromocriptine and cocaine use. Am J Obstet Gynecol, 162, 1065–1066.

Becker, G. & Hill, S. (1988). Midline granuloma due to illicit cocaine use. Arch Otolaryngol Head Neck Surg, 114, 90–1.

Boni, J. P., Barr, W. H. & Martin, B. R. (1991). Cocaine inhalation in the rat: pharmacokinetics and cardiovascular response. J Pharmacol Exp Ther, 257(1), 307–315.

Bouchi, J., el Asmar, B., Covetil, J. et al (1992). Alveolar hemorrhage after cocaine inhalation. Presse Medicale, 21 (22):1025–1026.

Brody, S., Anderson, C. & Gutman, J. (1988). Pneumomediastinum as a complication of "crack" smoking. Am J Emerg Med, 6 (241–243).

Buchanan, D.,Lam, D. & Seaton, A. (1981). Punk rocker's lung: pulmonary fibrosis in a drug snorting fire-eater. Br Med J, 283 (6307), 1661.

Bush, M., Rubenstein, R., Hoffman, I. & Bruno, M. (1984). Spontaneous pneumomediastinum as a consequence of cocaine use. NY State J Med (December), 618–619.

Chow, J., Robertson, A. & Stein, R. (1990). Vascular changes in the nasal submucosa of chronic cocaine addicts. Am J Forensic Med & Pathol, 11(2), 136–143.

Christou, T., Turnbull, T. & Cline, D. (1990). Cardiopulmonary abnormalities after smoking cocaine. South Med J, 83(3), 335–338.

Cohen, H. & Cohen, S (1984). Spontaneous bilateral pneumothorax in drug addicts. Chest, 86 (4), 645–647.

Cooper, C., Bai, T. & Heyderman, E. (1983). Cellulose granulomas in the lungs of a cocaine sniffer. Br Med J, 286, 2021–2022.

Cucco, R., Yoo, O., Cregler, L. & Chang, J. (1987). Nonfatal pulmonary edema after "freebase" cocaine smoking. Am Rev Respir Dis, 136, 179–181.

Daggett, R. B., Haghighi, P. & Terkeltaub, R. A. (1990). Nasal cocaine abuse causing an aggressive midline intranasal and pharyngeal destructive process mimicking midline reticulosis and limited Wegener's granulomatosis. J Rheumatol, 17(6), 838–840.

Douglas, R., Levison, M. (1980). Pneumothorax in drug abusers. An urban epidemic? Chest, 4, 613–617.

Deutsch, H. & Millard, D. J. (1989). A new cocaine abuse complex. Arch Otolaryngol Head Neck Surg, 115, 235–237.

Duberstein, J. & Kaufman, D. (1971). A clinical study of an epidemic of heroin intoxication and heroin-induced pulmonary edema. Am J Med, 51, 704–714.

Efferen, L., Palat, D. & Meisner, J. (1989). Nonfatal pulmonary edema following cocaine smoking. N Y State J Med(July), 415–416.

Forrester, J., Steele, A., Waldron, J. & Parsons, P. (1990). Crack lung: an acute pulmonary syndrome with a spectrum of clinical and histopathologic findings. Am Rev Respir Dis, 142 (2), 462–467.

Hamilton, A.M. (1894). A system of legal medicine. E.B. Treat and Company, New York, New York.

Hammer, J. & Villegas, O. (1969). The effect of coca leaf chewing on the buccal mucosa of Aymara and Quechua Indians in Bolivia. Oral Surg, 28, 287–295.

Hind, C.R, (1990). Pulmonary complications of intravenous drug misuse, part I. Thorax, 45, 891–898.

Hind, C.R., (1990). Pulmonary complications of intravenous drug misuse, part II. Thorax, 45, 957–961.

Hoffman, C. & Goodman, P. (1989). Pulmonary edema in cocaine smokers. Radiology, 172 (August), 463–465.

Hopkins, G. (1972). Pulmonary angiothrombotic granulomatosis in drug offenders. JAMA, 221(8), 909–911.

Hunter, J., Loy, H., Markovitz, L. & Kim, U. (1986). Spontaneous pneumomediastinum following inhalation of alkaloidal cocaine and emesis. Mt. Sinai J Med, 53(6), 491–493.

Itkonen, J., Schnoll, S. & Glassroth, J. (1984). Pulmonary dysfunction in 'free-base' cocaine users. Arch Intern Med, 144, 2195–2197.

Karch, S. (1990). Problems with high-dose epinephrine therapy. Am J For Med and Path, 11(2), 178–179.

Kline, J. & Hirasuana, J. (1990). Pulmonary edema after freebase cocaine smoking - not due to an adulterant. Chest, 97(4), 1009–1010.

Klinger, J., Bensadoun, E. & Corrao, W. (1992). Pulmonary complications from alveolar accumulation of carbonaceous material in a cocaine smoker. Chest, 101:1171–1173.

Kringsholm, B. & Christoffersen, P. (1987). Lung and heart pathology in fatal drug addiction. A consecutive autopsy study. Forensic Sci Int, 34, 39–51.

Kurachek, S. & Rockoff, M. (1985). Inadvertent intravenous administration of racemic epinephrine. JAMA, 253(10), 1441–1442.

Kurtzman, R.S., (1970). Complications of narcotic addiction. Radiology, 96, 23–30.

Leitman, B., Greengart, A. & Wasser, H. (1988). Pneumomediastinum and pneumopericardium after cocaine abuse. Am J Radiol, 151, 614.

Luque, M., Cavallaro, D., Torres, M. et al. (1987). Pneumomediastinum, pneumothorax and subcutaneous emphysema after alternate cocaine inhalation and marijuana smoking. Ped Emerg Care, 3, 107–110.

Lewis, J., Groux, N., Elliot, J. et al. (1980). Complications of attempted central venous injections performed by drug abusers. Chest, 74, 613–617.

Mcarroll, K. & Rozler, M. (1991). Lung disorders due to drug abuse. J Thorac Imaging, 6(1), 30–35.

Macklin, M. & Macklin, C. (1944). Malignant interstitial emphysema of the lungs and mediastinum as an important occult complication in many respiratory diseases and other conditions. Medicine, 23, 281–358.

Maier, H. W. (1926). Der Kokainismus (O.J. Kalant from the German 1926 edition, Trans.) Toronto: Addiction Research Foundation.

Merhar, G., Colley, D., Clark, R. (1981) Cervicothoracic complications of intravenous drug abuse. Comput Tomog, 5 (12), 271–282.

Mir, J.B., Galvette, JA., Plaza, MV. et al. (1986). Spontaneous pneumomediastinum after cocaine inhalation. Respiration, 50, 230–232.

Morris, J. & Shuck, J. (1985). Pneumomediastinum in a young male cocaine user. Ann Emerg Med, 14, 164–166.

Murray, R., Albin, R., Megner, W. & Criner, G. (1988). Diffuse alveolar hemorrhage temporally related to cocaine smoking. Chest, 93(2), 427–429.

Murray, R., Simalek, J., Golle, M. & Albin, R. (1989). Pulmonary artery medial hypertrophy without foreign particle microembolization in cocaine users. Chest, 94S, 48.

Murray, R., Simalek, J., Golle, M. & Albin, R. (1988). Pulmonary vascular abnormalities in cocaine users. Am Rev Respir Dis, 137(Suppl 4, part 2), 459.

Oh, P. and Balter, M. (1992). Cocaine induced eosinophilic lung disease. Thorax, 47:478–479.

Osler, W. (1880). Oedema of the left lung; morphia poisoning. Montreal Gen Hosp Rep, 1, 2291.

Oubeid, M., Bickel, J. T., Ingram, E. A. & Scott, G. C. (1990). Pulmonary talc granulomatosis in a cocaine sniffer. Chest, 98(1), 237–239.

Pace, B.W., Doscher, W. & Margolis, I.B. (1984). The femoral triangle: a potential death trap for the drug abuser. N. Y. State J med, 84, 596–598.

Patel, R., Dutta, D. & Schonfeld, S. (1987). Free-base cocaine use associated with bronchiolitis obliterans organizing pneumonia. Ann Int Med, 107(2), 186–187.

Pearman, K. (1979). Cocaine: a review. J Laryngol Otol, 93, 1191–1199.

Perreault, C., Allen, P., Hague, N. et al. (1989). Differential mechanisms of cocaine-induced depression of contractile function in cardiac versus vascular smooth muscle. Circulation, 80(4), II-15.

Ponn, R., Ruiz, R., Toole, A. & Stern, H. (1987). Pneumomediastinum from cocaine inhalation. Conn Med 51(6), 366–367.

Purdie, F. (1982). Therapy for pulmonary edema following IV "freebase" cocaine use. Ann Emerg Med, 11(4), 228–229.

Radow, S., Nachamkin, I., Morrow, C. et al. (1983). Foreign body granulomatosis: clinical and immunologic findings. Am Rev Respir Dis, 127(5), 575–580.

Rajs, J., Härm, T. & Ormstad, K. (1984). Postmortem findings of pulmonary lesions of older datum in intravenous drug addicts. Virchows Arch, 402, 405–414.

Robin, E., Wong, R. & Ptashne, K. (1989). Increased lung water and ascites after massive cocaine overdosage in mice and improved survival related to beta-adrenergic blockade. Ann Intern Med, 110(3), 202–207.

Roh, L. & Hamele-Bena, D. (1990). Cocaine-induced ischemic myocardial disease. Am J Forensic Med & Pathol, 11(2), 130–135.

Rose, A., Novitzky, D. & Cooper, D. (1988). Myocardial and pulmonary histopathologic changes. Transpl Proc, 20(5, Suppl 7), 29–32.

Salzman, G., Khan, F. & Emory, C. (1987). Pneumomediastinum after cocaine smoking. South Med J, 80(11), 1427–1429.

Savader, S., Omori, M. & Martinez, C. (1988). Pneumothorax, pneumomediastinum and pneumopericardium: complications of cocaine smoking. J Fla Med Assoc, 75, 151–152.

Schweitzer, V. (1986). Osteolytic sinusitis and pneumomediastinum: deceptive otolaryngologic complications of cocaine abuse. Laryngoscope, 96 (February), 206–210.

Seaman, M.E. (1989). Barotrauma related to inhalation drug abuse. J Emerg Med, 8,141–149.

Shesser, R., Davis, C. & Edelstein, S. (1981). Pneumomediastinum and pneumothorax after inhaling alkaloidal cocaine. Ann Emerg Med, 10(4), 213–215.

Shetty, P.C., Krasicky, G., Sharma & Berke, M. (1985). Mycotic aneurysms in intravenous drug abusers: the utility of intravenous digital subtraction angiography. Radiology, 155, 319–321.

Siegel, H. (1972). Human pulmonary pathology associated with narcotic and other addictive drugs. Hum Pathol, 3, 55–66.

Simpson, R. & Edwards, W. (1986). Pathogenesis of cocaine-induced ischemic heart disease. Arch Pathol Lab Med, 110, 479–484.

Steinberg, A. & Karliner, J. (1968). The clinical spectrum of heroin pulmonary edema. Arch Int Med, 122, 122–127.

Strichartz, G. (1987). Handbook of experimental pharmacology, Volume 81:Local Anesthetics. New York: Springer-Verlag.

Szakacs, J., Dimmette, R. & Cowart, E. (1959). Pathologic implications of the catecholamines epinephrine and norepinephrine. US Armed Forces Med J, 10, 908–925.

Talebzadeh, V., Chevrolet, J., Chatelain, P. et al. (1990). Myocardite à éosinophiles et hypertension pulmonaire chez une toxicomane. Ann Pathol, 10(1), 40–46.

Tomashefski, J. & Hirsch, C. (1980). The pulmonary vascular lesions of intravenous drug abuse. Human Pathol, 11, 133–145.

Tomashefski, J., Hirsch, C. & Jolly, P. (1981). Microcrystalline cellulose pulmonary embolism and granulomatosis. Arch Pathol & Lab Med, 105, 89–93.

Wolf, H., Moon, R., Mitchell, P. & Burger, P. (1990). Barotrauma and air embolism in hyperbaric oxygen therapy. Am J Forensic Med & Pathol, 11(2), 149–153.

Zorc, T., O'Donnell, A., Holt, R.W. et al. (1988). Bilateral pyopneumothorax secondary to intravenous drug abuse. Chest, 93, 645–647.

1.10.4 GASTROINTESTINAL DISORDERS

Most of the gastrointestinal problems associated with cocaine use are due to catechol mediated effects on blood vessels. However, cocaine metabolites, and possibly cocaine itself, may be directly toxic to the liver. Norcocaine is hepatotoxic in experimental animals as is cocaethylene, which is synthesized in the liver and has overall toxicity similar to that of cocaine itself, and binds to many of the same receptors that cocaine does. Presently there is no evidence that cocaine is hepatotoxic.

1.10.4.1 Ischemic injuries

Ischemic colitis due to cocaine abuse was first described in 1985 (Fishel, Hammamoto, Barbul et al., 1985). There have been regular reports ever since (Mizrahi, Laor & Stamler, 1988) (Nalbandian, Sheth, Dietrich & Georgiou, 1985) (Garfia, Valverde, Borondo et al., 1990) (Endress & King, 1990) (Riggs & Weibley, 1991) (Freudenberger, Cappell & Hutt, 1990) (Nathan & Hernandez, 1990) (Yang, Han & Mccarthy, 1991) (Endress, Gray & Wollschlaeger, 1992) (Hall, Zaninovic, Lewis et al., 1992). The case originally described by Fishel was a that of 37-year old with right lower quadrant pain and diarrhea. A right hemicolectomy was performed for removal of a mass that proved to be an inflamed cecum. Microscopic examination of the removed bowel disclosed "findings consistent with pseudomembranous colitis and some areas that were suggestive of ischemic colitis." In the case reported by Endress, the ilium had zones of hemorrhage and ulceration but no particularly distinctive features (Endress & King, 1990). A retrospective study of patients with gastroduodenal perforations suggests that "crack" cocaine smokers may constitute a specific subgroup of patients who develop their perforation on the basis of an acute ischemic event, rather than as a complication of chronic ulcer disease (Lee, LaMaute, Pizzi et al, 1990), and that perforation is more likely to be duodenal rather than gastric (Abramson et al. 1992).

The role of catechol excess in cocaine-related bowel disease is strongly suggested by the fact that bowel obstruction and ischemia with similar pathologic findings occurs in patients with pheochromocytoma. Khafagi et al. described a patient with extremely high catecholamine levels who developed pseudo bowel obstruction that rapidly resolved with intravenous phentolamine infusions (Khafagi, Lloyd & Gough, 1987). In fact, catechol mediated gastrointestinal lesions have been recognized since the 1930's, when treatment of asthmatics with nebulized epinephrine came into fashion. Occasionally treatment was complicated by tracheal hemorrhages and ulceration of the gastrointestinal mucosa (Galgaini, Proescher, Dock & Tainter, 1939).

Szakacs systematically studied the effects of chronic catechol administration in experimental animals and humans. He reported in the 1950's that fibrinoid degeneration and necrosis could be seen in the arteriolar walls of vessels both in the heart and in the gastrointestinal tract. Prolonged norepinephrine infusion induced endothelial proliferation, occasionally sufficient to cause "complete obstruction of small arteries of the gastrointestinal tract, leading to infarction and perforation of the bowel". Similar lesions were observed in experimental animals and in patients with pheochromocytoma (Szakacs, Dimmette & Cowart, 1959). Nearly forty years later, precisely the same lesion has been identified in cocaine users (Garfia et al., 1990). Thrombotic lesions have also been described, presumably caused by the same sequence of events that lead to thrombosis in the heart and other blood vessels.

1.10.4.2 Hepatic disease

Hepatocellular necrosis can be produced in animal models of cocaine toxicity, but the clinical significance is not clear. Clinical studies of chronic cocaine abusers are contradictory. One study found significant transaminase elevations in chronic cocaine users (Marks & Chapple, 1986), but other studies have failed to demonstrate liver function abnormalities, or showed only minimal enzyme changes (Kothur, Marsh & Posner, 1991). Normal liver function has been observed in both parenteral (Rippetoe, Phillips & Lange, 1991) and non-parenteral users, provided the users were not hepatitis B carriers (Tabasco-minguillan, Novick & Kreek, 1990).

The relative absence of cocaine-related liver disease has to do with the fact that oxidative cocaine metabolism plays a very minor role in man. In animals, however, cytochrome P450 and flavin adenine dinucleotide containing monooxygenase metabolize significant amounts of cocaine to norcocaine. Further enzymatic breakdown yields N-hydroxynorcocaine and norcocaine nitroxide (Shuster, Quimby, Bates & Thompson, 1977; Shuster, Casey & Welankiwar, 1983). Norcocaine nitroxide, once thought to be a highly reactive free radical, is now known to be stable. It reacts neither with proteins nor glutathione (Rauckman, Rosen & Cavagnaro, 1982). However, further oxidation to the norcocaine nitrosodium ion produces a compound that is highly reactive with glutathione. If glutathione stores fall below a certain level, lipid peroxidation is unopposed and cocaine metabolites bind to hepatic proteins, eventually leading to cell death (Evans, 1983) (Kloss, Rosen & Rauckman, 1984). Necrosis is worse if animals are pretreated with agents that induce P450 synthesis and is less if they are treated with P450 inhibitors. In animals, one of two different patterns may be observed. Fatty infiltration and periportal inflammation occur in association with periportal (Evans & Harbison, 1978) (Evans, 1983) or centrolobular necrosis (Shuster et al. 1977). Both types of necrosis can be prevented if the animal is pretreated with P450 inhibitors (Evans, 1983). In addition, cocaine given to mice cause depression of hepatic mitochondrial function, sometimes to a marked degree (León-Velarde et al. 1991), but whether this also occurs in humans is not known.

The situation is much more complex in humans. The first case of human hepatotoxicity to be reported was that of a polydrug abuser who had sustained a cardiac arrest. In addition to cocaine, his toxicology screen was positive for alcohol and barbiturates, but negative for acetaminophen. Examination of the liver disclosed a zone-1 type injury, with periportal necrosis and sparing of the centrozonal hepatocytes (Perino, Warren & Levine, 1987). A 24-year old with fulminant liver failure was

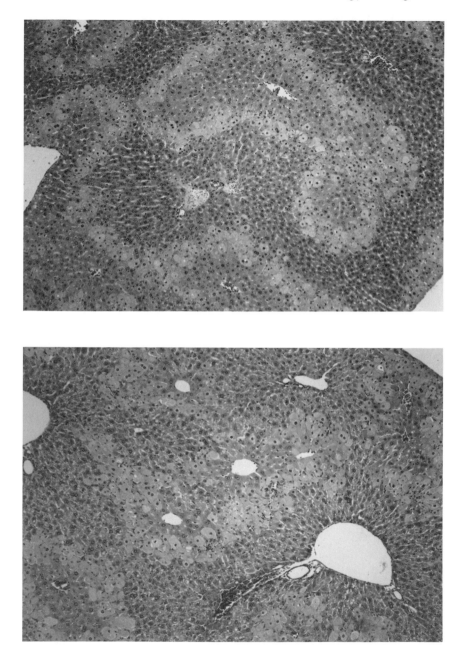

Figure 1.10.4.2 Effects of cocaine and cocaethylene on the rat liver
The microphotograph on top is from a rat treated with cocaine. Photograph on
bottom is from rat treates with cocaethylene; patterns of injury are the same.
Courtesy of Stephen M. Roberts, University of Florida, Center for Environmental
and Human Toxicology.

described in another report. His toxicology was negative for everything but cocaine. Morphologic features included coagulative-type perivenular and midzonal necrosis along with periportal microvesicular fatty change (Kanel, Cassidy, Shuster & Reynolds, 1990). Another report described a group of four patients, two with well-demarcated zone-3 necrosis identical to that seen in cases of acetaminophen poisoning (Wanless, Goponath, Tan et al., 1990). In a controlled autopsy study of cocaine-related deaths, the livers of the cocaine users showed no more sign of hepatotoxicity than did the control group (Copeland, 1989).

Because most cytochrome P450 activity is located in Zone 3, it is not surprising to find that acetaminophen and cocaine cause similar lesions. The difficulty in predicting a pattern of injury in humans is that humans use multiple drugs. The first patient described had used both alcohol and barbiturates. Both of these agents are capable of inducing the P450 system. Until more cases of liver injury have been reported, it would be unwise to consider any pattern of hepatic injury as diagnostic for cocaine toxicity. Conceivably a patient could develop hepatic failure secondary to acetaminophen ingestion and incidentally test positive for cocaine metabolism. The presence of zone-3 lesions would not then be proof of cocaine toxicity. Finally, in animals at least, there is also evidence for cocaine-induced lipid peroxidation and hepatic damage. The likelihood of hepatic injury is increased by concurrent retroviral infection (Odeleye, Lopez, Smith et al. 1992). If this alteration also occurs in humans, than the incidence of liver disorders in drug users should rise as HIV infection becomes more widespread.

An additional possibility to be considered is that hepatic injury could be secondary to cocaethylene production. This compound is produced in the liver, by transesterification, but only in the presence of ethanol (Hearn, Flynn, Hime et al., 1991). In animal experiments, cocaethylene is nearly as toxic as cocaine itself. When cocaethylene is given to mice it produces dose-dependent hepatic zone 2 (midlobular) necrosis. Pretreatment with cytochrome P450 inducers makes the necrosis worse and shifts the zone of necrosis to zone 1 in the periphery. Treatment with inhibitors such as cemitidine reduces toxicity. This is essentially the same pattern seen in mice given cocaine, suggesting that both cocaine and cocaethylene share common mechanisms of toxicity (Roberts, Roth, Harbison, James 1992) (Roth, Harbison, James et al 1992). In vivo studies are lacking, but the cytotoxic effects of cocaine on isolated human hepatocytes have been evaluated (Ponsoda, Jover, Castell & Gómez-Lechón, 1992). In this system, even low levels of cocaine cause decreases in the ability to synthesize urea, and in hepatic glycogen and glutathione content. In the presence of alcohol the cytotoxic effects become more pronounced.

References

Abramson, D., Gertler, J., Lewis, T. et al. (1992). Crack and gastroduodenal perforation. Gastroenterology, 102:1431–1438.

Copeland, A. (1989). The microscopic pathology of the liver in fatal cocaine intoxication. J Forensic Sci, 29, 185–189.

Endress, C. & King, G. (1990). Cocaine-induced small-bowel perforation. Am J Radiol, 154, 1346–1347.

Endress, C., Gray, D., Wollschlaeger, G. (1992). Bowel ischemia and perforation after cocaine use. Am J Roen, 159:73–75.

Evans, MA. (1983). Role of protein binding in cocaine-induced hepatic necrosis. J Pharmacol Exp Ther, 224, 73–79.

Evans, M. & Harbison, R. (1978). Cocaine-induced hepatotoxicity in mice. Toxicol Appl Pharmacol, 45, 739–754.

Fishel, R., Hamamoto, G., Barbul, A. et al. (1985). Cocaine colitis: is this a new syndrome? Dis Colon Rectum, 28, 264–266.

Freudenberger, R. S.,Cappell, M. S. & Hutt, D. A. (1990). Intestinal infarction after intravenous cocaine administration. Ann Intern Med, 113(9), 715–716.

Galgaini, J., Proescher, F., Dock, W. & Tainter, M. (1939). Local and systemic effects from inhalation of strong solutions of epinephrine. JAMA, 112, 1929–1933.

Garfia, A., Valverde, J., Borondo, J. et al. (1990). Vascular lesions in intestinal ischemia induced by cocaine-alcohol abuse: report of a fatal case due to overdose. J Forensic Sci, 35(3), 740–745.

Hall, T., Zaninovic, A., Lewis, D. et al (1992). Neonatal intestinal ischemia with bowel perforation: an in utero complication of maternal cocaine abuse. Am J Roent, 150(6):1303–1304.

Hearn, W. L., Flynn, D. D., Hime et al (1991). Cocaethylene - a unique cocaine metabolite displays high affinity for the dopamine transporter. J Neurochem, 56(2), 698–701.

Kanel, G., Cassidy, W., Shuster, L. & Reynolds, B. (1990). Cocaine-induced liver cell injury: comparison of morphological features in man and experimental models. Hepatology, 11, 646–651.

Khafagi, F., Lloyd, H. & Gough, I. (1987). Intestinal pseudo-obstruction in pheochromocytoma. Aust N Z J Med, 17 (2), 246–248.

Kloss, M., Rosen, G. & Rauckman, E. (1984). Cocaine-mediated hepatotoxicity: a critical review. Biochem Pharmacol, 33, 169–173.

Kothur, R., Marsh, F. & Posner, G (1991). Liver function tests in nonparenteral cocaine users. Arch Intern med, 151, 1126–1128.

Lee, H., LaMaute, H., Pizzi, W. et al. (1990). Acute gastroduodenal perforations associated with use of crack. Ann Surg, 211(1), 15–17.

León-Velarde, F., Huicho, L. and C. Monge. (1991). Effects of cocaine on oxygen consumption and mitochondrial respiration in normoxic and hypoxic mice. Life Sci, 50:213–218.

Marks, V. & Chapple, P. (1967). Hepatic dysfunction in heroin and cocaine users. Br J Addict, 62, 189–195.

Mizrahi, S., Laor, D. & Stamler, B. (1988). Intestinal ischemia induced by cocaine abuse. Arch Surg, 123, 394.

Nalbandian, H., Sheth, N., Dietrich, R. & Georgiou, J. (1985). Intestinal ischemia caused by cocaine ingestion: report of two cases. Surgery, 97(3), 374–376.

Nathan, L. & Hernandez, E. (1990). Intravenous substance abuse and a presacral mass. JAMA, 263(11), 1496.

Odeyleye, O., Lopez, M., Smith, B. et al. (1992). Cocaine hepatotoxicity during protein undernutrition of retrovirally infected mice. Can J Physiol Pharmacol, 70:338–343.

Perino, L., Warren, G. & Levine, J. (1987). Cocaine-induced hepatotoxicity in humans. Gastroenterology, 93, 176–180.

Ponsoda, X., Jover, R., Castell, J. & Gómez-Lechón, P. (1992). Potentiation of cocaine hepatotoxicity in human hepatocytes by ethanol. Toxic in Vitro, 6(2) 155–158.

Radin, D. (1992). Cocaine-induced hepatic necrosis: CT demonstration. J Comp Assist Tomography 16(1) 155–156.

Rauckman, E., Rosen, G. & Cavagnaro, J. (1982). Norcocaine nitroxide: a potential hepatotoxic metabolite of cocaine. Mol Pharmacol, 21, 458–463.

Riggs, D. and Weibley,R. (1991). Acute hemorrhagic diarrhea and cardiovascular collapse in a young child owing to environmentally acquired cocaine. Ped Emerg Care, 7(3) 154–155.

Rippetoe, L., Phillips, R. & Lange, W. (1991). No association between IV cocaine use and liver toxicity. In L. Harris (ed.) Committee for Problems of Drug Dependency, Annual Conference. Published in National Institute on Drug Abuse Monograph Series, in press.

Roberts, S., Roth, L., Harbison, R., James, R. (1992). Cocaethylene hepatotoxicity in mice. Biochem Pharmacol, 43:1989–1995.

Roth, L., Harbison, R., James R. et al (1992). Cocaine hepatotoxicity: influence of hepatic enzyme inducing and inhibiting agents on the site of necrosis. Hepatology, 15:934–940.

Shuster, L., Quimby, F., Bates, A. & Thompson, M. (1977). Liver damage from cocaine in mice. Life Sci, 20, 1035–1041.

Shuster, L., Casey, E. & Welankiwar, S. (1983). Metabolism of cocaine and norcocaine to N-hydroxynorcocaine. Biochem Pharmacol, 32, 3045–3051.

Szakacs, J., Dimmette, R. & Cowart, E. (1959). Pathologic implications of catecholamines epinephrine and norepinephrine. US Armed Forces Med J, 10, 908–925.

Tabasco-minguillan, J., Novick, D. & Kreek, M. (1990). Liver function tests in non-parenteral cocaine users. Drug Alcohol Depen, 26(2), 169–174.

Wanless, I., Goponath, D., Tan, J. et al. (1990). Histopathology of cocaine hepatotoxicity: report of four patients. Gastroenterology, 98(2), 497–501.

Yang, R. D., Han, M. W. & Mccarthy, J. H. (1991). Ischemic colitis in a crack abuser. Dig Dis Sci, 36(2), 238–240.

1.10.5 Neurologic Disorders

Reports of neurologic complications were published almost as soon as purified cocaine became widely available. The first cocaine-related stroke was described in 1886 (Catlett, 1886). Today, neurologic complaints are the most common manifestation of cocaine toxicity, at least in patients going to the emergency room (Derlet & Albertson,

1989). During the late 1980's, stroke reemerged as a significant medical problem, and in patients less than 35 years of age, drug abuse is the most commonly identified predisposing condition for stroke (Kaku, 1990) (Feldmann, 1991). The incidence of stroke in this age group is increasing, but very little is known about the pathology of cocaine related stroke, or, for that matter, the pathology of any other cocaine-related neurologic disorders. There are, nonetheless, clinical features of cocaine--related stroke that clearly separate it from cases where drug abuse is not a factor. Similarly, the clinical features of cocaine-associated psychiatric disorders, especially psychosis, appear to be different from those seen in true schizophrenia and different also from the pattern seen in amphetamine abusers. Another important feature which differentiates cocaine from amphetamine abuse is that neurotoxicity produced by some amphetamines, as evidenced by chemical measurements and morphologic observations, does not occur in conjunction with cocaine abuse (Yeh & Desouza, 1991).

1.10.5.1 Psychiatric syndromes

Cocaine-induced paranoid psychosis was recognized by the early workers in the field. Magnon (Saury, 1890), Maier (Maier, 1926), and Lewin (Lewin, 1931) all wrote on the topic and took pains to distinguish the cocaine psychosis from symptoms induced by alcohol and other drugs. More recent studies (Siegel, 1978) (Gawin, 1986) have tended to confirm the earlier observations. Transient or "binge" paranoia is common among heavy users. In one study the incidence was nearly 70% (Satel & Gawin, 1990). What distinguishes the cocaine-associated syndrome from the syndrome induced by amphetamines is that the paranoia occurs only for a very brief period. The development of paranoia in this group of abusers is unpredictable, and is not dose related. Some individuals appear to be more vulnerable, but why that should be is unclear. Cerebral glucose metabolism, as accessed by (18F)-fluorodeoxy-glucose positron tomography of cocaine abusers in early withdrawal, increases. This increase in glucose metabolism involves all areas of the brain but is particularly noticeable in the basal ganglia and orbitofrontal cortex. The increase in the latter two areas correlates with clinical measures of cocaine craving, and is consistent with the notion that the changes are due to changes in brain dopamine activity (Volkow, Fowler et al., 1991).

1.10.5.2 Cerebral infarction

In the non-drug using population, strokes are most often secondary to cerebral infarction. The principal causes of infarction are arterial thrombus formation, embolism, spasm, and circulatory compromise with secondary cerebral hypoperfusion. In non-drug related cases, hemorrhage is the etiology only fifteen percent of the time (subarachnoid 10%, intracerebral 5%). An occasional case may involve a child or young adult, but stroke has always been thought of as a disease affecting the elderly. In the past, over 80% of cases occurred in individuals over 65 years old (Adams, Corsellis & Duchen, 1984). As cocaine abuse has become more common, both the age distribution and the underlying etiology of stroke appear to have changed. Case reports, and there are now over 100, are almost equally divided between hemorrhage and infarction, and most of the affected individuals have been in their mid 30's.

There was a 100-year hiatus between the first reports of stroke in the 1880's, and Brust's report in 1977 (Brust & Richter, 1977), but now case reports appear with great frequency. Even the more exotic syndromes, such as thalamencephalic infarcts (Rowley, Lowenstein & Rowbotham, 1990), lateral medullary syndrome (Mody, Miller, McIntyre et al., 1988), anterior spinal syndrome (Mody et al., 1988), embolization from a left atrial thrombus (Petty, Brust, Tatemichi & Barr, 1990), retinal infarction (Devenyi, Schneiderman, Devenyi & Lawby, 1988), and massive cerebellar infarcts (Aggarawal & Byrne, 1991) have all been described. There are multiple reports of simple infarction (Golbe & Merkin, 1986) (Levine, Washington, Jefferson & al., 1987) (Levine & Welch, 1988) (Jacobs, Roszler, Kelly et al., 1989) (Klonoff, Andrews & Obana, 1989) (Engstrand, Daras, Tuchman et al., 1989) (Moore & Peterson, 1989) (Chasnoff, Bussey, Savich & Stack, 1986) (Rowbotham, 1988) (Seaman, 1990) (Daras, Tuchman & Marks 1991) (Kelly, Gorelick & Mirza, 1992).

Except for one instance of biopsy proven vasculitis (Krendel, Ditter, Frankel & Ross, 1990), and one case of apparent embolism (Petty et al., 1990), the etiology of most cocaine-associated strokes is obscure. Autopsy reports of infarction are rare (Klonoff et al., 1989) and the results unrevealing. Angiography has been equally unrewarding. The absence of hard data allows ample room for speculation. Pharmacologically induced vasospasm, resulting either from some direct action exerted by cocaine on cerebral blood vessels, or secondary to catechol elevation, is frequently suggested (Levine et al., 1987), however there is very little information to substantiate either contention, and a number of other mechanisms are possible. Increased platelet responsiveness has been proposed as a possible etiology, but has only been demonstrated in vitro, and not in the setting of cerebral infarction (Levine et al., 1987).

Another promising line of research involves the effects of cocaine metabolites on the cerebral vasculature. Cocaine directly applied to cat pial arterioles causes vasodilation, and this action can be prevented with ß blockade (Dohi, Jones, Hudak & Traystman, 1990), but other experiments with cat cerebral arteries have show up to 50% decreases in average cross-sectional area when arteries are perfused with benzoylecgonine (10-5M) (Madden & Powers, 1990). If benzoylecgonine also causes cerebral vasoconstriction in man, then it would explain why patients frequently present with symptoms some time after they have last used the drug. The elimination half-life of cocaine itself is less than one hour, but the half-life for benzoylecgonine is closer to seven hours, and benzoylecgonine can be detected in the brain for days after cocaine was last used. If benzoylecgonine is vasoactive, that would also explain why cocaine users have demonstrable reductions in cerebral flow for days after their last drug use (Volkow, Mullani, Gould, Adler & Krajewski, 1988). Nor is benzoylecgonine the only metabolite that might be implicated. Cocaethylene is nearly as toxic as cocaine itself, but its half-life is quite a bit longer than cocaine's, and it might still be present when cocaine itself isn't detectable.

Of the usual risk factors associated with cerebral infarction, the most likely seems to be cerebral hypoperfusion. Cocaine causes both acute and chronic alterations in cerebral blood flow (CBF). Flow studies with single photon emission computed tomography (SPECT) have shown mild reductions in flow and, frequently, multiple small superficial cortical areas of hypoperfusion. Frontal lobe hypoperfusion is also common (Mena, Giombetti, Moody et al., 1990) (Volkow et al., 1988). Thus cocaine users may be subject to decreased cerebral flow, even in the face of a normal cardiac output. Although atherosclerotic lesions are uncommon among individuals in their mid-thirties, some have argued that cocaine leads to accelerated atherogenesis (Dressler, Malekzadeh & Roberts, 1990) (Kolodgie, Virmani, Cornhill et al., 1990; Kolodgie, Virmani, Cornhill et al., 1991). If cardiac output is reduced, blood pressure fluctuations could also lead to infarction, especially in the face of preexisting atherosclerotic lesions. Cocaine associated cardiomyopathy (Duell, 1987) (Wiener, Lockhart & Schwartz, 1986) (Chokshi, Moore, Pandian & Isner, 1989) (Karch & Billingham, 1988) and arrhythmias (Young & Glauber, 1947) (Boag & Havard, 1985) (Crumb, Clarkson, Xu & Kadowitz, 1989; Crumb, Kadowitz, You-Qoi & Clarkson, 1990) (Duke, 1986) (Neely, Urthaler & Walker, 1989) (Ruben & Morris, 1952) (Temesy-Armos, Fraker & Wilkerson, 1989) (Williams, 1990) (Lathers, Tyau, Spino & Agarwal, 1988) are both recognized occurrences and either could result in sudden blood pressure fluctuations. A sudden drop in blood pressure, combined with asymptomatic stenotic lesions, could lead to infarction. One recent report described a woman with cardiomyopathy (presumably cocaine related) who sustained a cerebral embolism (Petty et al., 1990). The situation is somewhat analogous to cocaine-associated myocardial infarction. The presence of preexisting lesions may exacerbate transient flow decreases which would have otherwise been asymptomatic.

1.10.5.3 Cerebral vasculitis

The frequency with which cerebral vasculitis causes stroke in cocaine users is unclear. The process has been documented only in two patients. A biopsy from one patient showed small vessels within an area of infarction with transmural infiltration by both acute and chronic inflammatory cells. Occasional multinucleated giant cells were also present. In the other case there was also lymphocytic infiltration of the small vessel walls with multiple cystic, necrotic and gliotic areas in the cerebral white matter, especially in the frontal lobes. Multinucleated giant cells were seen in the gliotic areas. The process was most intense in the frontal lobes (Krendel et al., 1990). Data is scanty, but if cocaine does cause vascular inflammation, then it probably does so by virtue of some direct toxic effect, unrelated to catechol toxicity. Patients with pheochromocytoma and animals treated with exogenous catecholamines have no signs of CNS inflammation. Small perivascular hemorrhages can be induced in animals by giving large amounts of epinephrine (Stief & Tokay, 1935), but cerebral vessel wall necrosis and infiltrates do not occur.

Necrotizing anigiitis, a form of periarteritis nodosa associated with the abuse of amphetamine and other stimulant drugs (Citron, Halpern, McCarron et al., 1970) (Kessler, Jortner & Adapon, 1978) (Bostwick, 1981) has never been seen in cocaine users, except insofar as they used cocaine along with intravenous amphetamines and heroin. This disorder was first described in the early 1970's, but its incidence seems to have steadily declined over the last 20 years. The fact that this disorder has essentially disappeared, while intravenous amphetamine abuse has not, suggests that the disorder may have been due to a contaminant that had been introduced into the amphetamine during the course of manufacture and/or distribution. Quality control is nonexistent in illicit labs, and the potential for introducing agents with novel sorts of toxicity is quite real.

1.10.5.4 Subarachnoid and intraventricular hemorrhage

About half the strokes associated with cocaine abuse are due to either intracerebral (Lehman, 1987) (Green, Kelly, Gabrielson et al., 1990) (Mercado, Johnson, Calver & Sokol, 1989) (Nolte & Gleman, 1989) (Caplan, Hier & Banks, 1982) (Lichtenfeld, Rubin & Feldman, 1984) (Schwartz & Cohen, 1984) (Wojak & Flamm, 1987) (Lowenstein, Massa, Rowbotham, Collins et al, 1987) (Mody et al, 1988) (Tardiff, Gross, Wu et al, 1989) (Mittleman & Wetli, 1987) (Jacobs et al., 1989) (Rowley et al., 1990) (Klonoff et al., 1989) (Green et al., 1990) or subarachnoid hemorrhage (Lundberg, Garriott, Reynolds, Carvey & Shaw, 1977) (Chynn, 1975) (Levine & Welch, 1988) (Lichtenfeld et al., 1984) (Schwartz & Cohen, 1984) (Rogers, Henry, Jones et al., 1986) (Cregler & Mark, 1987) (Wojak & Flamm, 1987) (Lowenstein et al., 1987) (Altes-Capella, Cabezudo-Artero & Forteza-Rei, 1987) (Tardiff et al., 1989) (Mittleman & Wetli, 1987) (Jacobs et al., 1989) (Klonoff et al., 1989). Subarachnoid hemorrhage is more common than intracerebral hemorrhage by a ratio of 4:3.

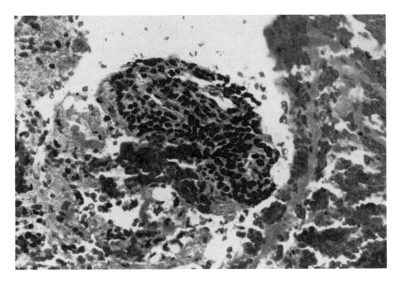

Figure 1.10.5.3 (1) Cerebral vasculitis in a cocaine user
Biopsy specimen from patient surviving episode of vasculitis. Transmural infiltration of a small cortical vessel. Both acute and chronic inflammatory cells are present. Original magnification 800x. Courtesy of Dr. David A. Krendel, Section of Neurology, The Emory Clinic.

As is the case with cocaine related infarction, individuals are in their mid-thirties. Most (80%) subarachnoid hemorrhages have been related to the presence of angiographically proven saccular aneurysms. Of the 22 cases reported to date, nine involved the anterior communicating artery, six were in the posterior communicating system and the remainder scattered through out the cerebral circulation. Underlying lesions were found in only half the reported intracerebral hemorrhages. Most often the cause was an underlying arteriovenous malformation. The other half of this group had no demonstrable underlying lesions and there was a propensity to bleed into the basal ganglia and thalamus (Green et al., 1990).

Bleeding at these sites is often from small saccular aneurysms. Saccular aneurysms involving the arteries at the base of the brain occur in 1–2% of the adult population, and are often found incidentally at autopsy. Usually they are located at arterial bifurcations. They form as a result of multiple factors, including atheroma and degenerative changes, and secondary flow abnormalities (Sekhar & Heros, 1980). The role of hypertension in the formation and rupture of saccular aneurysms is still unclear (Graham, 1989). The role of hypertension in cocaine-associated subarachnoid bleed, though frequently assumed, has not been established.

Intracerebral hemorrhage is usually due to hypertension, although in some series the number of cases due to vascular malfor-

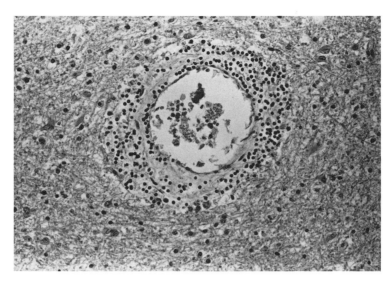

Figure 1.10.5.3. 2 Cerebral vasculitis in a cocaine user
Autopsy specimen from another patient with cerebral vasculitis. Illustration
shows a lymphocytic infiltrate around a small cerebral vessel. Original magnification 800x. Courtesy of Dr. David A. Krendel, Section of Neurology, The Emory
Clinic.

mation roughly equals the number due to hypertension (Gras et al.,
1991). By far the most common site for hypertensive hemorrhage is the
basal ganglia, outnumbering the second most common site, the cerebral
white matter, by a ratio of 7:1 (Adams et al., 1984). Hemorrhage in the
white matter is usually a result of amyloid angiopathy, and probably has
little do with hypertension. Hemorrhage in the basal ganglia is
classically associated with microaneurysm formation and atherosclerosis
in the small basal perforating arteries. Microaneurysms have not been
observed in cocaine users or experimental animals. It also seems unlikely
that the intermittent, transient elevations of blood pressure associated
with cocaine use could produce typical hypertensive changes in the cerebral vasculature. On the other hand, it is reasonable to suppose that
transient elevations could lead to the rupture of preexisting malformations, or bleeding into a tumor (Yapor & Guiterrez, 1992), and that
process no doubt accounts for much of the reported pathology.
Hemorrhage in individuals without underlying lesions remains
unexplained.

1.10.5.5 Seizures

Seizures in cocaine users may be a consequence of stroke or
intracerebral hemorrhage, or even of massive overdose. They may also
be a manifestation of a preexisting seizure disorder that was exacerbated

by cocaine use. Various series have placed the incidence of this complication at somewhere between 2 and 10% (Lowenstein et al. 1987) (Derlet and Albertson, 1989). In one series of nearly 1,000 patients with acute medical complications of cocaine use, seizures were noted in nearly 10 per cent. Only 4 of these patients had status epilepticus, and all of them were victims of massive overdose (Dhuna et al. 1991). Interestingly, seizures were three times as common in women as in men (18.4% vs 6.2%). This finding is consistent with the results of other studies that suggest pregnancy and other hormonal alterations can exacerbate cocaine toxicity (Plessinger and Woods, 1990) (Sharma et al., 1991).

"Kindling" is a term used to describe the eventual development of generalized convulsions in response to repeated subconvulsive brain stimuli in animals. Whether this process also occurs in humans has been debated for some time, particularly in cases where cocaine is involved, because cocaine-induced kindling has been demonstrated in animals. It has been speculated, but without proof, that kindling, or some similar process, is the mechanism responsible for seizures in chronic cocaine abusers. The fact that kindling does occur in humans is suggested by one well-described case of a 37-year-old woman who initially experienced generalized tonic-clonic seizures immediately after smoking crack, but who went on to develop generalized seizures even when she was not using the cocaine (Dhuna et al. 1991).

References

Adams, J., Corsellis, J. & Duchen, L. (Ed.). (1984). Greenfield's Neuropathology (4th ed.) London: Edward Arnold.

Aggarwal, S and B Byrne. (1991). Massive ischemic cerebellar infarction due to cocaine use. Neuroradiology, 33:449–450.

Altes-Capella, J., Cabezudo-Artero, J. & Forteza-Rei, J. (1987). Complications of cocaine abuse. Ann Intern Med, 107, 940–941.

Boag, F. & Havard, C. (1985). Cardiac arrhythmia and myocardial ischaemia related to cocaine and alcohol consumption. Post Grad Med J, 61, 997–999.

Bostwick, D. (1981). Amphetamine induced cerebral vasculitis. Hum Pathol, 12, 1031–1033.

Brust, J. & Richter, R. (1977). Stroke associated with cocaine abuse? NY State J Med, 77, 1473–1475.

Caplan, L., Hier, D. & Banks, G. (1982). Current concepts of cerebrovascular disease-stroke: stroke and drug abuse. Stroke, 13 (6), 869–872.

Catlett, G. (1886). Cocaine: what was its influence in the following case. Medical Gazette (February 6), 166.

Chasnoff, I., Bussey, M., Savich, R. & Stack, C. (1986). Perinatal cerebral infarction and maternal cocaine use. J Pediatrics, 108, 456–459.

Chynn, K.C. (1975). Acute subarachnoid hemorrhage. JAMA, 233, 55–56.

Chokshi, S., Moore, R., Pandian, N. & Isner, J. (1989). Reversible cardiomyopathy associated with cocaine intoxication. Ann Intern Med, 111, 1039–1040.

Citron, B., Halpern, M., McCarron, M. et al., (1970). Necrotizing angiitis associated with drug abuse. N Engl J Med, 283, 1003–1011.

Cregler, L. & Mark, H. (1987). Relation of stroke to cocaine abuse. N Y State J Med, 87, 128–129.

Crumb, W., Clarkson, C., Xu, Y. & Kadowitz, P. (1989). Electrocardiographic evidence for cocaine cardiotoxicity in cats. Circulation, 80(4), II–132.

Crumb, W., Kadowitz, P., You-Qui, X. & Clarkson, C. (1990). Electrocardiographic evidence for cocaine cardiotoxicity in the cat. Canadian J Physiol and Pharmacol, 68(5), 622–625.

Daras, M., Tuchman, A., Marks, S. (1991). Central nervous system infarction related to cocaine abuse. Stroke, 22 (10) 1320–1325.

Derlet, R. & Albertson, T. (1989). Emergency department presentation of cocaine intoxication. Ann Emerg Med, 18(2), 182–186.

Devenyi, P., Schneiderman, J., Devenyi, R. & Lawby, L. (1988). Cocaine induced central retinal artery occlusion. Canad Med Assn J, 138, 129–130.

Dhuna, A., Pascual-Leone, A., and F. Langendorf (1991). Chronic, habitual cocaine abuse and kindling-induced epilepsy: a case report.

Dohi, S., Jones, M. D., Hudak, M. L. & Traystman, R. J. (1990). Effects of cocaine on pial arterioles in cats. Stroke, 21(12), 1710–1714.

Dhuna, A, Pascual-Leonem Am Langendorf, F. and Anderson, C. (1991). Epileptogenic properties of cocaine in humans. Neurotoxicology, 12:621–626.

Dressler, F., Malekzadeh, S. & Roberts, W. (1990). Quantitative analysis of amounts of coronary arterial narrowing in cocaine addicts. Am J Cardiol, 65(5), 303–308.

Duell, P. (1987). Chronic cocaine abuse and dilated cardiomyopathy. Am J Med, 83, 601.

Duke, M. (1986). Cocaine, myocardial infarction and arrhythmias - a review. Conn Med, 50, 440–442.

Engstrand, B., Daras, M., Tuchman, A. et al. (1989). Cocaine-related ischemic strokes. Neurology, 39 Suppl 1, 186.

Feldmann, E. (1991). Intracerebral hemorrhage (Reprinted from Current Concepts of Cerebrovascular Disease and Stroke, Vol 25, Pg 31–35, 1990). Stroke, 22(5), 684–691.

Gawin, FH, Kleber, HD. (1986). Abstinence symptomology and psychiatric diagnosis in cocaine abusers. Arch Gen Psychiatry, 43:107–113.

Golbe, L. & Merkin, M. (1986). Cerebral infarction in a user of free-base cocaine ("crack"). Neurology, 36, 1602–1604.

Graham, F. (1989). Morphologic changes during hypertension. Am J Cardiol, 63, 6C–9C.

Gras, P, Arveux, P., Giroude, M. et al. (1991). Les Hémorrhagies intracérébrales spontanées du sujet jeune. Rev Neurol (Paris), 147(10) 653–657.

Green, R., Kelly, K.,Gabrielson, T. et al. (1990). Multiple intracerebral hemorrhages after smoking "crack" cocaine. Stroke, 21, 957–962.

Jacobs, I., Roszler, M., Kelly et al. (1989). Cocaine abuse: neurovascular complications. Radiology, 170, 223–227.

Kaku, D.A. & Lowenstein, D.H. (1990). Emergence of recreational drug abuse as a major risk factor for stroke in young adults. Ann Intern Med, 113 (11),821–827.

Karch, S. & Billingham, M. (1988). The pathology and etiology of cocaineinduced heart disease. Arch Pathol Lab Med, 112, 225–230.

Kelly, M., Gorelick, P., Mirza (1992). The role of drugs in the etiology of stroke. Clin Neuropharmacol, 15:249–275.

Kessler, J., Jortner, B. & Adapon, B. (1978). Cerebral vasculitis in a drug abuser. J Clin Psych, 39, 559–564.

Klonoff, D., Andrews, B. & Obana, W. (1989). Stroke associated with cocaine use. Arch Neurol, 46, 989–993.

Kolodgie, F., Virmani, R., Cornhill, JF. et al. (1990). Cocaine: an independent risk factor of atherosclerosis. Circulation, 82, Supplement III(4), III-447.

Kolodgie, F. D., Virmani, R., Cornhill, J. F.,et al (1991). Increase in atherosclerosis and adventitial mast cells in cocaine abusers - an alternative mechanism of cocaine-associated coronary vasospasm and thrombosis. J Am Coll Cardiol, 17(7), 1553–1560.

Krendel, D. A., Ditter, S. M., Frankel, M. R. & Ross, W. K. (1990). Biopsyproven cerebral vasculitis associated with cocaine abuse. Neurolog, 40(7), 1092–1094.

Lathers, C., Tyau, L., Spino, M. & Agarwal, I. (1988). Cocaine-induced seizures, arrhythmias and sudden death. J Clin Pharmacol, 28, 584–593.

Lehman, L. (1987). Intracerebral hemorrhage after intranasal cocaine use. Hosp Physician, July, 69–70.

Levine, S., Washington, J., Jefferson, M. et al. (1987). "Crack" cocaine associated stroke. Neurology, 37, 1849–1853.

Levine, S. & Welch, K. (1988). Cocaine and Stroke. Stroke, 19(6), 779–783.

Lewin, L. (1931). Phantastica: narcotic and stimulating drugs, their use and abuse (P.H.Wirth, Ph.C, B.Sc., Trans.). (Second English edition ed.). New York: E.P. Dutton & Company.

Lichtenfeld, P., Rubin, D. & Feldman, R. (1984). Subarachnoid hemorrhage precipitated by cocaine snorting. Arch Neurol, 41, 223–224.

Lowenstein, D., Massa, S., Rowbotham et al.(1987). Acute neurologic and psychiatric complications associated with cocaine abuse. Am J Med, 83, 841–846.

Lundberg, G., Garriott, J., Reynolds, P.,et al (1977). Cocaine-related death. J Forensic Sci, 22, 402–408.

Madden, J. & Powers, R. (1990). Effect of cocaine and cocaine metabolites on cerebral arteries in vitro. Life Sciences, 47(13), 1109–1114.

Maier, H. W. (1926). Der Kokainismus (O.J. Kalant from the German 1926 edition, Trans.). Toronto: Addiction Research Foundation.

Mena, I., Giombetti, R., Mody, C. et al. (1990). Acute cerebral blood flow changes with cocaine intoxication. Neurology, 40, Suppl 1, 179.

Mercado, A., Johnson, G., Calver, D. & Sokol, R. (1989). Cocaine, pregnancy and postpartum intracerebral hemorrhage. Obst and Gynecol, 73(3), 467–468.

Mittleman, R. & Wetli, C. (1987). Cocaine and sudden "natural" death. J Forensic Sci, 32(1), 11–19.

Mody, C., Miller, B., McIntyre, H. et al. (1988). Neurologic complications of cocaine abuse. Neurology, 38, 1189–1193.

Moore, P. & Peterson, P. (1989). Nonhemorrhagic cerebrovascular complications of cocaine abuse. Neurology, 39, Suppl 1, 302.

Neely, B., Urthaler, F. & Walker, A. (1989). Cocaine enhances spontaneous SR calcium release in length-clamped ferret papillary muscles. Circulation, 80(4), II–16.

Nolte, K. & Gelman, B. (1989). Intracerebral hemorrhage associated with cocaine abuse. Arch Pathol Lab Med, 113, 812–813.

Petty, G. W., Brust, J. C. M., Tatemichi, T. K. & Barr, M. L. (1990). Embolic stroke after smoking 'crack' cocaine. Stroke, 21(11), 1632–1635.

Plessinger, MA and Woods, J. (1989). Progesterone increases cardiovascular toxicity to cocaine in nonpregnant ewes. Am J Obstet Gynecol, 163(5), 1659–1664.

Rogers, J., Henry, T., Jones, A. et al. (1986). Cocaine-related deaths in Pima County, Arizona, 1982-1984. J Forensic Sci, 31(2), 1404–1408.

Rowbotham, M., Root, RK, Boushey, HA, Warnock, DG, Smith, LH, (1988). Neurologic aspects of cocaine abuse. West J Med, 149, 442–448.

Rowley, H., Lowenstein, D. & Rowbotham, M. (1990). Thalmomesencephalic strokes after cocaine abuse. Neurology, 39, 428–430.

Ruben, H. & Morris, M. (1952). Effect of cocaine on cardiac automaticity in the dog. J Pharm Exp Ther, 55–64.

Satel, S. & Gawin, F. (1990). Seasonal cocaine abuse. Am J Psychiatry, 146(4), 534–535.

Schwartz, K. & Cohen, J. (1984). Subarachnoid hemorrhage precipitated by cocaine snorting. Arch Neurol, 41, 705.

Seaman, M. (1990). Acute cocaine abuse associated with cerebral infarction. Ann Emerg Med, 19(1), 34–37.

Sekhar, L. & Heros, R. (1980). Origin, growth and rupture of saccular aneurysms: a review. Neurosurgery, 8 (2), 248–260.

Sharma, A. Plessinger, M., Sherer, D. et al. (1992) Pregnancy enhances cardiotoxicity of cocaine - role of progesterone. Toxicol Appl Pharmacol, 113 (1):30–35.

Siegel, R. (1978). Cocaine hallucinations. Am J Psychiatry, 135:309-314.

Stief, A. & Tokay, L. (1935). Further contributions to histopathology of experimental adrenalin intoxication. J Nerv and Ment Dis, 81, 633–648.

Tardiff, K., Gross, E., Wu, J. et al. (1989). Analysis of cocaine-positive fatalities. J Forensic Sci, 34(1), 53–62.

Temesy-Armos, P., Fraker, T. & Wilkerson, R. (1989). Cocaine causes delayed cardiac arrhythmias in conscious dogs. Circulation, 80(4), II-132.

Volkow, N., Mullani, N., Gould, K. et al. (1988). Cerebral blood flow in chronic cocaine users: a study with positron emission tomography. Br J Psych, 152, 641–648.

Volkow, N. D., Fowler, J. S., Wolf et al. (1991). Changes in brain glucose metabolism in cocaine dependence and withdrawal. Am J Psychiatry, 148(5), 621–626.

Wiener, R., Lockhart, J. & Schwartz, R. (1986). Dilated cardiomyopathy and cocaine abuse: report of two cases. Am J Med, 81, 699–701.

Williams, S. (1990). A FASEB sampler: cocaine's harmful effects. Science, 248, 166.

Wojak, J. & Flamm, E. (1987). Intracranial hemorrhage and cocaine use. Stroke, 18, 712–715.

Yapor, W. and F. Gutierrez. (1992). Cocaine-induced intratumoral hemorrhage: case report and review of the literature. Neurosurgery, 30(2) 288–291.

Yeh, S. Y. & De Souza, E. B. (1991). Lack of neurochemical evidence for neurotoxic effects of repeated cocaine administration in rats on brain monoamine neurons. Drug Alcohol Depend, 27(1), 51–61.

Young, D. & Glauber, J. (1947). Electrocardiographic changes resulting from acute cocaine intoxication. Am Heart J, 34, 272–279.

1.10.6 RENAL DISEASE

Infarction (Sharff, 1984), thrombosis (Wohlman, 1987) and even hemolytic-uremic syndrome (Tumlin, Sands & Someren, 1990) have been reported as complications of cocaine use, however the most common renal problem in cocaine users is rhabdomyolysis and acute tubular necrosis. Rhabdomyolysis was recognized as a complication of both narcotic (Richter, Challenor, Pearson et al., 1971) and stimulant abuse (Kendrick, Hull & Knopchel, 1977) long before the current wave of cocaine popularity. The first case directly related to cocaine was described in 1987 (Merrigan et. al. 1987). The mechanism in cases of narcotic abuse is no better understood than the underlying process by which stimulant drugs produce rhabdomyolysis. In some cases the relationship to prolonged seizure activity is clear, however, seizures have been absent in most of the cocaine-associated cases. In a few instances, pressure-related injury seems to be the most likely explanation (Singhal & Faulkner, 1988). Cocaine-induced vasospasm leading to myocyte necrosis has been proposed as a mechanism (Roth et al., 1988). A common thread in many, but not all cases, is hyperthermia (Campbell, 1988) (Loghmanee & Tobak, 1986) (Lomax & Daniel, 1990) (Menashe & Gottlieb, 1988) (Rosenberg, Pentel, Pond et al., 1986) (Pogue & Nurse, 1989). The histologic changes accompanying the process are uncharacterized. In one study of two cases the skeletal muscle was necrotic, but with no sign of vasculitis. There were no polarizable foreign bodies, and no specific lesions though contraction band necrosis was very prominent in some fibers (Nolte, 1991). Even if a satisfactory explanation for the occurrence of rhabdomyolysis could be found, it would not necessarily explain why some individuals go on to develop renal failure while others do not. It seems likely that some other cofactor besides cocaine use is required before full-blown rhabdomyolysis develops (Enriquez 1991).

The etiology for cocaine-associated tubular necrosis is multifactorial. Hypovolemia, renal arterial vasoconstriction and myoglobinuria all combine to produce the syndrome. In spite of a number of case reports, morphologic alterations in cocaine users have not been characterized. (Anand, Siami & Stone, 1989; Brody, Wrenn, Wilber & Slovis, 1990; Herzlich, Arsura, Pagala & Grob, 1988; Jandreski, Bermes, Leischner & Kahn, 1989; Justiniani, Cabeza & Miller, 1990; Kokko, 1990; Krohn, Slowman-Kovacs & Leapman, 1988; Lombard, Wong & Young, 1988;

Menashe & Gottlieb, 1988; Merigian & Roberts, 1987; Parks, Reed & Knochel, 1989; Reinhart & Stricker, 1988; Roth, Alarcon, Fernandez et al, 1988; Rubin & Neugarten, 1989; Schwartz & McAfee, 1987; Singhal, Horowitz, Quinones et al., 1989; Singhal, Rubin, Peters et al., 1990; TabascoMinguillan, Novick & Kreek, 1990; Welch & Todd, 1990; Welch, Todd & Krause, 1991). These patients could be expected to have the same morphologic changes as anyone else with acute tubular necrosis, with granular reddish or brown myoglobin casts in the distal tubules and collecting ducts. Since histologic studies have been limited to two patients (Nolte 1991), further speculation is pointless.

Renal failure without rhabdomyolysis also occurs (Tumlin et al., 1990). A 28-year old woman with nausea, vomiting and severe abdominal pain developed anuria, hemolytic anemia and thrombocytopenia (known as the HUS or Hemolytic-Uremic syndrome). Renal biopsy showed patchy areas of cortical necrosis, associated with the characteristic changes of thrombotic microangiopathy. Electron microscopy demonstrated extensive detachment of the endothelium from the basement membrane with the accumulation of electron lucent material and red cell debris in the subendothelial area. Catechol toxicity, thromboxane generation and acute hypertensive reactions are well known sequelae of cocaine use, and any or all could lead to HUS syndrome. After the initial endothelial injury intravascular coagulation and the other elements of the HUS syndrome could result.

The focal type of glomerulonephritis associated with heroin related nephrotic syndrome has not been seen in cocaine or stimulant abusers. The presence of such lesions in cocaine abusers should raise the suspicion of HIV infection, since the most common renal lesion in AIDS patients is a similar sort of focal segmental glomerulosclerosis. (Sanders & Marshall, 1989)

Congenital abnormalities of the genitourinary tract have been attributed to intrauterine cocaine exposure (Chavez, Mulinare & Cordero, 1989), but there is little evidence for any increase in congenital defects when the incidence is compared in controlled studies. Tissue studies are not available, but one prospective study using ultrasound evaluated 100 consecutive infants exposed to cocaine in utero and failed to find any consistent teratogenic effect (Rosenstein, Wheeler & Heid, 1990).

References

Anand, V., Siami, G. & Stone, W. (1989). Cocaine-associated rhabdomyolysis and acute renal failure. Souther Med J, 82(1), 67–69.

Brody, S., Wrenn, K., Wilber, M. & Slovis, C. (1990). Predicting the severity of cocaine-associated rhabdomyolysis. Ann Emerg Med, 19(10), 1137–1143.

Campbell, B. (1988). Cocaine abuse with hyperthermia, seizures and fatal complications. Med J Australia, 149(7), 387–389.

Chavez, G., Mulinare, J. & Cordero, J. (1989). Maternal cocaine use during early pregnancy as a risk factor for congenital urogenital anomalies. JAMA, 262(6), 795–798.

Enriquez, R, Palacios, F., González et al. (1991). Skin vasculitis, hypokalemia and acute renal failure in rhabdomyolysis associated with cocaine. Nephron, 59:336–337.

Herzlich, B., Arsura, E., Pagala, M. & Grob, D. (1988). Rhabdomyolysis related to cocaine abuse. Ann Intern Med, 109, 335–336.

Jandreski, M., Bermes, E., Leischner, R. & Kahn, S. (1989). Rhabdomyolysis in a case of free-base cocaine ("crack") overdose. Clin Chem, 35(7), 1547–1549.

Justiniani, F., Cabeza, C. & Miller, B. (1990). Cocaine-associated rhabdomyolysis and hemoptysis mimicking pulmonary embolism. Am J Med, 88, 316–317.

Kendrick, W., Hull, A. & Knochel, J. (1977). Rhabdomyolysis and shock after intravenous amphetamine administration. Ann Int Med, 86, 381–387.

Kokko, J. (1990). Metabolic and social consequences of cocaine use. Am J Med Sci, 299 (6), 361–365.

Krohn, K., Slowman-Kovacs, S. & Leapman, S. (1988). Cocaine and rhabdomyolysis. Ann Intern Med, 108, 639–640.

Loghmanee, F. & Tobak, M. (1986). Fatal malignant hyperthermia associated with recreational cocaine and ethanol use. Am J Forensic Med Pathol, 7, 246–248.

Lomax, P. & Daniel, K. A. (1990). Cocaine and body temperature in the rat - effect of exercise. Pharmacol Biochem Behav, 36(4), 889–892.

Lombard, J., Wong, B. & Young, J. (1988). Acute renal failure due to rhabdomyolysis associated with cocaine toxicity. Western J Med, 148(4), 466–468.

Menashe, P. & Gottlieb, J. (1988). Hyperthermia, rhabdomyolysis and myoglobinuric renal failure after recreational use of cocaine. Southern Med J, 81(3), 379–380.

Merigian, K. & Roberts, J. (1987). Cocaine intoxication: hyperpyrexia, rhabdomyolysis and acute renal failure. J Toxicol Clin Toxicol, 25, 135–148.

Nolte, KB. (1991). Rhabdomyolysis associated with cocaine abuse. Hum Pathol, 22(11) 1141–1145.

Parks, J., Reed, G., and J. Knochel. (1989). Case report: cocaine associated rhabdomyolysis. Am J Med Sci, 297:334–336.

Pogue, V. & Nurse, H. (1989). Cocaine associated-myoglobinuric renal failure. Am J Med, 86, 183–189.

Reinhart, W. & Stricker, H. (1988). Rhabdomyolysis after intravenous cocaine. Am J Med, 85, 579.

Richter, R., Challenor, Y., Pearson, J. et al. (1971). Acute myoglobinuria associated with heroin addiction. JAMA, 216, 1172–1176.

Rosenberg, J. ,Pentel, P., Pond, S. et al. (1986). Hyperthermia associated with drug intoxication. Crit Care Med, 14(11), 964–969.

Rosenstein, B., Wheeler, J. & Heid, P. (1990). Congenital renal abnormalities in infants with in utero cocaine exposure. J Urol, 144, 110–112.

Roth, D., Alarcon, F., Fernandez, J. et al. (1988). Acute rhabdomyolysis associated with cocaine intoxication. N Engl J Med, 319, 673–677.

Rubin, R. & Neugarten, J. (1989). Cocaine-induced rhabdomyolysis masquerading as myocardial ischemia. Am J Med, 86(5), 551–553.

Sanders, M. & Marshall, A. (1989). Acute and chronic toxic nephropathies. Ann Clin and Lab Sci, 19(3), 216–220.

Schwartz, J. & McAfee, R. (1987). Cocaine and rhabdomyolysis. J Fam Pract, 24 (2), 209.

Sharff, J. (1984). Renal infarction associated with intravenous cocaine use. Ann Emerg Med, 13(12), 1145–1147.

Singhal, P. & Faulkner, M. (1988). Myonecrosis and cocaine abuse. Ann Int Med,109:843.

Singhal, P., Horowitz, B., Quinones, M. et al. (1989). Acute renal failure following cocaine abuse. Nephron, 52, 76–79.

Singhal, P. C.,Rubin, R. B.,Peters, A.,et al. (1990). Rhabdomyolysis and acute renal failure associated with cocaine abuse. J Toxicol-Clin Toxic, 28(3), 321–330.

Tabasco-Minguillan, J., Novick, D. & Kreek, M. (1990). Liver function tests in non-parenteral cocaine users. Drug Alcohol Depen, 26(2), 169–174.

Tumlin, J., Sands, J. & Someren, A. (1990). Special feature: hemolytic-uremic syndrome following crack cocaine inhalation. Am J Med Sciences, 229(6), 366–371.

Welch, R. & Todd, K. (1990). Cocaine-associated rhabdomyolysis. Ann Emerg Med, 19(4), 449.

Welch, R., Todd, K. & Krause, G. (1991). Incidence of cocaine-associated rhabdomyolysis. Ann Emerg Med, 20, 154–157.

Wohlman, R. (1987). Renal artery thrombosis and embolization associated with intravenous cocaine injection. Southern Med J, 80(7), 928–930.

1.10.7 HEMATOLOGIC ABNORMALITIES

Thrombocytopenic purpura was recognized in heroin users more than a decade before the spread of HIV infection (Adams, Rufo, Talarico et al., 1978). What the etiology was then is not really known, but now thrombotic thrombocytopenic purpura in heroin users is almost always linked to HIV infection (Karpatkin, 1990). For the moment, at least, that does not appear to be the case among cocaine users. One study described seven HIV-seronegative intravenous cocaine abusers with extensive cutaneous petechiae, ecchymoses and heme positive stools. Their bone marrows all had normal or increased numbers of megakaryocytes and their platelet counts all improved promptly after steroid administration. No other etiology for their condition could be identified. As with many of the other cocaine associated syndromes, possible etiologies include toxic contaminants or metabolites, as well as immune reactions to the cocaine itself. There are many other ways cocaine could effect platelet function. Circulating catecholamines are elevated in cocaine users and elevated catechol levels can alter α and β receptor densities in both circulating lymphocytes and platelets (Maki, Kontula & Harkonen, 1990). In vitro studies have shown that cocaine can cause increased thromboxane generation in vitro, however that observation has never been confirmed clinically (Tonga, Tempesta, Tonga et al, 1985). Other studies have failed to show that cocaine has any effect on platelet aggregation or granule release (Kugelmass & Ware, 1992).

Another hematologic abnormality associated with cocaine use, at least indirectly, is methemoglobinemia. Street-level cocaine is occasionally diluted with benzocaine or other related local anesthetics, and oxidation of ferrous (Fe^2) hemoglobin to the ferric (Fe^3) state is a well-recognized complication of benzocaine administration. One case report described a 27-year-old man with a massive overdose (urine levels were 106 mg/L, along with 3.8 mg/L of benzocaine - blood levels weren't measured) who developed classic methemoglobinemia (McKinney, Postiglione & Herold, 1992). Cocaine itself has never been implicated as a cause of this disorder.

References

Adams, W., Rufo, R., Talarico, L. et al. (1978). Thrombocytopenia and intravenous heroin use. Ann Intern Med, 89, 207–211.

Karpatkin, S. & Nardi, M. (1988). Immunological thrombocytopenic purpura in human immunodeficiency virus-seropositive patients with hemophilia. J Lab Clin Med, 111(4), 441–448.

Kugelmass, A. & Ware, J.(1992). Cocaine and coronary artery thrombosis. (letter). Ann Intern Med, 116(9) 776–777.

Maki, T., Kontula, K. & Harkonen, M. (1990). The beta-adrenergic system in man - physiological and pathophysiological response - regulation of receptor density and functioning. Scand J Clin Lab Invest, 50(S201), 25–43.

Karpatkin, S. (1990). HIV-1 related thrombocytopenia. Hematol Oncol Clin North Am, 4, 193–218.

McKinney, C., Postiglione, K, and Herold, D. (1992). Benzocaine-adulterated street cocaine in association with methemoblobinemia. Clin Chem, 38(4) 596–597.

Orser, B. (1991). Thrombocytopenia and cocaine abuse. Anesthesiology, 74(1), 195–196.

Tonga, G., Tempesta, E., Tonga, A. et al. (1985). Platelet responsiveness and biosynthesis of thromboxane and prostacyclin in response to in vitro cocaine treatment. Haemostasis, 15, 100–107.

1.10.8 HORMONAL ALTERATIONS

Over and above cocaine's local effects on catechol reuptake, cocaine also causes increased release of epinephrine and norepinephrine from the adrenal medulla (Gunne & Jonsson, 1964) (Chiueh & Kopin, 1978) (Trouve, Nahas & Manger, 1990). Unfortunately, catechol metabolism in cocaine abusers remains largely uncharacterized. On the other hand, abnormalities of prolactin secretion have been demonstrated both in man and in experimental animals. Acute administration of cocaine causes an initial drop in prolactin levels, followed later by rebound hyperprolactinemia (Mello, Mendelson, Drieze & Kelly, 1990) (Mendelson, Mello, Teoh et al., 1989). Prolactin secretion is regulated by dopaminergic pathways and it is thought that cocaine somehow affects dopaminergic neurons in the basal hypothalamus, leading to inadequate dopaminergic suppression of prolactin secretion. In a controlled study of eight men, aged 24–26, who were chronic cocaine abusers, doses of 0.5 to 2.0 grams were given both intranasally and as smoked free base, and serial prolactin and luteinizing hormone levels were compared over a 6-hour period. Four of the 8 men developed significant hyperprolactinemia (>25 ng/mL), and all of the cocaine users had higher levels of prolactin than the controls. At the same time, the cocaine users had significant lower leuteinizing hormone levels, indicating that the hyperprolactinemia in cocaine users is associated with suppression of leuteinizing hormone activity (Mendelson, 1989).

Clinically, alterations in circulating prolactin levels may not be of very great significance. Under normal circumstances the hormone's main function is the stimulation of lactation in the post partum period. It does not appear to play a role in normal gonadal function, but its secretion can be altered in different physiologic states. Many drugs, especially those that are dopamine antagonists, cause changes in prolactin secretion. Measuring changes in prolactin levels may be of some forensic value. Markedly depressed levels are a good confirmation of recent drug use. High levels, which have been noted in detoxification patients, are consistent with withdrawal. It has been suggested that very high levels may be a marker for those detoxification patients who subsequently fail treatment and resume drug use (Teoh, Mendelson, Mello et al, 1990).

References

Bagasra, O. & Forman, L. (1989). Functional analysis of lymphocyte subpopulations in experimental cocaine abuse. I. Dose-dependent activation of lymphocyte subsets. Clin Exp Immunol, 77, 289–293.

Chao, C. C., Molitor, T. W., Gekker, G.,et al. (1991). Cocaine-mediated suppression of superoxide production by human peripheral blood mononuclear cells. J Pharmacol Exp Ther, 256(1), 255–258.

Chiueh, C. & Kopin, I. (1978). Centrally mediated release by cocaine of endogenous epinephrine and norepinephrine from the sympathoadrenal medullary system of unanesthetized rats. J Pharmacol Exp Ther, 205 (1), 148–154.

Gunne, L. & Jonsson, J. (1964). Effects of cocaine administration on brain, adrenal and urinary adrenaline and noradrenaline in rats. Psychopharmacologia, 6(2), 125–129.

Mello, N. K., Mendelson, J. H., Drieze, J. & Kelly, M. (1990). Acute effects of cocaine on prolactin and gonadotropins in female rhesus monkey during the follicular phase of the menstrual cycle. J Pharmacol Exp Ther, 254(3), 815–823.

Mendelson, J., Mello, N., Teoh, S. et al. (1989). Cocaine effects on pulsatile secretion of anterior pituitary, gonadal and adrenal hormones. J Clin Endocrinol Metab, 69, 1256–1260.

Mendelson, J.H., Teoh, S.K., Lange, U. et al. (1988). Anterior pituitary, adrenal, and gonadal hormones during cocaine withdrawal. Am J Psychiatry, 145, 1094–1098.

Mendelson, J.H. (1991). Plasma prolactin levels and cocaine abuse. Am J Psychiatry, 148(3), 397.

Ou, D., Shen, M. & Luo, Y. (1989). Effects of cocaine on the immune system of Balb/c mice. Clin Immunol Immunopathol, 52, 305–312.

Teoh, S. K., Mendelson, J. H., Mello, N. K. et al. B. (1990). Hyperprolactinemia and risk for relapse of cocaine abuse. Biol Psychiatry, 28(9), 824–828.

Tonga, G., Tempesta, E., Tonga, A. et al. (1985). Platelet responsiveness and biosynthesis of thromboxane and prostacyclin in response to in vitro cocaine treatment. Haemostasis, 15, 100–107.

Trouve, R., Nahas, G. & Manger, W. (1990). Cocaine, catecholamines, and cardiac toxicity. Acta-Anesthesiol Scand, 94 (suppl) 77–81.

Watson, E., Murphy, J., ElSohly, H. et al. (1983). Effects of the administration of coca alkaloids on the primary immune responses of mice: Interaction with 9-tetrahydrocannabinol and ethanol. Toxicol Appl Pharmacol, 71, 1–13.

1.10.9 IMMUNE SYSTEM ABNORMALITIES

Chronic use of cocaine has effects on the immune system, but the exact mechanisms remain to be characterized. Current thinking favors the notion that cocaine's effects on the immune system are probably mediated via the central nervous system and the neuroendo-crine axis. Mice chronically treated with cocaine are less able to resist some types of viral infection than are controls (Starec et al. 1991). Mice chronically treated with cocaine also manifest increased natural killer-cell activity, which is further increased in the presence of retroviral infection (Poet et al. 1991). Other studies have shown that cocaine treatment can suppress the secretion of gamma interferon from mice leukocytes (Watzl, Chen, Scuderi et al 1992). The fact that cocaine modulates natural killer activity and interferon secretion may well have a bearing on the high rate of HIV seropositivity seen in HIV infected patients (Anthony et al. 1991).

In humans, both phagocytic activity and T suppressor cell acti-vity are suppressed (Ou, Shen & Luo, 1989) (Bagasra & Forman, 1989). Inhibition of delayed type hypersensitivity has also been demonstrated (Watson, Murphy, ElSohly et al., 1983). Cocaine use also leads to abnor-mal cytokine production. Peripheral blood lymphocytes from cocaine users have higher levels of interleukin-2, and there is a positive corre-lation between cocaine concentrations and interleukin-2 levels (Chen et al. 1991)

Cultured human peripheral mononuclear cells lose much of their ability to produce superoxide anion (which is how they attack intracellular pathogens), and the effects seem to be dose related (Chao, Molitor, Gekker et al 1991). Many intravenous opiate abusers have antiplatelet antibodies (7S immunoglobulin G) and signs of increased platelet destruction by the reticuloendothelial system, but this process has not been demonstrated in cocaine users (Karpatkin & Nardi, 1988). The findings in the cocaine-related cases of thrombocytopenia have suggested that an immune mechanism is also operative (Orser, 1991).

References

Anthony, J., Vlahov, D., Nelson, K. et al. (1991). New evidence on intravenous cocaine use and the risk of infection with human immunodeficiency virus type 1, Am J Epidemol, 134(10):1175–1189.

Bagasra, O. & Forman, L. (1989). Functional analysis of lymphocyte subpopulations in experimental cocaine abuse. I. Dose-dependent activation of lymphocyte subsets. Clin Exp Immunol, 77, 289–293.

Chen, G-J., Pillai, R., Erickson, J. et al. (1991). Cocaine immunotoxicity: abnormal cytokine production in Hispanic drug users. Toxicology Letters, 59:81–88.

Chao, C. C., Molitor, T. W., Gekker, G.,et al (1991). Cocaine-mediated suppression of superoxide production by human peripheral blood mononuclear cells. J Pharmacol Exp Ther, 256(1), 255–258.

Karpatkin, S. & Nardi, M. (1988). Immunological thrombocytopenic purpura in human immunodeficiency virus - seropositive patients with hemophilia. J Lab Clin Med, 111(4), 441–448.

Maki, T., Kontula, K. & Harkonen, M. (1990). The beta-adrenergic system in man - physiological and pathophysiological response - regulation of receptor density and functioning. Scand J Clin Lab Invest, 50(S201), 25–43.

Ou, D., Shen, M. & Luo, Y. (1989). Effects of cocaine on the immune system of Balb/c mice. Clin Immunol Immunopathol, 52, 305–312.

Poet, T., Pillai, R., Wood, S and Watson, R. (1991). Stimulation of natural killer cell activity by murine retroviral infection and cocaine. Toxicol Let, 59:147–152.

Starec, M., Rouveix, B, Sinet, M. et al. (1991). Immune status and survival of opiate- and cocaine-treated mice infected with Friend virus. J Pharmacol Exp Ther, 259(2) 745–750.

Tonga, G., Tempesta, E., Tonga, A. et al. (1985). Platelet responsiveness and biosynthesis of thromboxane and prostacyclin in response to in vitro cocaine treatment. Heamostasis, 15, 100–107.

Watson, E., Murphy, J., ElSohly, H. et al. (1983). Effects of the administration of coca alkaloids on the primary immune responses of mice: Interaction with 9-tetrahydrocannabinol and ethanol. Toxicol Appl Pharmacol, 71, 1–13.

Watzl, B., Chen, G., Scuderi, P. et al. (1992). Cocaine-induced suppression of interferon-gamma secretion in leukocytes from young and old C57BL/6 mice. Int J Immunopharmac, 14:1125–1131.

1.10.10 FETAL PATHOLOGY

From the outset a great deal of attention has been focused on this problem, but answers are elusive. Prospective and retrospective studies have claimed there was evidence for increased incidence of fetal demise (Ahmed, Spong, Geringer et al., 1989) (Neerhof, MacGregor et al., 1989) (Ryan, Ehrlich & Finnegan, 1987) (Bingol, Fuchs, Diaz et al, 1986), spontaneous abortion (Neerhof et al., 1989) (Chasnoff, Burns, Schnoll et al., 1985) (MacGregor, Keith et al., 1987), abruption (Chasnoff, Griffith, MacGregor et al., 1989) (Ahmed et al., 1989), congenital malformations (Chasnoff et al., 1989) (Bingol et al., 1986), and prematurity (Chasnoff et al., 1989) (Cherukuri, Minkoff, Feldman et al., 1988) (Ahmed et al., 1989) (Neerhof et al., 1989). None of these claims are supported by anatomic studies, though ultrasonography has been used in two large series which (1) failed to demonstrate renal abnormalities and (2) suggested an increased incidence of septal defects in children born to cocaine-using mothers (Lipshultz, Frassica & Orav, 1991) (Shaw, Malcoe, Lammer & Swan, 1991) (Shepard, Fantel & Kapur, 1991). One of the more interesting case reports described a newborn with a single right ventricle. After a meticulous dissection of the heart it appeared that coronary spasm may have occurred in utero, producing an infarct which destroyed the right ventricle (Shepard et al., 1991).

The notion that maternal cocaine can cause vasospasm, thereby inducing ischemia and subsequent reperfusion injury, is plausible (Fantel, Barber, Carda et al.). However, the analysis of case control data from several large databases indicates that, since 1968, there has been no upward trend in the number of infants born with single ventricle, even though the number of cocaine using mothers has increased drastically during that time (Martin & Khoury, 1992). This suggests that, even if maternal cocaine use can cause single ventricle, most cases are due to something else.

Cocaine use does increase the risk of small-for-gestational-age births (Handler, Kistin, Davis & Ferre, 1991), and possibly for preterm delivery. There certainly are no lesions or patterns of injury which are in any way diagnostic. In the case of the cardiovascular system, at least, there are some fairly good reasons not to expect changes. There is down regulation, or at least uncoupling, of ß receptors at birth (Karch & Billingham, 1986). If that is the case, then the newborn should be relatively resistant to the toxic effects of catechol excess.

References

Ahmed, M., Spong, C., Geringer, J. et al. (1989). Prospective study on cocaine
    use prior to delivery (abstract). JAMA, 262, 1880.

Bingol, N., Fuchs, M., Diaz, V. et al. (1986). Teratogenicity of cocaine in
    humans. Pediatr Res, 20(4 (part 2)), 337A.

Chasnoff, I., Burns, W., Schnoll, S. et al. (1985). Cocaine use in pregnancy. N
    Engl J Med, 313, 666–669.

Chasnoff, I., Griffith, R., MacGregor, S. et al. (1989). Temporal patterns of
    cocaine use in pregnancy: perinatal outcome. JAMA, 261, 1741–1744.

Cherukuri, R., Minkoff, H., Feldman, J. et al. (1988). A cohort study of alka-
    loidal cocaine ("crack") in pregnancy. Obstet Gynecol, 72, 147–151.

Fantel, A., Barber, C., Mackler, B. (1992). Ischemia/Reperfusion - a new
    hypothesis for the developmental toxicity of cocaine. Teratology,
    46:285–292.

Handler, A., Kistin, N., Davis, F. & Ferre, C. (1991). Cocaine use during
    pregnancy: perinatal outcomes. Am J Epidemiol, 133(8), 818–825.

Karch, S. & Billingham ME (1986). Myocardial contraction bands revisited. Hum
    Pathol, 17, 9–13.

Lipshultz, S., Frassica, J. & Orav, E. (1991). Cardiovascular abnormalities in
    infants prenatally exposed to cocaine. J Pediatr, 118, 44–51.

MacGregor, S., Keith, L., Chasnoff, IJ et al. (1987). Cocaine use during preg-
    nancy: adverse perinatal outcome. Am J Obstet Gynecol, 157, 686–690.

Martin, L. and Khoury, M. (1992). Cocaine and single ventricle: a population
    study. Teratology, 46:267–270.

Neerhof, M., MacGregor, Retzky, S. et al. (1989). Cocaine abuse during preg-
    nancy: peripartum prevalence and perinatal outcome. Am J Obstet
    Gynecol, 161, 633–638.

Ryan, L., Ehrlich, S. & Finnegan, L. (1987). Cocaine abuse in pregnancy: effects
    on the fetus and newborn. Neurotoxicol Teratol, 9, 295–299.

Shaw, G. M., Malcoe, L. H., Lammer, E. J. & Swan, S. H. (1991). Maternal use
    of cocaine during pregnancy and congenital cardiac anomalies. J
    Pediatr, 118(1), 167–168.

Shepard, T. H., Fantel, A. G. & Kapur, R. P. (1991). Fetal coronary thrombosis
    as a cause of single ventricular heart. Teratology, 43(2), 113–117.

Volpe, J. (1992). Mechanisms of disease, effect of cocaine use on the fetus. N
    Engl J. Med, 327:399–407.

Young, S., Vosper, H., Phillips, S. (1992). Cocaine: its effects on maternal and
    child health. Pharmacotherapy, 12:1–17.

1.11 WHEN IS COCAINE THE CAUSE OF DEATH?

Cocaine-related deaths pose a forensic problem of considerable
and increasing importance. If cocaine is listed as the cause of death, that
means the death is accidental. While many insurance policies exclude
death by the self-administration of drugs, double indemnity claims can
still occur if death is deemed accidental, and insurance companies may
well object to the diagnosis. In criminal cases the role of cocaine toxicity
can be equally important. Over and above civil and criminal consider-

ations, the social stigma associated with the diagnosis of drug-related death is also an important issue which should not be ignored.

Cause of death is easy to determine when the cocaine blood level is 1,000 ng and there is florid pulmonary edema. Such cases are not uncommon, but even in the absence of obvious changes, there may be subtle histologic alterations that are equally diagnostic. To make an appropriate determination, three factors need to be considered. These determinations have been incorporated in an algorithm. Quantitation of cocaine blood levels is not required for actual decision making. Knowledge of exact cocaine and benzoylecgonine levels does allow one to estimate when and perhaps how much drug was taken, but the presence of any drug at all, in conjunction with appropriate historical and autopsy findings, is sufficient to determine causality. Blood levels of over 5,000 ng/mL have been observed as incidental findings, and there is no upper limit that can be guaranteed fatal. Cocaine levels may be low or nonexistent at the time of death. Accordingly, cocaine levels are of historic interest only and can't be counted on to rule in or out cocaine as a cause of death. Most states (California is an exception) simply list the cause of death as "drug related". Such a designation covers all deaths which are considered not to be suicide, but rather unexpected complications of chronic drug usage. There need be no attempt to make the artificial separation between toxicity and poisoning. Literally hundreds of studies and case reports have amply demonstrated that cocaine related deaths are generally not dose related (Smart & Anglin, 1986).

The acute and chronic effects of cocaine abuse alter the heart and the way the heart conducts electrical impulses. As discussed in the section on sudden death, cocaine elevates circulating catecholamines and elevated catecholamines produce contraction band necrosis. Contraction band necrosis heals by fibrosis. Accordingly, the presence of patchy microfocal fibrosis suggests earlier healed bouts of contraction band necrosis and earlier episodes of cocaine abuse. Eosinophilic and lympho-cytic infiltrates, which have been reported in cocaine users, are con-sistent with subacute injury (Isner, Estes, Thompson et al., 1986) (Virmani, Rabinowitz & Smialek, 1987). None of these tissue responses is unique. Contraction band necrosis is observed in many disorders, ranging from cobalt poisoning to electrocution and aggressive resuscita-tion with catecholamines (Karch & Billingham, 1986), but the constella-tion of microfocal fibrosis, contraction band necrosis, and cellular infiltrate is seen in only one setting: chronic exposure to high levels of circulating catecholamines. The only differential is damage secondary to chronic abuse of some other sympathomimetic such as amphetamine or pheochromocytoma (Kline, 1961) (Buda, Jones, LeMire et al., 1986) (Ro-senbaum, Billingham, Ginsburg et al., 1987). Small pheochromocytomas may occur in other organs beside the adrenals. Chromaffin cells are also located in the trigone of the bladder and behind the aorta in the Organ

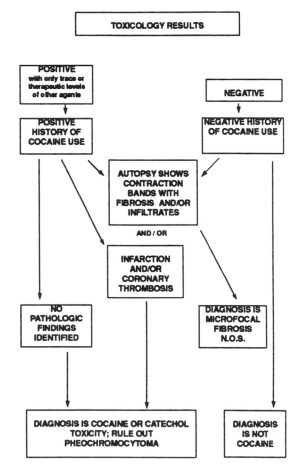

Figure 1.11 When is cocaine the cause of death?
Whether or not cocaine is the cause of death cannot be determined by toxicologic results alone; historical and anatomic findings must also be taken into account. This flow diagram illustrates possible approaches to making the diagnosis. If classic anatomic findings are present, and there is a strong history of chronic coaine abuse, then negative toxicology testing does not rule out the diagnosis.

of Zuckerkandel and can, on occasion, be very difficult to identify at autopsy. Thus the diagnosis of cocaine-related death cannot be made on the basis of pathologic findings alone. There must also be a positive history or drug test.

Myocardial infarction due to coronary spasm may occur in individuals with otherwise normal arteries, and if the infarction causes death, and is associated with positive toxicology testing, then the cause of death is cocaine toxicity. The same would apply to patients with existing lesions who infarct because of the increased work load cocaine imposes on the myocardium. Increasingly, it appears that cocaine may lead to accelerated atherogenesis (Dressler, Malekzadeh & Roberts, 1990) (Kolodgie, Virmani, Cornhill et al., 1991). Even if it doesn't, the extra work load cocaine use imposes on an already diseased heart can, in fact, be the cause of death. Without the occurrence of coronary spasm or infarction, cocaine, like all local anesthetics, has toxic effects on the myocardium and can cause marked depression of cardiac output (Rhee, Valentine & Lee, 1990) (Strichartz, 1987) and that too can lead to infarction.

The third, and final, component of the algorithm is the history. If there is a strong history of cocaine abuse and typical myocardial pathology is observed, the case should be signed out as cocaine-induced sudden death, even in the face of negative toxicology testing. On the other hand, if typical pathologic findings are present, but toxicology and history are both negative, the diagnosis must be microfocal fibrosis, etiology "not otherwise specified". In the event that additional information becomes available at a later date, the diagnosis can be revised, but the presence of isolated myocardial alterations is not sufficient for diagnosis. It may not always be possible to reach a firm diagnosis, but in today's society, the evaluation of sudden death in young people should begin with a consideration of the possible role of cocaine or other stimulant abuse.

References

Buda, A., Jones, C., LeMire, M. et al. (1986). Cardiac abnormalities in pheochromocytoma: a catecholamine-induced cardiotoxicity (abstract). Circulation, 74 (Suppl), 449.

Dressler, F., Malekzadeh, S. & Roberts, W. (1990). Quantitative analysis of amounts of coronary arterial narrowing in cocaine addicts. Am J Cardiol, 65(5), 303–308.

Isner, J., Estes, N., Thompson, P. et al. (1986). Acute cardiac events temporarily related to cocaine abuse. N Engl J Med, 315, 1438–1443.

Karch, S. & Billingham ME (1986). Myocardial contraction bands revisited. Hum Pathol, 17, 9–13.

Kline, I. (1961). Myocardial alterations associated with pheochromocytomas. Am J Pathol, 38(5), 539–552.

Kolodgie, F. D., Virmani, R., Cornhill, J. F. et al. (1991). Increase in atherosclerosis and adventitial mast cells in cocaine abusers: an alternative mechanism of cocaine-associated coronary vasospasm and thrombosis. J Am Coll Cardiol, 17(7), 1553–1560.

Rhee, H. M., Valentine, J. L. & Lee, S. Y. (1990). Toxic effects of cocaine to the cardiovascular system in conscious and anesthetized rats and rabbits - evidence for a direct effect on the myocardium. Neurotoxicology, 11(2), 361–366.

Rosenbaum, J., Billingham, M., Ginsburg, R. et al. (1987). Cardiomyopathy in a rat model of pheochromocytoma: morphological and functional alterations. J Pharmacol Exp Ther, 241, 354–360.

Smart, R. & Anglin, R. (1986). Do we know the lethal dose of cocaine? J Forensic Sci, 32(2), 303–312.

Strichartz, G. (1987). Handbook of experimental pharmacology, Volume 81: Local Anesthetics. New York: Springer-Verlag.

Virmani, R., Rabinowitz, M. & Smialek, J. (1987). Cocaine-associated deaths: absence of coronary thrombosis and a high incidence of myocarditis. Lab Invest, 56, 83.

2 Other Naturally Occurring Stimulants

Cocaine is not the only plant that contains psychoactive alkaloids. At least four other species contain alkaloids capable of producing amphetamine-like effects. Absinthe abuse ceased being a problem at the turn of the century, and khat abuse is confined to the sub-Sahara, but the xanthine derivatives, especially caffeine, are the world's most widely abused drugs. The other important alkaloid is ephedrine. Ephedrine abuse can lead to psychosis, but the principal importance of this compound is its role in the illicit production of amphetamines. Little is known about the actions of these compounds in man, and still less about the pathologic changes associated with their abuse.

2.1 ABSINTHE

2.1.1 HISTORY

Absinthe is French for wormwood (*Artemisia absinthium* and *Artemisia pontica*). A perennial herb related to sage (*Salvia officinalis*), wormwood grows to a height of two to three feet. Plants have leafy stems and tiny, greenish yellow flowers. The Egyptians used wormwood for medical purposes. Pliny, in the first century A.D., recommended it as a vermifuge, and wormwood was mentioned in several of Shakespeare's plays. Late in the 1700's, techniques for the mass production of grain alcohol were introduced, and shortly afterward herb-based liqueurs appeared on the market. In the early 1800's Henri-Louis Pernod ushered in the era of absinthe abuse when he opened his factory in Pontarlier. Pernod's liquor, which was immensely popular in France and throughout Europe, was a distillate of herbs. The recipe included wormwood, anise, fennel (which were responsible for its green color), hyssop and lemon balm (Arnold 1989).

Absinthe drinking became very popular just a few years before Mariani started selling his coca fortified wines, and the popularity of both coca and absinthe seemed to rise almost in parallel. During the 1860's and 70's Degas and Manet immortalized images of absinthe drinking. Toulouse-Lautrec painted van Gogh with a glass of absinthe just three years after Freud published "Über Coca". Baudelaire used both cocaine and absinthe, but wrote about only the latter. Valentine Magnan

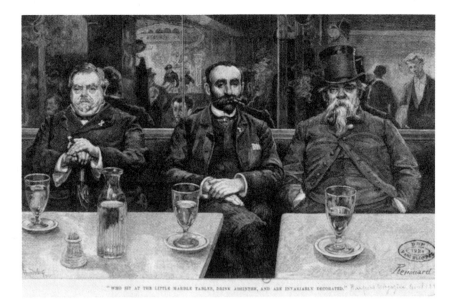

"WHO SIT AT THE LITTLE MARBLE TABLES, DRINK ABSINTHE, AND ARE INVARIABLY DECORATED."

Figure 2.1 Absinthe drinkers
These gentlemen were obviously intoxicated, but whether from the terpenes or
the alcohol in their drinks is not entirely clear. Some evidence suggests that the
active ingredients in this drink may have been very similar to those in
marijuana.

studied the medical complications of both drugs (Magnan 1874, Magnan
and Saury 1889), and sounded warnings about the potential toxicity of
each.

Just as the manufacturers of cocaine-containing patent medicines
minimized the medical problems associated with cocaine use, so did the
manufacturers of absinthe cordials. At first, the manufacturers were
successful. During the period from 1875 to 1913 annual consumption of
absinthe per French citizen increased by 1,500%. In 1912, just two years
before the Harrison Narcotic Act banned cocaine from patent medications in the United States, the French government passed legislation
limiting the alcohol and absinthe content of commercial products. In
1915 the sale and manufacture of absinthe was banned entirely. There
was some resistance at first, but the prohibition stood, and absinthe
abuse is now only a historical curiosity, while cocaine is enjoying a
renaissance. Why one drug, but not the other, should have entirely
disappeared, is probably explained by simple logistics. A few million
dollars' worth of cocaine can be smuggled in a suitcase, while a few
million dollars worth of absinthe would fill up a large tanker!

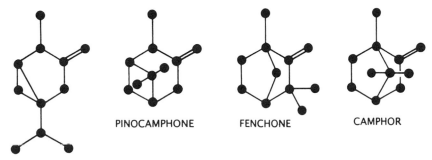

THUJONE   PINOCAMPHONE   FENCHONE   CAMPHOR

Figure 2.1.2 Terpenes
Absinthe contained many different compounds; thujone was the principal agent.

2.1.2 CLINICAL AND AUTOPSY STUDIES

The compounds found in absinthe are terpenes, structural isomers of camphor. The structure of thujone, the principal terpene extracted from wormwood, was published in 1900. Modern clinical studies of thujone are all but nonexistent. Studies from the 1920's and 1930's suggest that its effects are indistinguishable from those of camphor. Camphor is a potent CNS stimulant and, before the introduction of electroconvulsant therapy, camphor was used to treat depression. It has been suggested that, because the structure of the thujones is very similar to that of tetrahydrocannabinol, both produce similar psychological effects (del Castillo, Anderson, and Rubottom 1975), and that absinthe drinkers were not getting much more than a marijuana "high."

Small doses of camphor cause stimulation and euphoria, but ingestion of larger amounts (>30 mg/kg) can result in convulsions, coma, and death. Without knowing the thujone content of the absinthe being consumed at the turn of the century, it is hard to say how much thujone absinthe drinkers were actually getting, let alone whether that amount was sufficient to cause toxicity, but it seems likely that it was far less than 30 mg/kg. Blood and tissue levels in camphor-associated deaths have never been reported, and autopsy information is limited to observations in the older literature (Amory 1868) and one slightly more recent case (Smith and Margolis 1954). Absinthe abuse is now nonexistent, but camphor is still a common ingredient in many over-the-counter medications (Camphophenique™, Mentholatum™, Vicks Vaporub™, Sloan's Liniment™, etc.) and is responsible for occasional episodes of toxicity.

References

Amory, R. (1868). Absinthe. Boston Medical and Surgical Journal :68.
Arnold, WN. (1989). Absinthe. Scientific American (6):112–117.

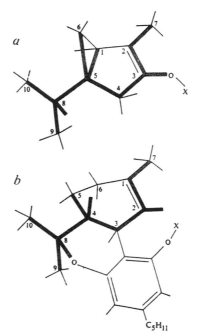

Figure 2.1.3 Similarities between absinthe and marijuana?
The backbone of the terpene molecule bears a striking resemblance to the
backbone of the THC molecule.

Magnan, V. (1874). On the comparative action of alcohol and absinthe. Lancet 2:2664
(September 19):410–412.
Magnan, V. and Saury, R. (1889). Trois cas de cocainisme chronique. Compt Rend Soc
Biol (Paris) 1:60.
Smith, A G, and G Margolis (1954). Camphor poisoning: anatomical and pharmacologic
study; report of a fatal case; experimental investigation of protective action
of barbiturate. Am J Pathol 30:857–868.

2.2 CAFFEINE

2.2.1 HISTORY

Caffeine is the world's most widely used stimulant drug. Annual
consumption of caffeine is thought to be well over 100,000 tons. It is
estimated that over 80% of the US population drink coffee or tea. In
addition, formidable amounts are also consumed in soft drinks, cold
medications, and pain relief formulas. One study placed the average
American's caffeine consumption at 2.4 mg/kg/day for adults and half
that amount for children between the ages of 5 and 18. European consumption is thought to be even higher - 3.5 mg/kg/day (Commission of
the European Communities 1983). An average cup of coffee contains
40–100 mg of caffeine. The content of cola drinks is lower, ranging from

30 to 50 mg. A dedicated coffee drinker can easily ingest more than a gram of caffeine per day. Per capita consumption was not always so high.

Caffeine can radically improve performance during athletic competitions. In a controlled study, elite marathon runners given 9 mg/kg of caffeine before testing were able to increase the time they were able to run on a treadmill by an average of 70% (Graham and Spriet 1991)! Equally important, they were able to achieve this improvement without evidence of toxicity and without being disqualified for exceeding the International Olympic Committee's requirement that testing reveal no more than 12 μg/mL of caffeine. These results are sure to prompt further experimentation with doses high enough that they do produce toxicity.

The origins of coffee drinking are something of a mystery. According to legend, the prior of a Muslim convent observed that goats eating berries from certain trees tended to stay up all night. He thought that using the beans might help him and his followers stay awake during their prayer vigils in the mosque, so he brewed a beverage called *kahweh* and was said to have been quite pleased with the results. The first substantial evidence of widespread popularity is from the sixteenth century. In 1511, when a new Egyptian governor arrived in Mecca, he noticed people sitting around the mosques drinking coffee. He asked what they were doing and he was told that they were drinking coffee in order to get the energy they needed to pray all night. The governor had his doubts, and so he convened a meeting of clerics and elders to discuss whether or not coffee might not be some sort of intoxicating agent, and therefore prohibited by the Koran. The assembly concluded that coffee was indeed an intoxicant, and therefore should be banned. Sales of coffee were prohibited and stocks were burned. Had the new governor bothered to check with his superiors, he would have found that the Sultan of Cairo was an avid coffee drinker; the Sultan promptly overruled the governor's decision, and coffee drinking in Mecca has been legal ever since. Venetian traders introduced coffee to Europe. The first coffee house in London was opened in 1652; it was located in St. Michael's Alley, Cornhill. Its owner, Pasqua Rosee, advertised extensively, making mostly medicinal claims for the drink. According to Rosee, coffee was "a very good help to the digestion...and makes you fit for business (Thompson 1928). In spite of Rosee's claims, coffee drinking was at first suspect. Coffee drinkers were said to have a haggard appearance and to be "subject to fits of agitation and depression." Coffee drinking had been introduced into France nine years earlier, and by 1690 there were 250 registered coffee houses; by 1782 that number had risen to 1,800. Some of the coffee houses were quite opulent, with marble tables and crystal chandeliers. Like the English, the French also had some doubts about the habit. Medical literature from that period contains reports both praising and condemning coffee's effects. It was

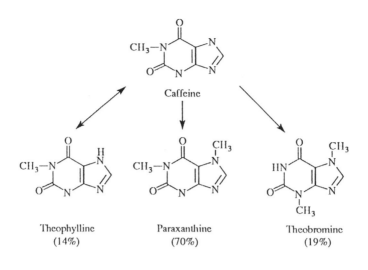

Figure 2.2.2 Caffeine metabolism
Assuming an average caffeine intake of roughly 500 mg per day, 70% will be excreted as paraxanthine, 20% as theobromine, and 14% as theophylline. The results may be quite different in smokers and patients with cirrhosis.

alleged that coffee caused inflammation of the liver and spleen, and even that it caused renal colic.

Suspicions that coffee drinking is unhealthy have never entirely disappeared. Even Virchow classified caffeine, along with alcohol, as an addictive substance. Lewin, who generally thought that coffee drinking was a good thing, accepted reports of "delirium, vertigo, trembling, and even convulsions" as an occupational disease in coffee roasters (Lewin 1931). In modern times epidemiologic investigations have focused on possible links between caffeine intake and myocardial infarction, sudden death, and fibrocystic disease. Alleged links to cancer have never been proven (Stavric 1992). The histopathologic changes associated with caffeine abuse have been studied only in animals (Strubelt et al. 1976).

2.2.2 CHEMICAL CONSTANTS AND TISSUE DISPOSITION

Caffeine is 3,7,-Dihydro-1,3,7-trimethyl-1H-purine-2,6-dione or 1,3,7,-trimethylxanthine. Other older names were methyltheobromine and thein. Its formula is $C_8H_{10}N_4O_2$, and it has a molecular weight of 194.19. It is composed of 49.5% carbon, 5.2% hydrogen, 28.9% nitrogen, and 16.5% oxygen. Purified caffeine crystallizes into hexagonal prisms with a melting point of 238°C. It is a basic alkaloid with a pKa of 0.8.

Caffeine is a methylated purine derivative, and like cocaine, is classified as an alkaloid. The term was originally introduced to described compounds which could be extracted from plants and whose salts were crystallizable. Caffeine is found in naturally occurring plants, including kola nuts, cocoa beans, and tea. Chemical extraction of roasted coffee beans yields from 8 to 20 mg of caffeine per gram of coffee (Zuskin, Duncan, and Douglas 1983). Measurements made one hour after drinking two cups of coffee showed a peak caffeine value of 5.3 μgm/mL (Marks and Kelly 1973), but in general peak levels can be expected anywhere from 15 to 45 minutes after ingestion. The half-life is extremely variable. In healthy adults, reported half-lives have been anywhere between 3 and 7 hours (Levy and Zylber-Katz 1982). Caffeine is almost entirely metabolized by the liver to other xanthines, including theophylline, which is then excreted in the urine. On average, 14% of ingested caffeine is excreted as theophylline and 70% as paraxanthine. The latter is not found in nature, but is found as a metabolite in many different species (Ullrich, Compagnone, Münch et al 1992).

2.2.3 CLINICAL AND AUTOPSY STUDIES

For a drug that is so widely taken, surprisingly little is known about its chemistry or toxicology. Caffeine is very similar in structure to theophylline and shares a common mechanism of toxicity, but on a weight-for-weight basis theophylline is a good deal more toxic than caffeine. Since theophylline, paraxanthine and caffeine are all present after ingestion, assessing caffeine's toxic potential becomes quite difficult. Theophylline and caffeine are interconvertible in humans. The ratio of plasma theophylline to caffeine after caffeine administration is 8.6. After theophylline administration, the ratio of theophylline to caffeine is nearly the same (Stavric 1988).

Little data about tissue disposition is available, and kinetics have been studied only at low doses in healthy volunteers. Recent studies in rats have shown that, after dosing with caffeine, concentrations of caffeine and theophylline are equal in most tissues except the brain, where caffeine levels are 25% higher than theophylline levels (Ståhle, Segersvärd, Ugersted 1992). This differential may partly explain the difference in clinical profile between the two drugs.

However, since newborns, like adults, are able to interconvert caffeine and theophylline, some useful information can be derived from studies on how infants metabolize aminophylline. In three newborns treated with therapeutic doses of intravenous aminophylline, the highest levels were in the blood and then the brain. Decreasing levels were found in heart, liver, lung and kidney. Brain theophylline levels ranged from 6 to 30 μg/gram, while caffeine levels ranged from 2.1 to 3.7 μg/gram. Caffeine can be detected in most biofluids, including saliva, semen and breast milk (Bonati et al. 1982), but levels have not been systematically studied.

After ingesting 24 grams of caffeine in an unsuccessful suicide attempt, one woman had a caffeine blood level was 200 μg/mL, while her theophylline level was 17.2 μ/mL (Benowitiz et al. 1982). Severe, but not lethal, toxicity can be seen with much lower blood levels. Toxicity in a 58-year old was associated with a blood level of only 33 μg/mL (Iverson et al. 1984). Blood levels in cases of fatal intoxication have ranged from 79 mg/L to 1,560 mg/L (McGee 1980) (Mrvos et al. 1989). Infants born to heavy coffee drinkers have elevated caffeine levels at birth (Khanna and Somani 1984), but there is no evidence that the elevation results in toxicity in these children.

Two special situations are of clinical and forensic interest. In infants the plasma half-life of caffeine is 17 times longer than in healthy adults (Labow 1983). Accordingly, infants being treated with aminophylline run a real risk of toxicity from caffeine, which continues to accumulate in their blood as aminophylline is converted to caffeine. Similar results can occur in patients with liver insufficiency or decreased cardiac output (Lacroix et al. 1985). Treatment with aminophylline under these circumstances runs a risk of caffeine toxicity. Measurement of both theophylline and caffeine levels in individuals at risk would be prudent.

TABLE 2.2.2.1
HALF LIFE OF CAFFEINE VS. AGE

Age	Half life of caffeine
Premature, at birth	65 – 102 hours
Term, at birth	82 hours
3 – 4.5 months old	14.4 hours
5 – 6 months old	2.6 hours
Adult	3 – 7.5 hours

All methylxanthines, including caffeine, are phosphodiesterase inhibitors. Excessive use causes typical symptoms of sympathetic stimulation. Coffee ingestion increases plasma catecholamine levels, but only to a very modest degree. Early studies demonstrated that caffeine stimulates the release of catecholamines from the adrenal medulla, and there have been clinical reports suggesting fairly substantial catechol elevations (Benowitiz et al. 1982) (Robertson et al. 1978). But in one study, human volunteers given a mean dose of 250 mg had statistically insignificant increases in catecholamines (Cameron, Modell, and Hariharan 1990). This limited rise in catecholamines is in contrast with the other naturally occurring psychostimulants and may explain why, even though enormous quantities of caffeine are consumed, few histologic abnormalities have been reported.

Caffeine's physiologic effects include decreases in cerebral blood flow and transient increases in systolic blood pressure (Cameron, Modell, and Hariharan 1990) (Mathew and Wilson 1991). A dose of 250 mg (approximately 2.5 cups of coffee) is enough to reduce cerebral blood flow for 90 minutes. The decrease in cerebral flow is unexplained. It is not due to changes in the general circulation or in CO_2 levels, but it might be the result of caffeine's ability to block adenosine receptors. Adenosine is a powerful cerebral vasodilator and it may be that adenosine receptor blockade results in decreased cerebral flow. Interactions with the adenosine receptor have also been suggested as a possible mechanism in caffeine-related seizures, though this suggestion remains unproven (Morgan and Durcan 1990). Caffeine increases myocardial contractility by increasing the release of Ca2+ from the sarcoplasmic reticulum and elevating intracytosolic calcium concentration (Petersen 1991). A relationship between caffeine intake and ventricular ectopy has always been presumed, but electrophysiologic studies of patients with recurrent ventricular tachycardia have failed to confirm any such action. In fact, some patients with ventricular ectopy have fewer extra beats after they are given coffee (Chelsky 1990). There is also evidence that caffeine can inhibit plasma cholinesterase. Since few, if any, of the symptoms associated with caffeine toxicity are similar to those seen with cholinesterase deficiency, the significance of this observation also remains to be seen (Karadsheh, Kussie, and Linthicum 1991).

2.2.4 BLOOD LEVELS IN FATAL CASES

There is one report of a 22-year-old woman who committed suicide by taking an unknown number of caffeine tablets. She died of an apparent cardiac arrhythmia. Blood obtained during attempted resuscitation had 1,560 mg of caffeine per liter. Autopsy findings consisted mainly of pulmonary edema and visceral congestion (Mrvos et al. 1989). A second woman, age 19, also died of a ventricular arrhythmia. At autopsy her caffeine blood level was 181 mg/L. No histopathologic alterations were identified. In 1985 Garriott reported on five fatalities, three of combined caffeine/ephedrine, and two cases of caffeine only. In these cases blood levels ranged from 130 to 344 mg/L. The report didn't comment on histologic findings, if any. Fatalities have also been associated with much lower levels. A 1980 case report described two patients who expired after using repeated coffee enemas. Both had underlying diseases and both appeared to have succumbed to fluid and electrolyte abnormalities. Both of these women had negligible caffeine levels at the time of death (Eisele and Reay 1980). Aside from blood levels, data on the tissue distribution of caffeine is so sparse as to prohibit any generalization.

2.2.5 AUTOPSY FINDINGS

Based on the very limited data available, it appears that caffeine-related deaths in humans are usually arrhythmic and are not accompanied by any distinct histologic changes. In studies designed to access caffeine cardiotoxicity, caffeine infusions of 0.5 mg/kg in miniswine produced neither EKG changes nor myocardial lesions (Vick et al. 1989). However, when the same amount of caffeine was infused along with low doses of isoproterenol (1 μg/kg/min, a dose that is too low to produce EKG changes or necrosis in this model), myocardial necrosis and arrhythmias were easily demonstrated. In one overdose, with a caffeine level of 113.5 mg/L, there was acute heart failure with right atrial dilation, acute pulmonary edema, and passive congestion of the liver, but no specific lesions in the heart were identified (Bryant 1981). A second case, with even higher caffeine levels (181 mg/L) had no evident anatomic cause for death (McGee 1980). In a third case, where blood levels were not measured, pulmonary edema and passive congestion of the liver were observed (Alstott, Miller, and Forney 1973). The failure to demonstrate myocardial lesions is consistent with the fact that caffeine toxicity is not associated with marked elevations in circulating catecholamines. It may be that caffeine's modest sympathomimetic activities are sufficient to produce toxicity only in the presence of some other ß agonist (Strubelt et al. 1976).

References

Alstott, R., A. Miller and R. Forney (1973). Report of a human fatality due to caffeine. J Forensic Sci 18 (2):135–137.

Benowitiz, N., J. Osterloh, N. Goldschlager et al. (1982). Massive catecholamine release from caffeine poisoning. JAMA 248 (9):1097–1098.

Bonati, M., R. Latini, F. Galletti et al. (1982). Caffeine disposition after oral doses. Clin Pharm Ther 32:98–106.

Bryant, J. (1981). Suicide by ingestion of caffeine. Arch Pathol Lab Med 105:685–686.

Cameron, O., J. Modell, and M. Hariharan (1990). Caffeine and human cerebral blood flow: a positron emission tomography study. Life Sci 47 (13): 1141–1146.

Chelsky, L., Cutler, J., Griffith, K. et al. (1990). Caffeine and ventricular arrhythmias: an electrophysiologic approach. JAMA (17):2236–2240.

Commission of the European Communities (1983). Report of the Scientific Committee for Food on Caffeine. Office for Official Publications of the European Communities.

Eisele, J. and D. Reay (1980). Deaths related to coffee enemas. JAMA 244 (14): 1608–1609.

Graham, T. and Spriet, L. (1991). Performance and metabolic responses to a high caffeine dose during prolonged exercise. J Appl Physiol, 71 (6) 2292–2298.

Iversen, S., P. Murphy, T. Leakey et al. (1984). Unsuspected caffeine toxicity complicating theophylline therapy. Hum Toxicol 3 (6):509–512.

Karadsheh, N., P. Kussie and D. Linthicum (1991). Inhibition of acetylcholinesterase by caffeine, anabasine, methyl pyrolidine and their derivatives. Toxicology Letters 55 (3):335–342.

Khanna, N. and S. Somani (1984). Maternal coffee drinking and unusually high concentration of caffeine in newborn. J Clin Toxicol 22(5) 473–483.

Labow, R. (1983). Effects of caffeine being studied for treatment of apnea in newborns. Can Med Ass J 129:230–231.

Lacroix, C., J. Nouveau, G. Laine et al. (1985). Interaction théophylline-caféine chez des brochopathes atteints d'insuffisance cardiaque et hépatique. Press Méd 14:1340.

Levy, M. and E. Zylber-Katz (1982). Caffeine metabolism and coffee attributed sleep disturbances. Clin Pharmacol Ther 33:770–775.

Lewin, Louis (1931). Phantastica: narcotic and stimulating drugs, their use and abuse. Second English edition, translated by P.H.Wirth, Ph.C, B.Sc. New York: E.P. Dutton & Company.

Marks, V. and J. Kelly (1973). Absorption of caffeine from tea, coffee, and coca cola. Lancet 1:827.

Mathew, R. and W. Wilson (1991). Substance abuse and cerebral blood flow. Am J Psychiatry 148 (3):292–305.

McGee, M. (1980). Caffeine poisoning in a 19-year old female. J Forensic Sci 25 (1): 29–32.

Morgan, P. and M. Durcan (1990). Caffeine-induced seizures: apparent proconvulsant activity of n-ethyl carboxamidoadenosine (NECA). Life Sci 47 (1):1–8.

Mrvos, R., P. Reilly, B. Dean et al. (1989). Massive caffeine ingestion resulting in death. Vet Hum Toxicol 31 (6):571–572.

Petersen, O. (1991). Actions of caffeine. News Physiol Sci 6 (APR):98–99.

Robertson, D., J. Frölich, R. Carr et al. (1978). Effects of caffeine on plasma renin activity, catecholamines and blood pressure. N Engl J Med 298 (4):181–186.

Ståhle, L., Segersvärd, S. and Ungersted, U. (1992). Drug distribution studies with microdialysis III: caffeine and theophylline in blood, brain and other tissues in rats. Life Sci, 49:1843–1852.

Stavric, B. (1988). Methylxanthines: toxicity to humans. 2. Caffeine. Fd Chem Toxic 26 (7):645–662.

Stavric, B. (1992). An update on research with coffee/caffeine (1989–1990). Fd Chem Tox, 30:533–555.

Strubelt, O., A. Hoffman, C. Siegers and J. Sierra-Callejas (1976). On the pathogenesis of cardiac necrosis induced by theophylline and caffeine. Acta Pharmacol Toxicol 39:383–392.

Thompson, C. (1928). The quacks of old London. New York, London, Paris: Brentano's Ltd.

Ullrich, D., Compagnone, D., Münch, B. et al (1992). Urinary caffeine metabolites in man. Age-dependent changes and pattern in various clinical situations. Euro J Clin Pharmacol, 43:167–172.

Vick, J., V. Whitehurst, E. Herman and T. Balazs (1989). Cardiotoxic effects of the combined use of caffeine and isoproterenol in the minipig. J Toxicol and Environ Health 26:425–435.

Zuskin, E., P. Duncan and J. Douglas (1983). Pharmacological characterization of extracts of coffee dusts. Br J Ind Med 40:193–198.

2.3 KHAT

2.3.1 History

Khat is an evergreen that grows at high altitudes in East Africa and on the Arabian peninsula. Its leaves contain a naturally occurring psychostimulant, closely related in structure to both ephedrine and amphetamine. Khat first came to the notice of Europeans in 1762, when the botanist Peter Forskal found it growing on the mountain slopes in Yemen (Pantelis et al. 1989). The habit of chewing Khat leaves is, however, much older. There are historical references as far back as the thirteenth century, when the Arab physician Naguib Ad-Din gave Khat leaves to soldiers to relieve fatigue (Giannini et al. 1986). Ad-Din might not have been the first ever to give soldiers psychostimulants, but he was certainly one of the earliest to experiment with performance-enhancing drugs. Since Ad-Din's pioneering experiments the practice has been repeated many times. Aschenbrant gave cocaine to Prussian recruits during the Franco Prussian war; Japan and the Allies issued amphetamines to their troops during World War II.

In 1852 James Vaughn, an English surgeon, published illustrations along with an account of Khat chewing in the *Pharmaceutical Gazette* (Vaughn 1852). Figure 2.3.1 is from Vaughn's paper. Vaughn speculated that the principal reason for khat's popularity was the fact that, unlike alcohol, its use was not forbidden by the Koran. Khat chewing is usually a social event, sessions often lasting for hours. In some areas of Africa where Khat chewing is still popular (the WHO estimates that there are still millions of khat users), houses often have a special room, called a *muffraj*, just for Khat chewing. The normal dose consumed at any one time is 100 to 200 grams of leaves and stems are chewed over a 3 to 4 hour period (Max, 1991). An occasional solitary individual will chew to increase his work capacity. Users describe increased feelings of alertness and an improved ability to concentrate. Use is also said to make people friendlier and improve the flow of ideas (Kennedy, Teague, and Fairbanks 1980). Nonetheless, use of this material conforms to most definitions of addiction. Chewers attempting to secure their daily supply of leaves will to so to the exclusion of all other activities. In Yemen 4% of all arable land is used to grow khat, and in Djibouti, 10% of the country's revenues is derived from taxes on khat (Max, 1991). Anecdotal reports from Somalia suggest that soldiers from warring clans dose themselves liberally with khat before going into combat.

2.3.2 Chemistry and Clinical Studies

Cathinone is (s)-2-Amino-1-phenyl-1-propanone. Its formula is $C_9H_{11}NO$, with a molecular weight of 165.23. It is composed of 72.5%

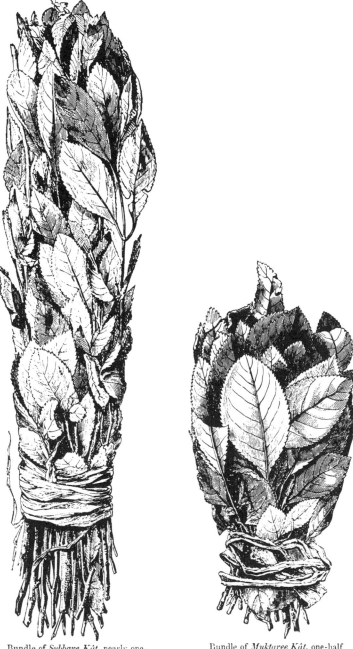

Bundle of *Subbare Kát*, nearly one-half the natural size.

Bundle of *Muktaree Kát*, one-half the natural size.

Figure 2.3.1 Khat leaves
This drawing from 1852 was the first illustration of Khat to appear in the English literature. Khat abuse is still a problem in some parts of Africa, where some of the gratuitous violence in areas such as Somalia is attributed to Khat abuse.

carbon, 7.4% hydrogen, 9.4% nitrogen, and 10.7% oxygen. The hydrochloride crystals ($C_9H_{11}ClNO$) have a melting point of 189–190°C.

If many of the mood alterations induced by Khat sound like those produced by amphetamine, it is not by chance. The active ingredient, cathinone, has the same basic configuration as amphetamine. A second active component, cathine, is much less active because its lipid solubility is much lower than cathinone's. With the passage of time cathinone is rapidly converted to cathine, and the result is a considerable loss of potency. Only fresh leaves have any commercial value, and the fragile nature of the product probably explains why it is not more widely distributed (Giannini 1986) (Critchlow 1987).

Other than knowing that Khat is rapidly absorbed across the oral mucosa, that it is mainly metabolized by the liver (WHO Advisory Group 1980), and that very little is excreted in the urine (Kalix and Braenden 1985), not much else is known about the pharmacokinetics of this compound. Urine levels were measured in six volunteers, 2, 4, 6 and 8 hours after taking 0.5 mg/kg of optically pure (S)-(-)cathinone. Resultant levels were from 0.2 to 3.8 μg/mL for the parent compound, 7.2 to 46 μg/mL for (R,S)-(-)norephedrine, and 0.5 to 2.5 μg/L for (R,R)-(-) norpseudoephedrine (Mathys and Brenneisen 1992). It is not known if the normal antibody-based screening tests for amphetamine would be sufficiently cross-reactive to detect this compound, but it seems unlikely.

Khat chewing produces symptoms consistent with sympathetic activation. There are both positive inotropic and chronotropic effects. Chewing khat causes elevations in blood pressure, temperature and respiratory rate, with inconsistent effects on heart rate. In isolated heart preparations, cathinone causes increased release of norepinephrine (Wagner, 1982). Khat also causes chronic constipation and reduced milk production in nursing mothers. Most of these effects are transient. There have been reports that in some parts of Saudi Arabia the only patients seen with oral cancers are those with long histories of khat chewing (Soufi, Kameswaran and Maltani 1991).

Papers in the older literature described cerebral hemorrhage, myocardial ischemia and pulmonary edema (Halbach 1972). Animal studies have shown that cathinone releases dopamine and, at very high concentrations, blocks dopamine uptake (Wagner 1982). Cathinone has never been evaluated for neurotoxicity in animals and, lacking autopsy information, the situation in humans remains unclear.

There have been no published autopsy studies. Khat's cardiovascular effects appear to be catechol related, but plasma catecholamines have not been measured. Urinary catechol excretion is increased after Khat chewing. Unlike acute cocaine abuse, where prolactin levels are depressed (see section 1.10.8 on cocaine's hormonal effects), and in spite of reports of decreased lactation, Khat chewing seems not to affect prolactin levels (Nencini et al. 1983). Because the absorption of cathinone

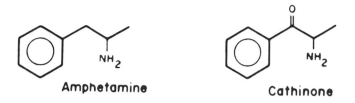

Amphetamine   **Cathinone**

Figure 2.3.2 Cathinone molecule
Many of Khat's effects are similar to those produced by amphetamine. The structures of both molecules bear strong resemblances to each other.

from chewed leaves is relatively slow, and because the breakdown of cathinone to cathine is relatively rapid, blood levels tend to plateau, which may explain why episodes of florid toxicity seem to be uncommon (Max, 1991).

Khat rapidly loses its potency, so its widespread use is doubtful outside of the sub-Sahara. However, air transport is possible and home cultivation isn't very difficult, no doubt explaining sporadic reports of Khat-associated psychosis in the UK or U.S. For all physiologic and pathologic purposes, Khat's effects are basically those of amphetamine. Since amphetamine is abundant and inexpensive in the United States, Khat is unlikely to become an important drug of abuse any time soon.

References

Critchlow, S. and Siefert, R. (1987). Khat-induced paranoid psychosis. Br J Psychiat 150:247–249.

Giannini, AJ, H Burge, JM Shaheen and WA Price (1986). Khat: another drug of abuse. J Psychoactive Drugs 18 (2):155–158.

Group, WHO Advisory (1980). Review of the pharmacology of khat. Bulletin on Narcotics 31:83–99.

Halbach, H. (1972). Medical Aspects of the chewing of khat leaves. Bull Wld Hlth Org 47:21–29.

Kalix, P. and O Braenden (1985). Pharmacological aspects of the chewing of khat leaves. Pharm Rev 37:149–164.

Kennedy, JG, J Teague and L Fairbanks (1980). Qat use in North Yemen and the problem of addiction: a study in medical anthropology. Culture, Med and Psych 4:311–344.

Mathys, K. and Brenneisen, R. (1992). Determination of (S)-(-)cathinone and its metabolites (R,S)-K(-)norephedrine and (R,R)-(-) norpseudoephedrine in urine by high-performance liquid chromatography with photodiode--array detection. J Chromatogr 593:1–2.

Max, B. (1991). This and that: the ethnopharmacology of simple phenethyl-amines, and the question of cocaine and the human heart. Trends Pharm Sci 12:320–333.

Nencini, P, MC Anania, AM Ahmed et al. (1983). Physiological and neuroen-docrine effects of Khat in man. In Proceedings of First International

Conference on Khat: Health and socio-economic aspects of Khat use. Edited by B. Shahander, R. Geadah, A. Tounge and J. Rolli. 148–152. Lausanne: International Council on Alcohol and Addictions.

Pantelis, C, CG Hindler and JC Taylor (1989). Use and abuse of khat (Catha edulis): a review of the distribution, pharmacology, side effects and a description of psychosis attributed to khat chewing. Psychological Med 19:657–668.

Soufi, HE, Kameswaran, M. and Malatani, T. (1991). Khat and oral cancer. J Laryngol and Otology, 105 (8) 643–645.

Vaughn, J. (1853). Notes upon the drugs observed at Aden, Arabia. Pharm J:268–271.

Wagner, GC. Preston, K, Ricaurte, GA et al. (1982). Neurochemical similarities between *d,l.-* cathinone and *d*-amphetamine. Drug Alcohol Depend 9:279–284.

2.4 EPHEDRINE

2.4.1 HISTORY

Ephedrine is a naturally occurring stimulant with medically useful properties. Like amphetamine, it is a mixed-acting agent. It is an adrenergic receptor agonist, and it also causes the increased release of catecholamines. When first introduced, purified ephedrine was thought to be too toxic for clinical use, but in 1930 Chen and Schmidt published a comprehensive paper recommending ephedrine in the treatment of asthma (Chen and Schmidt 1930), and ephedrine was soon very much in demand. It quickly replaced epinephrine, which was the only effective agent available at the time. Ephedrine rapidly became the first-line drug against asthma, and as it became more popular concerns arose about its availability. The possibility of an ephedrine shortage fostered research on ways to synthesize it. Amphetamines were created largely as a byproduct of those efforts. The anticipated ephedrine shortage never emerged, but ephedrine is still in use today as a component of some asthma and headache medications. Its most important use, however, is not medicinal. Clandestine laboratories use ephedrine as a precursor in the manufacture of methamphetamine, and many states now restrict ephedrine distribution.

Naturally occurring ephedrine is obtained from Ma Huang (*Ephedra vulgaris*), a herb that has been used by Chinese physicians for at least 5,000 years. Fifteenth-century Chinese texts recommend it as an antipyretic and antitussive, and it was used in Russia to treat arthritic symptoms. Indians and Spaniards in the Southwest used it to treat venereal diseases (Grinspoon and Hedblom 1975). *Ephedra* species are found around the world, but the ephedrine content may vary quite considerably. Herbal teas are still brewed from it and have been referred to by a variety of names including teamsters' tea, Mormon tea and chaparral tea (Max 1991).

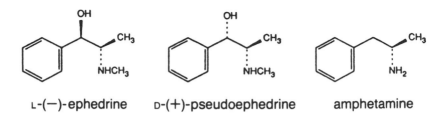

L-(−)-ephedrine   D-(+)-pseudoephedrine   amphetamine

Figure 2.4 Ephedrine and pseudoephedrine
Ephedrine's principal importance is as a precursor in the illicit production of methamphetamine, however, ephedrine is a potent stimulant in its own right and has significant abuse potential.

When compared to other stimulants, ephedrine has relatively greater peripheral effects and, in theory, less ability to produce central stimulation. In therapeutic doses it, and its optical isomer pseudo-ephedrine, are used as nasal decongestants and bronchodilators chiefly because they are thought to be free of CNS side effects. Ephedrine's CNS stimulating properties are, nonetheless, quite considerable and it is somewhat surprising that it is not more widely abused (Martin et al. 1971). Filipinos have, for many years, smoked a mixture of ephedrine and caffeine called Shabu. In the late 1980's Shabu smoking gave way to the practice of smoking methamphetamine ("ice").

2.4.2 CHEMISTRY AND METABOLISM

Ephedrine is alpha-[1-(Methylamino)ethyl]benzene-methanol. Its formula is $C_{10}H_{15}NO$, with a molecular weight of 165.23. It is composed of 72.7% carbon, 9.2% hydrogen, 8.5% nitrogen, and 9.7% oxygen. Isomeric forms include (±) ephedrine and (±)pseudoephedrine. The two naturally occurring isomers are (-)ephedrine and (+)pseudoephedrine. Racemic (±) ephedrine forms whitish crystals with a melting point of 79°C. Both ephedrine and pseudoephedrine are weak bases, with pKa's of 9.6 and 9.4 respectively. Both agents share properties with cocaine and with the amphetamines because they (1) stimulate beta receptors directly and (2) also cause the increased release of norepinephrine. As a result, both drugs have ß1 and ß2 activity. The number of beta receptors on human lymphocytes decreases rapidly after the administration of ephedrine. The density of binding sites drops to 50% of normal after 8 days of treatment, which may explain why there is a gradual loss of bronchodilator efficacy when ephedrine is taken chronically. Receptor density returns to normal five to seven days after the drug has been withdrawn (Neve and Molinoff 1986). The down regulation of receptors that occurs with ephedrine use is in marked contrast to cocaine, where chronic exposure appears not to affect receptor density at all (Costard-Jackle et al. 1989). Blood and tissue levels of ephedrine are poorly characterized. Most of a given dose is excreted unchanged in the urine, where it can be detected by a number of tests.

The International Olympic Committee, while not entirely banning ephedrine consumption, has ruled that urine levels of over 0.5 μg/mL indicate abuse and are grounds for disqualification. Unlike amphetamines, acidification of the urine has no effect on ephedrine excretion (Beckett and Wilkinson 1965). Ephedrine's elimination half-life is nearly 6 hours (Welling et al. 1971). The 5 μg level set by the IOC is probably unrealistically low. In a recent study healthy volunteers, given realistic doses of ephedrine-containing nasal spray (roughly 14 mg), were found to have urine levels ranging from 0.09 to 1.65 μg/mL.

2.4.3 CLINICAL STUDIES

The most frequently reported complications of ephedrine abuse are behavioral. Episodes of ephedrine-induced psychosis have been observed with some regularity (Herridge and A'Brook 1968) (Roxanas and Spalding 1977), but other sorts of medical complications are rare. There have been scattered reports of pseudoephedrine-associated hypertension (Mariani 1986), coronary artery spasm (Weiner et al. 1990), cardiomyopathy (To et al. 1980), and intracranial hemorrhage in association with ephedrine and pseudoephedrine overdose (Loizou et al. 1982) (Rutstein 1963) (Wooten et al. 1983). There are no reported autopsy studies. Baselt and Cravey mention the case of a young woman who died several hours after ingesting 2.1 grams of ephedrine combined with 7.0 grams of caffeine, but tissue findings weren't described. Her blood ephedrine level was 5 mg/L, while the concentration in the liver was 15 mg/kg (Baselt and Cravey 1989).

References

Baselt, R. and B. Cravey. Disposition of toxic drugs and chemicals in man. 3rd ed., Chicago, London: Year Book Medical Publishers, 1989.

Beckett, A. and G. Wilkinson (1965). Urinary excretion of (-)-methylephedrine, (-)-ephedrine, and (-)-norephedrine in man. J Pharm Pharmac 17 suppl: 107S–108S.

Costard-Jäckle, A., S. Jackle, Kates, R. and M. Fowler. Electrophysiological and biochemical effect of chronic cocaine administration. Circulation 80 (4 1989): II:15.

Grinspoon, L and P Hedblom. The Speed Culture: Amphetamine use and abuse in America. Cambridge, Mass and London, England: Harvard University Press, 1975.

Herridge, C. and M. A'Brook (1968). Ephedrine psychosis. Br Med J 2:160.

Lefebvre, R., Surmont, F., Bouckaert, J., and Moerman, E. (1992). Urinary excretion of ephedrine after nasal application in healthy volunteers. J Pharm Pharmacol, 44:672–675.

Loizou, L, J. Hamilton and S. Tsementzis (1982). Intracranial hemorrhage in association with pseudoephedrine overdose. J Neurol Neurosurg and Psychiat 45: 471–472.

Mariani, P. (1986). Pseudoephedrine induced hypertensive emergency treatment with labetalol. Am J Emerg Med 4:141–142.

Martin, W, J Sloan, J Sapira, and D Jasinski (1971). Physiologic, subjective and behavioral effects of amphetamine, methamphetamine, ephedrine, phenmetrazine and methylphenidate in man. Clin Pharmacol and Ther 12:245–248.

Max, B. (1991). This and that: the ethnopharmacology of simple phenethylamines, and the question of cocaine and the human heart. Trends Pharm Sci 12:329–333.

Neve, K. and P. Molinoff (1986). Effects of chronic administration of agonists and antagonists on the density of beta-adrenergic receptors. Am J Cardiol 57: 17F–22F.

Roxanas, M. and J. Spalding (1977). Ephedrine abuse psychosis. Med J Aust 2:639–640.

Rutstein, H. (1963). Ingestion of pseudoephedrine. Hypertension and unconsciousness following: report of a case. Arch Otolaryngol 77:145–147.

To, L., J. Sangster, D. Rampling et al. (1980). Ephedrine-induced cardiomyopathy. Med J Aust 2:35–36.

Weiner, I, A. Tilkian, and M. Palazzolo (1990). Coronary artery spasm and myocardial infarction in a patient with normal coronary arteries: temporal relationship to pseudoephedrine ingestion. Cath and Cardiovas Diag 20:51–53.

Welling, P., K. Lee, J. Patel et al. (1971). Urinary excretion of ephedrine in man without pH control following oral administration of three commercial ephedrine sulfate preparations. J Pharm Sci 60:1629–1634.

Wooten, M., M. Khangure and M. Murphy (1983). Intracerebral hemorrhage and vasculitis related to ephedrine abuse. Ann Neurol 13:337–340.

3 Synthetic Stimulants

3.1 AMPHETAMINE AND METHAMPHETAMINE

3.1.1 HISTORY

During the 1930's, there were concerns that the supply of naturally occurring ephedrine might not be sufficient to meet the needs of asthma sufferers. Several laboratories set out to synthesize ephedrine. A graduate student at UCLA, Gordon Alles, was assigned the task of synthesizing ephedrine as his thesis project. Alles reviewed the older literature and discovered research by Edeleano, who had synthesized and characterized the basic properties of the phenylisopropylamine molecule in 1887. Alles took the phenylisopropylamine molecule as a starting point, and tried to synthesize ephedrine from it. Alles never was able to synthesize ephedrine, but he did discover that phenylisopropylamine, later called dextroamphetamine, had novel stimulant properties. He gave samples to laboratory animals, and when he saw little evidence of toxicity, he tried it on himself. Amphetamine's mood-altering properties quickly became apparent. At an even earlier date, a Japanese chemist named Ogata had also started working on the same problem. He ended up synthesizing a different amphetamine. He called the result d-phenylisopropylmethylamine hydrochloride, later known as methamphetamine. Ephedrine was finally synthesized by Emde in 1929, but the anticipated ephedrine shortage never occurred.

Ogata licensed his method for producing methamphetamine to the Burroughs Wellcome Company, which sold methamphetamine in the United States under the brand name Methedrine™ until it was taken off the market in 1968. In 1932 Smith, Kline and French began to market a nasal inhaler containing Benzedrine™, their patent name for racemic ß-phenylisopropylamine (dl-amphetamine). The inhaler effectively relieved nasal congestion, but very soon after its introduction it became apparent that Benzedrine™ also relieved drowsiness and fatigue. Exaggerated claims by both drug manufacturers and the popular press led to wide-spread interest and even wider-spread amphetamine abuse.

The medical community responded to the introduction of amphetamine in almost exactly the same way it had responded to the introduction of cocaine 50 years earlier. Amphetamines were recommended for the same assortment of unrelated conditions that had been treated with cocaine at the turn of the century. Given what is known

EPIDEMIC OBESITY

your patients need
your kinds of help

The slender willpower of the obese patient is no match for the heavyweight forces of commercial temptation. Millions of dollars are spent to obsess him with the fattening, forbidden foods that have made obesity "epidemic" . . . while more millions promote the latest fads in diets. No wonder the patient, bedeviled and bewildered, loses the struggle against temptation . . .

For willpower alone is not enough. Your kinds of help are sorely needed. You alone can meet the patient's individual need for authoritative diagnosis and advice in the struggle against overweight. You alone can help the patient deal with underlying emotional factors and establish sensible eating habits.

It can be a difficult task. Temptation sometimes triumphs. But not as often, when your kinds of help include your selective use of . . .

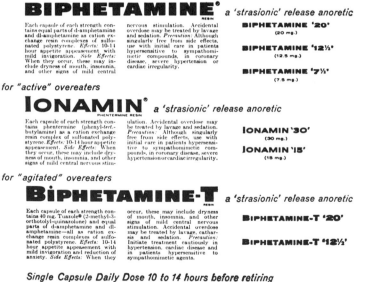

for "sedentary" overeaters

BIPHETAMINE®
a 'strasionic' release anoretic

Each capsule of each strength contains equal parts of d-amphetamine and dl-amphetamine as cation exchange resin complexes of sulfonated polystyrene. *Effects:* 10-14 hour appetite appeasement with mild invigoration. *Side Effects:* When they occur, these may include dryness of mouth, insomnia, and other signs of mild central nervous stimulation. Accidental overdose may be treated by lavage and sedation. *Precaution:* Although singularly free from side effects, use with initial care in patients hypersensitive to sympathomimetic compounds, in coronary disease, severe hypertension or cardiac irregularity.

BIPHETAMINE '20'
(20 mg.)

BIPHETAMINE '12½'
(12.5 mg.)

BIPHETAMINE '7½'
(7.5 mg.)

for "active" overeaters

IONAMIN®
PHENTERMINE RESIN
a 'strasionic' release anoretic

Each capsule of each strength contains phentermine (phenyl-tert.-butylamine) as a cation exchange resin complex of sulfonated polystyrene. *Effects:* 10-14 hour appetite appeasement. *Side Effects:* When they occur, these may include dryness of mouth, insomnia, and other signs of mild central nervous stimulation. Accidental overdose may be treated by lavage and sedation. *Precaution:* Although singularly free from side effects, use with initial care in patients hypersensitive to sympathomimetic compounds, in coronary disease, severe hypertension or cardiac irregularity.

IONAMIN '30'
(30 mg.)

IONAMIN '15'
(15 mg.)

for "agitated" overeaters

BIPHETAMINE-T
RESIN
a 'strasionic' release anoretic

Each capsule of each strength contains 40 mg. Tuazole® (2-methyl-3-orthotolyl-quinazolone) and equal parts of d-amphetamine and dl-amphetamine—all as cation exchange resin complexes of sulfonated polystyrene. *Effects:* 10-14 hour appetite appeasement with mild invigoration and reduction of anxiety. *Side Effects:* When they occur, these may include dryness of mouth, insomnia, and other signs of mild central nervous stimulation. Accidental overdose may be treated by lavage, cathartis and sedation. *Precaution:* Initiate treatment cautiously in hypertension, cardiac disease and in patients hypersensitive to sympathomimetic agents.

BIPHETAMINE-T '20'

BIPHETAMINE-T '12½'

Single Capsule Daily Dose 10 to 14 hours before retiring

STRASENBURGH

Figure 3.1 Medical use of amphetamine
For many years amphetamine was promoted as a treatment for obesity. When first introduced to the market, amphetamine was claimed to be something of a wonder drug. The same claims were made for amphetamine as were made for cocaine when it was first introduced. This advertisement was published in a 1961 issue of JAMA.

today, some of the earlier recommended uses for the amphetamines seem quite bizarre. At one point amphetamine was even recommended as a "valuable adjunct" in the treatment of seizures and schizophrenia. Bearing in mind that amphetamine-induced psychosis is thought, by some, to be a useful model for the study of schizophrenia, it's difficult to imagine just what sorts of reactions clinicians of the time were observing! Amphetamines were also said to be useful in treating barbiturate overdose, "caffeine mania", smoking, multiple sclerosis, myasthenia, head injuries, cerebral palsy, migraine, urticaria, sea sickness, dysmenorrhoea, ureteral colic, obesity, irritable colon, radiation sickness, Ekbom's syndrome, and other seemingly unrelated conditions, including loss of libido (Bett 1946).

It should be no surprise then, that amphetamine was also recommended for the treatment of morphine addiction. Freud's disastrous experiments of 1885 had apparently been quite forgotten by the mid 1940's. Troops of both the Allied and Axis forces were supplied with amphetamines during the war and, perhaps as a result, demand for amphetamine rapidly increased when the war was over. Laws limiting the distribution of amphetamine were enacted during the 1940's, but a regulatory lapse allowed the continued sale of Smith Kline's inhaler; inside each inhaler were eight folded-paper sections impregnated with 250 mg of amphetamine. Abusers opened the inhaler and chewed the papers. Friends mailed the strips to prison inmates and abuse within the prison system became a problem (Monroe and Drell 1947). In an escalating battle with would-be abusers, amphetamine manufacturers tried adding denaturants, such as emetine and picric acid to the strips, but abusers found ways to extract the amphetamine, or simply put up with the transient side effects.

Because of all the difficulties associated with their product, Smith, Kline and French reformulated it in 1949 and changed its name to Benzedrex™. The new formulation contained propylhexedrine, also a potent vasoconstrictor, but with only 1/12 the CNS stimulant potency of amphetamine. Smith Kline and French's patents expired in 1953, and almost immediately Wyeth, Rexall, Squibb, Eli Lilly, and WS Merrell entered the market with competing products. Abuse continued, and in 1959 the amphetamine inhaler was finally classified a prescription item.

The first amphetamine-related deaths were reported within a few years of amphetamine's introduction. The serious complications associated with amphetamine abuse are essentially the same as for cocaine: arrhythmic sudden death, stroke, psychosis, and rhabdomyolysis. There are no controlled studies to confirm the fact, but it seems that psychotic behavior is more common among amphetamine users than among cocaine users. Based on the number of case reports, cardiomyopathy also seems to be more common than in cocaine users, while myocardial infarction is a less common event. Most of these case reports are in the older literature, and mentions of toxicity were uncommon during the 1980's. Today amphetamine abuse is a relatively minor problem compared to cocaine. Amphetamine accounted for less than 1 per cent of drug related emergency room visits, and less than 2% of drug-related deaths reported in the DAWN survey for 1990. Cocaine, on the other hand, accounted for 22% of visits and 43% of the deaths (National Institute on Drug Abuse, 1992)

   With the appearance of smokable "ice," a pure form of (+) meth-amphetamine hydrochloride, case reports of toxicity began reappearing. Methamphetamine becomes "ice" when it crystallizes out of a saturated solution. Depending on how methamphetamine is prepared, and there are a number of possible ways, solvent is captured within the structure of the crystals. The type of solvent is a clue to what processes were used in the manufacture and may suggest where the illicit drug was made. The volatility of the solvent in which the methamphetamine is dissolved determines how large the resultant crystals will be. With very volatile solvents, like freon, crystallization is rapid and only very small crystals form. With less volatile solvents, such as methanol, larger crystals are produced. No matter the size of the crystals, they are all equally smokable.

   The first illicit "ice" labs were Japanese. They began operations in the early 1980's. Enforcement efforts by police convinced the illegal chemists to transfer their operations out of Japan to Korea. To this day, Korea remains the principal manufacturer of "ice." At first the market for this form of amphetamine was confined to Taiwan, Japan and the Philippines. Japanese and Korean abusers took it intravenously, but the Filipinos began smoking it. They were already used to smoking stimulants, having smoked Shabu (a mixture of ephedrine and caffeine) for years, and "ice" became immensely popular. Demand within the Filipino community was responsible for the introduction of "ice" into Hawaii. In the late 1980's Korean chemists emigrated and established illicit laboratories in Portland and Los Angeles. Most of their production was shipped back to the Philippines. In 1988 there were sporadic seizures of "ice" across the US. No labs were seized in 1989, but in 1990 the DEA seized 7 in California alone.

   Anecdotal reports suggest that cocaine users (crack smokers) don't particularly like "ice" because the high isn't as intense and it lasts too long. There has been very little cross-over between cocaine and amphetamine abusers, and that may explain why no real "ice" epidemic ever occurred. In addition to "ice", there are other structurally related compounds such as fenfluramine and phenylpropanolamine that share some common mechanisms of action and toxicity with methamphetamine. A few of these synthetic agents also have a potential for neurotoxicity that is not associated with methamphetamine use.

3.1.2 ILLICIT MANUFACTURE

   In 1958, the annual legal production of amphetamine was 75,000 pounds. By 1970 it had risen to over 200,000 pounds, enough to make

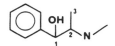

(+) pseudoephedrine

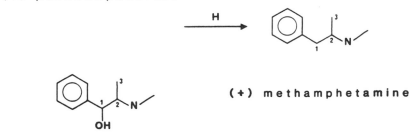

(+) methamphetamine

(-) ephedrine

Figure 3.1.2   Making methamphetamine
The most popular formula for making methamphetamine starts with ephedrine
and uses red phosphorus as a catalyst. Ephedrine used to be cheap and easily
available, but now its sales are controlled.

10 billion 5-mg tablets (Kaplan, 1985). Consumption today is difficult to
gauge. As the indications for amphetamine use became fewer and fewer,
and more complications were recognized, legal production fell off. As
legal manufacturers pulled out of the market, illegal labs began to fill the
void. In 1980, 150 illicit methamphetamine (as opposed to "ice") labs
were seized in the United States; by 1989 that number had risen to 650.
The increase has been driven by both increased demand and the lure of
quick profits. The lure must be very great, since at the current street
price of $500 a gram, an initial investment in $700 worth of chemicals
could yield a net profit of $2,500,000.

   During the 1970's the preferred method among "meth cooks"
began with phenyl-2-propanone (P2P) as the precursor. When P2P itself
became a controlled substance, clandestine chemists were also forced to
synthesize it. P2P can be synthesized in a number of ways: the most
frequently used approach starts with phenylacetic acid, acetic anhydride
and sodium acetate. P2P is then converted to methamphetamine by reductive amination. Methylamine, aluminum foil, mercuric chloride,
diethyl ether and isopropanol are required. Fairly high yields can be
obtained via this synthetic route. The reaction product is a racemic
mixture. Since the (+) form of methamphetamine is five times as potent
as the (-) isomer, the potency and yield of the final product can be quite
variable.

   Not only may the potency vary, but an assortment of contaminants may be introduced. Some of the contaminants have strong stimulant properties themselves (Soine 1986), while others may be quite toxic,

possibly more toxic than amphetamine, but the declining popularity of this synthetic route has diminished their importance (Van der Ark et al. 1978). Lead poisoning occurs in illicit amphetamine users (Allcott et al. 1987). Mercury in trace amounts can also be found (Soine 1988). Some samples have been analyzed which contained over 1,300 ppm of mercury, but unlike the cases of lead contamination, mercury-related illnesses have not been reported in amphetamine users.

Of late, interest has shifted to another route of synthesis. Either (-)-ephedrine or (+)-pseudoephedrine is converted to methamphetamine by reductive dehalogenation using red phosphorus as a catalyst. If (-)ephedrine is used as the starting point, the process generates (+) methamphetamine. Pseudoephedrine also yields dextro-methamphetamine. No matter what the isomer produced, contaminants will be present. As is true with the P2P route, some of these contaminants, particularly 2-(phenylmethyl)phenethylamine, may also be toxic in their own right. Unfortunately, the subject has not been studied in any detail (Soine, 1989). Red phosphorus synthesis has rapidly become the most popular way to manufacture illegal methamphetamine, and this has created an increased market demand for the main precursor, ephedrine. Until the red phosphorus route became popular, ephedrine was a non-prescription item, easily obtained from vitamin and organic food vendors. However, demand is now so great that many states are moving to restrict sales of ephedrine. Increasingly, large quantities are being purchased from Canada where the sale of amphetamine precursors is not controlled.

3.1.3 CHEMISTRY

Possible chemical designations include N,alpha-Dimethyl benzeneethanamine, d-N,alpha-dimethylphenethylamine, and d-deoxyephedrine. The drug has been sold under many proprietary names (Desoxyn, Hiropon, Isophen, Methedrine to name a few). Its formula is $C_{10}H_{15}N$, and its molecular weight is 149.2. It is 18.48% carbon, 10.13% hydrogen and 9.39% nitrogen, with a melting point of 170–175°C. The low melting point permits it to be smoked, regardless of the crystal size (Sekine and Nakahara 1987). Crystals have a bitter taste and are soluble in water, alcohol chloroform, and freon. Methamphetamine is not soluble in ether. Manipulation of the amphetamine's phenyl ring yields fenfluramine, a widely proscribed anorectic. Manipulation of the side chain has led to a the synthesis of a series of compounds with varying degrees of sympathomimetic activity.

3.1.4 ROUTES OF ADMINISTRATION

Methamphetamine can be swallowed, injected, smoked or "snorted." In spite of the publicity accorded to "ice" smoking, most users still prefer to inject it intravenously or take it orally. There is very

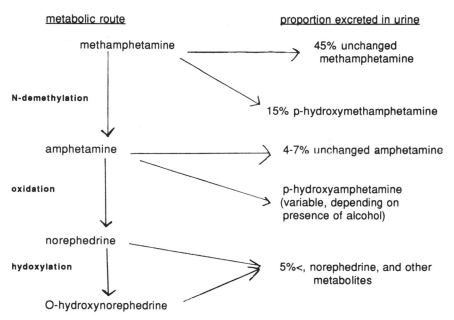

Figure 3.1.5.1 Methamphetamine metabolism
Metamphetamine is demethylated to produce amphetamine. Ephedrine and other analogues are not converted to amphetamine. Thus the presence of amphetamine in a sample containing methamphetamine is proof that methamphetamine, and not some harmless analogue, was taken.

little data regarding the blood levels that result from the different routes of administration. In one study a 10-mg dose given orally produced 30 ng/mL levels one hour later (Lebish et al. 1970), while a second study of 10 subjects given 12.5 mg found peak levels of 20 ng/mL at two hours, decreasing to 10 ng/mL at 24 hours (Driscoll et al. 1971). Similar studies on amphetamine produced comparable results, at least in terms of resultant blood levels. The problems with these observations is that they were done in relatively naive users. Tolerance to amphetamines quickly develops: intravenous abusers may inject several grams a day. The kinetics of large-dose intravenous abuse have not been evaluated, nor is there any data available on resultant blood levels after smoking, but in one study 160–200 mg of amphetamine given intravenously produced a one-hour plasma concentration of 269 ± ng/mL (Änggård et al. 1970). Measurements in methamphetamine users with obvious signs of behavioral toxicity have yielded comparable results. In Lebish's study of 7 patients with evidence of amphetamine toxicity, blood levels ranged from 105 ng/mL to 560 ng/mL (Lebish et al. 1970).

3.1.5 METABOLISM

Methamphetamine has a long half-life, nearly 12 hours. It is cleared from the blood by multiple routes. Roughly 20% is N-demethylated to form amphetamine and ephedrine derivatives which are also psychoactive (Caldwell et al. 1972) (Cho and Wright 1978). These compounds are further metabolized by a combination of deamination, p-hydroxylation and conjugation. Demethylation to amphetamine has evidentiary significance. Only minute amounts of (-)- methamphetamine are converted in this fashion, and other related compounds such as ephedrine are not converted at all. Accordingly, the presence of amphetamine in methamphetamine-containing specimens is confirmatory evidence that the restricted, psychoactive drug methamphetamine is being detected, and not some harmless analog. Current National Institute on Drug Abuse regulations prohibit the reporting of methamphetamine in a urine specimen unless (1) the methamphetamine level is over 500 ng/mL and (2) there is more than 200 ng/mL of amphetamine present.

Over a period of several days, up to 40% of a given dose of methamphetamine will appear unchanged in the urine. If the urine is acid, that amount may increase to over 75%. On the other hand, when the urine is extremely alkaline the amount excreted unchanged may drop to as low as 2% (Beckett and Rowland 1965). C^{14} tracer studies done in two volunteers disclosed that 23% of a given dose appeared in the urine within the first 24 hours. Other metabolites also appear in substantial quantities, including 4-hydroxymethamphetamine, norephedrine, and 4-hydroxynorephedrine (Caldwell et al. 1972). The (+) isomer of amphetamine is metabolized more rapidly than the (-) isomer. If the urine is acid the difference isn't of much consequence because then the major route of elimination is renal excretion. Evidently the general public is quite unaware of the fact that acidification of the urine hastens methamphetamine excretion. The underground press recommends drinking vinegar as a way to foil urine drug testing. Obviously, acidifying the urine will increase the probability of being caught. If the urine is alkaline, the difference in metabolic rate between the two assumes significance, because the (+) form is cleared about 5 hours more rapidly than the (-) isomer (17 hours vs. 12.7 hours) (Wan et al. 1978).

The metabolism of the amphetamine analogs varies considerably. After methamphetamine and amphetamine, the analog most likely to be encountered is methylphenidate (Ritalin™). Like the other amphetamines, it is rapidly absorbed after oral administration, reaching peak levels between 1 and 3 hours after ingestion (Dayton et al. 1970) (Wargin et al. 1983). In therapeutic settings, peak levels may be as high as 0.07 mg/L (Gualtieri et al. 1984). Unlike methamphetamine, methylphenidate has a short half-life of only 2 to 4 hours. First-pass hydrolysis to ritalinic acid occurs in the intestine, and about 80% of a given dose will appear in the

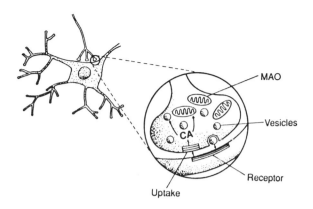

Figure 3.1.5.2 Effects of amphetamine on nerve endings
The effects of amphetamine on catechol metabolism are more complex than those of cocaine. In addition to blocking reuptake, amphetamine also causes increased release of neurotransmitters. Courtesy of Dr. Arthur K. Cho, Department of Pharmacology, UCLA School of Medicine.

urine as ritalinic acid. The peak plasma levels of both ritalin and ritalinic acid occur at the same tame. Another significant difference between methylphenidate and the other amphetamines is that the former has no effect on either dopamine or serotonin levels (Wagner et al. 1980)

3.1.6 TISSUE DISPOSITION

In the handful of autopsied dextroamphetamine deaths that have been reported, blood and tissue levels seems to be slightly higher than reported levels for methamphetamine (blood levels of 7 mg/L in Van Hoff's case and 11 mg/L in the case reported by Richards), though there are too few cases to permit any conclusions (Richards and Stephens 1973) (Von Hoof et al. 1974). In rabbits sacrificed one hour after intravenous methamphetamine injection, levels of methamphetamine in the liver were twice as high as levels in the blood. Levels of amphetamine, measured at the same time, were 8 times higher in the liver than in the blood. In the rabbit model, concentrations of both methamphetamine and amphetamine in skeletal muscle were equal to the concentration in the liver (Nagata 1990).

There is one case report of a woman with narcolepsy, maintained on 20 mg per day of amphetamine, who carried a child to term uneventfully. Amphetamine appears to concentrate in breast milk. Measurements made in the mother at 10 and 42 days after delivery demonstrated that amphetamine concentrations were much higher in the breast milk than in her plasma (Steiner, Envill, Hallberg, Rane 1984).

There is little data on the disposition of amphetamines in the fetus, though there is now a good experimental model. In pregnant ewes (125 days gestation is the equivalent of a 34-week human pregnancy), methamphetamine has been shown to quickly cross the placenta, appearing in fetal tissues 2.5 minutes after intravenous injection into the mother. Methamphetamine's half-life in ewes given 1.2 mg/kg is 39 minutes. The peak level in the ewe was 10.2 mg/L in and 7.2 mg/L in the fetus. Fetal half-life for methamphetamine was considerably longer than for the mother. Two hours after injection, levels were actually higher in the fetus than in the ewe. In this same study, tissue levels measured at 2 hours were, in every instance, higher than blood levels. The highest concentrations, both in ewe and fetus, were found in the intestine and lung, while the lowest concentrations were found in the brain and heart (Burchfield et al. 1991). This is exactly the opposite of the pattern observed with cocaine.

The results of two human studies are consistent with the experimental model. In one case a 24-year chronic amphetamine abuser delivered a premature, low Apgar, 2-pound, 7.5-ounce child that expired at 4 hours. Autopsy findings were consistent with intrauterine anoxia. Both methamphetamine and amphetamine levels were quite low (0.246 μg/g to 0.857 μg/g and, 0.030 μg/g to 0.120 μg/g). Methamphetamine concentration was highest in the lungs and lowest in the liver. The concentration in the lungs was nearly three times that in the blood (Garriott and Spruill 1973). In another case, an amphetamine-abusing mother, who had been using intravenous amphetamine a few hours prior to delivery, gave birth to twins that died 1 to 2 hours after birth. The highest levels were in the kidney and liver and the lowest levels were in the blood and brain. Methamphetamine levels ranged from 4.53 mg/kg to 11.0 mg/kg. Amphetamine levels were less than 15% of the methamphetamine levels, ranging from 0.18 mg/kg to 1.40 mg/kg (Bost et al. 1989). Decreases in birth weight, length, head circumference and gestational age have all been described as consequences of maternal amphetamine abuse (Gillogley et al. 1990). Tissue level measurements in adult deaths are extremely limited.

As is true with almost all of the abused drugs, the phenomenon of tolerance makes tissue and blood levels all but impossible to interpret. Methamphetamine levels in fatal cases have ranged from less than 1 mg/L to over 14 mg/L with associated amphetamine levels that are usually less than one tenth as high (Cravey and Reed, 1970) (Kojima, Une, Yashiki, 1983) (Matoba, Onishi, Shikata 1985) (Baselt, Cravey 1989) (Yamamoto, Watanabe, Ukita et al. 1992).

Detection of methamphetamine in the blood, urine, or liver is not, however, always proof of drug abuse. Selegiline (Eldepryl™, Deprenyl™) is a MAO inhibitor used in the treatment of parkinsonism. It is a derivative of phenethylamine, and two of its principal metabolites are amphetamine and methamphetamine. Both may accumulate in substantial amounts in patients receiving anti-parkinson therapy. In such cases, the clinical history will be necessary to make the correct diagnosis. Data on the tissue disposition of the amphetamine analogs is also sparse. A woman who died after injecting 40 mg of methylphenidate intravenously had a blood concentration of 2.8 mg/L (Levine et al. 1986). In that same case the concentration in the liver was 2.1 mg/kg, while the bile contained 5.7 mg/L and the kidneys 3.0 mg/kg. There is little accumulation of methylphenidate in the body. The blood level of a woman who died during a caesarean section, and who had presumably not had any drug for a number of hours, was only 9 ng/mL (Lundquest et al. 1987).

3.1.7 Interpreting Amphetamine Levels

Methamphetamine levels are difficult, if not impossible, to interpret and so are of little clinical value. Long-term methamphetamine use sets in train a complicated series of interactions affecting both blood levels and behavioral responses. As is true in cases of cocaine abuse, death may be associated with very low or very high levels. Unlike alcohol, but like cocaine, blood levels do not correlate well with impairment. Since tolerance occurs, very high levels should not be surprising (Von Hoof et al. 1974) (Kojima et al. 1983; Kojima et al. 1984) (Zalis and Parmley 1963) (Cravey and Reed 1970) (Orrenius and Maehly 1970). Were it not for the problems associated with tolerance, it seems likely that blood levels would parallel those associated with cocaine toxicity. In the past it was thought that cocaine levels in the range of 5 mg/L were uniformly fatal. With more experience it has become clear that levels many times higher may be observed as incidental findings at autopsy. Since the degree of tolerance for any drug is impossible to determine at autopsy, attributing any significance to isolated levels is unwise. Low levels, sometimes thought to be incidental findings in association with traumatic deaths, are hard to interpret. Very low levels (0.7 μg/mL) have been observed in patients dying of what could only be described as classic stimulant toxicity, with agitation, hypertension, tachycardia and hyperthermia (Fukunaga et al. 1987b).

In animal studies methamphetamine and amphetamine are stable in most tissues, no matter the degree of environmental exposure. Nagata found the concentrations of both drugs in whole blood, liver, and skeletal muscle were nearly unchanged after two years of storage in sealed tubes, and only decreased by half in samples of bone exposed to the air over a 2-year period. The amphetamine content of marrow submerged in tap water for 2 years hardly decreased from baseline. Levels in blood and urine stains did decrease very significantly with storage, but not to below detectable levels (Nagata 1990).

In NIDA regulated testing programs, a urine screening test is not considered to be positive for amphetamine unless immunologic screening tests demonstrate that the specimen contains amphetamine or methamphetamine in concentrations of 1,000 ng/mL or more, and subsequent GC/MS analysis shows a concentration of at least 500 ng/mL. First-generation amphetamine screening tests often cross reacted with compounds such as ephedrine, phenylpropanolamine, and diet pills such as phenteramine (Wayamine), phenmetrazine (Preludin), and fenfluramine (Pondimin). The Vicks decongestant inhaler contains the levo rotatory isomer of methamphetamine. This isomer has minimal CNS activity, but on both screening and confirmatory tests it may be confused with methamphetamine, unless special steps are taken. Newer generation screening tests, such as the EMIT d.a.u. monoclonal immunoassay were supposed to have solved this problem, but false positive screening tests still can occur. Agents structurally dissimilar to the amphetamines, such as chlorpromazine and brompheniramine, have been noted to cause positive reactions which are not confirmed by subsequent GC/MS testing (Olsen et al. 1992). Even though manufacturers do extensive premarketing tests to rule out cross reactivity of their reagents with other compounds, perforce they are unable to test all of the possible metabolites. For that reason, among others, the results of screening tests can never be accepted without a confirmatory test that utilizes a different technology.

In addition to problems separating isomers of methamphetamine, confusion with other compounds is also possible. Because specimens containing high levels of ephedrine were incorrectly analyzed as containing methamphetamine (Anon, 1990), NIDA issued a regulation requiring that, even if CG/MS showed > 500 ng/mL of methamphetamine, specimens do not qualify as a positive unless amphetamine is also detected in the sample. The reasons for the confusion relate to the analytic process itself. In some instances contaminants in a derivitizing agent (heptaflurobutyric anhydride, also referred to as HFBA) were responsible for the confusion, while in other cases the temperature at which samples were injected played a role (Wu et al. 1992). Whatever the cause for the error, humans do not metabolize ephedrine to amphetamine, so the presence of amphetamine in a specimen is additional proof that methamphetamine and not ephedrine, was responsible for the positive test result (DHHS,1990).

3.1.8 Toxicity by Organ System

3.1.8.1 Cardiovascular

Amphetamine's adverse effects on the heart are well established. For the most part, amphetamine toxicity shares common mechanisms with cocaine toxicity. In both instances, the underlying mechanism seems to be catechol excess. There are, however, some differences. Considering the vast numbers of individuals who have taken amphetamines, especially in the past, the reported incidence of cardiac events is lower than with cocaine. More than 50 years have passed since amphetamine became commercially available, and there are still fewer cases of amphetamine-associated infarction in the literature than reports of cocaine related myocardial infarction. On the other hand, cardiomyopathy seems to be a complication of amphetamine abuse more often than does cocaine abuse.

Amphetamines and other phenylisopropylamines such as pseudoephedrine (Sudafed™), phenylpropanolamine (multiple cold and diet pills) and propylhexedrine (Benzedrex™) have a more complicated mechanism of action than cocaine. Cocaine and the amphetamines both cause norepinephrine to accumulate in the synaptic cleft, secondarily producing elevated levels of norepinephrine in the blood stream. But amphetamines exert multiple other effects. Amphetamine is also transported into the presynaptic terminal, where it inhibits monoamine oxidase and prevents further storage of catecholamines within the nerve ending (Cho 1990). These actions taken together lead to increased sympathetic stimulation and increased circulating levels of catecholamines in the periphery (Fukunaga et al. 1987a).

High circulating catecholamine levels are cardiotoxic, no matter what the underlying cause. The very same morphologic alterations produced by amphetamine abuse have also been seen in patients with pheochromocytoma (Szakacs and Cannon A 1958), cocaine abuse (Tazelaar et al. 1987), and catechol infusions (Rona 1985). Based on the number of case reports published, amphetamine cardiotoxicity seems to be manifested most often as arrhythmic sudden death. Reports of amphetamine-related sudden death were first published shortly after amphetamine became commercially available. In 1939 the *Journal of the American Medical Association* carried a report describing a student who had collapsed during an examination and could not be resuscitated. He had taken a 10-mg tablet of dextroamphetamine shortly before the examination had begun. The only finding at autopsy was visceral congestion (Smith 1939).

In Japan, where amphetamine abuse has been a problem since it was first invented, methamphetamine induced arrhythmic sudden death is a recognized entity. Autopsy studies have shown typical catechol injuries in a pattern that is impossible to distinguish from that seen in cocaine abusers with sudden death. Myocardial alterations have included focal subendocardial hemorrhage, usually surrounding areas of myocyte disruption, sometimes with lymphocytic infiltrates (Fukunaga et al. 1987b). Just as in cocaine abusers, interstitial fibrosis can be a prominent finding. Granularity of myocyte fibers and occasional myocyte hypertrophy with disarray has also been seen. Medial hypertrophy of the arterioles has been also been observed (Matoba et al. 1985) (Fukunaga et al. 1987b). Other proven cases have been associated only with pulmonary and visceral congestion (Cravey and Reed 1970). The changes were not necessarily associated with very high blood levels.

There is evidence that just about all phenylisopropylamines can cause catechol mediated cardiotoxicity. Phenylpropanolamine given to rats produces a typical pattern of injury indistinguishable from the pattern seen after infusions of isoproterenol or norepinephrine (Pentel et al. 1987). Clinical studies have demonstrated increased creatinine kinase and MB isoenzyme levels, along with ventricular arrhythmias and repolarization abnormalities in patients taking phenylpropanolamine containing decongestant and appetite suppressant formulations (Pentel et al. 1982). Propylhexedrine (Benzedrex™) associated sudden deaths, which in the past were fairly common, are frequently accompanied by myocardial fibrosis (Anderson et al. 1979). The histologic changes in propylhexedrine related deaths are more difficult to interpret than with the other amphetamines. Most of the reported deaths were in intravenous drug abusers with pulmonary granulomas and pulmonary hypertension. Myocardial fibrosis is common in that subpopulation, making the role of stimulant abuse more difficult to access (Kringsholm and Christoffersen 1987).

Morphologic alterations, similar to those observed in cases of methamphetamine-related sudden death, are reproducible in animal models of amphetamine poisoning. Unanesthetized dogs, given 10 mg/kg of amphetamine and autopsied 1.5 to 22 hours later, had subendocardial hemorrhages. In some cases the hemorrhages were extensive enough to disrupt the conduction system. There was also myocardial fiber necrosis scattered throughout both ventricles, and many of the myocytes appeared eosinophilic and granular. In short, all the features associated with catechol toxicity were reproduced. In more extreme cases, hemorrhage into the mitral valve leaflets and in the papillary muscles occurs (Zalis et al. 1967). This pattern of bleeding into the leaflets and papillary muscles can be produced by infusing large amounts of norepinephrine. The connection was first recognized by over thirty years ago (Szakacs and Cannon, 1958) (Szakacs et al. 1959).

In spite of convincing laboratory evidence of amphetamine induced cardiotoxicity, and the fact that chest pain related to amphetamine ingestion was noted as early as 1936 (Anderson and Scott 1936), myocardial infarction has only rarely been observed. Infarcts have been reported after "snorting" methamphetamine (Furst et al. 1990), after intravenous injection (Packe et al. 1990) (Lam and Goldschlager 1988) (Carson et al. 1987), and after the oral use of various amphetamine analogs, including propylhexedrine (Marsden and Sheldon 1972), dextrofenfluramine (Evrard et al. 1990), pseudoephedrine (Wiener, 1990). None of these reports have been accompanied by autopsy studies, but in several cases angiography was done and it was normal. The absence of fixed lesions in these patients suggests that the infarcts were due to coronary spasm, but the underlying mechanism is not known. Any or all of the same factors cited in the case of cocaine-related spasm could also be involved in amphetamine-related spasm.

Stimulant-related cardiomyopathy has occurred in association with amphetamine (Smith et al. 1976) (Call et al. 1982) (Jacobs 1989), (+) methamphetamine (Matoba et al. 1985) (Hong et al. 1991) propylhexedrine (Croft et al. 1982), and methylphenidate (Stecyk et al. 1985) use. In one case endomyocardial biopsy showed patchy interstitial fibrosis with scattered mononuclear cells (Jacobs 1989). Another report described a 45-year-old oral amphetamine abuser who died of heart failure. Her heart was enlarged (530 grams) and the coronary arteries were widely patent. Histologic examination revealed widespread interstitial edema with scattered lymphocytic and histocytic infiltrates. There was degeneration of individual fibers and patchy myocardial fibrosis. Electron microscopic studies showed myofilaments with rupture and disarray. The mitochondria contained many large electron-dense granules (Smith et al. 1976). This particular finding is associated with mitochondrial calcium overload, which is the myocytes' response to both ischemia and to excessive catechol stimulation. In another case, patchy myocardial fibrosis, without infiltrates, was observed in the heart of a young "ice" smoker who died of an acute posterior wall infarct (Hong et al. 1991). "Reversible" cardiomyopathy has been reported as a complication of both amphetamine and cocaine use (Call et al. 1982) (Chokshi et al. 1989) (Henzlova et al. 1991) (Jacobs 1989). In all cases, there was acute onset of heart failure associated with decreased cardiac output and increased wedge pressure that eventually resolved with medical therapy. Since the patients survived, the underlying morphologic changes, if any, remain uncharacterized. It should be emphasized that the term "cardiomyopathy" is often misused. The diagnosis should be reserved for only those patients with normal coronary arteries and specific myocyte changes demonstrable on biopsy or autopsy.

The most perplexing aspect of amphetamine related cardiotoxicity is the infrequency with which it is reported. It may be that less florid lesions are not being seen at autopsy, but that would still not explain the relative absence of clinical case reports. The situation may be analogous to what occurs with cocaine abuse. When cocaine is "snorted" absorption is gradual and peak blood levels are much lower than those achieved after cocaine is smoked. Perhaps oral use of amphetamines prevents most people from developing cardiotoxic levels. Another possibility to consider is that tolerance develops so quickly that users are, in some way, protected.

3.1.8.2 Pulmonary toxicity

Pulmonary congestion may or may not be seen in acute fatalities (Von Hoof et al. 1974) (Richards and Stephens 1973), but the sort of pattern seen in classic narcotic related deaths has not been reported. The most commonly reported finding in the lung of stimulant abusers is thromboembolic arteriopathy. When drug tablets are crushed and injected intravenously, the insoluble fillers (microcrystalline cellulose, cornstarch or cotton fibers) contained in the tablet become trapped in the pulmonary microvasculature. Small vessels thrombose, and foreign body granulomas form. Eventually some of the foreign material will work its way into the perivascular spaces, leading to further granuloma formation and more fibrosis (Tomashefski and Hirsch 1980) (Tomashefski et al. 1981). If injections are repeated often enough, there is a net reduction in the size of the pulmonary vascular bed and an increase in pulmonary vascular resistance. At autopsy organizing and recanalizing thrombi will be seen, along with easily identifiable birefringent material (Rajs et al. 1984). Histologically, this sort of pulmonary hypertension can be distinguished from the much rarer primary variety by the presence of plexiform lesions at branching points of the obstructed small arteries (Pietra and Rüttner 1987) (Pietra et al. 1989). This complication seems to be associated more with some abused drugs than with others. In general, heroin abusers are much more prone to thromboembolic arteriopathy than stimulant abusers. Of the commonly abused stimulants, methylphenidate (Ritalin™) is the agent most often associated with pulmonary complications.

Granuloma formation and pulmonary fibrosis have been recognized as complications of methylphenidate abuse for many years (Hahn et al. 1969) (Lewman 1972) (Arnett et al. 1976) (Waller et al. 1980) (Levine et al. 1986), and clinical reports suggest that a newer dosage form of methylphenidate (Ritalin -SA™) is particularly likely to be associated with pulmonary symptoms in intravenous abusers. In one study more than 90% of the patients were found to have abnormalities of pulmonary function (both obstructive and restrictive) (Parran and Jasinski 1991). However, if there is anything unique about the histopathology of methylphenidate abuse, it remains to be identified. Presumably the deposition of birefringent material contained in the methylphenidate preparations is followed by a granulomatous inflammatory reaction and focal thrombosis (Byers et al. 1975). The situation has never been studied experimentally, and there is nothing to distinguish this finding in an amphetamine abuser from the same alterations seen in opiate addicts.

Intravenously injected methylphenidate, but not other stimulants, can produce obstructive lung disease. Panacinar emphysema, more pronounced in the lower lung fields, has been described in a group of young intravenous Ritalin™ abusers who died of severe obstructive lung disease (Sherman et al. 1987) (Schmidt et al. 1991). Autopsy findings included variable degrees of vascular involvement by talc granulomas, but no interstitial fibrosis. X-rays of these individuals show a distinctive picture with prominent, or even massive, fibrosis in the upper lobes and with translucence and bullae formation in the lower lobes (Paré et al. 1989). In most respects the clinical and pathologic findings are the same as those associated with alpha-1-antitrypsin deficiency, though tests for that disorder are negative. Obstructive lung disease is an uncommon complication of intravenous drug abuse, no matter the type, and its mechanism remains to be evaluated (Groth et al. 1972) (Vevaina et al. 1974) (Paré et al. 1989). It is unclear whether the apparent connection with methylphenidate has to do with the drug itself, or with the way it is compounded.

Even more difficult to explain is the occurrence of pulmonary hypertension in some individuals using therapeutic doses of amphetamine analogs, especially fenfluramine (Douglas et al. 1981) (McMurray et al. 1986) (Gaul et al. 1982) (Pouwels et al. 1990), but also propylhexedrine, phenformin (Fahlen et al. 1973), phenmetrazine and methylenedioxyamphetamine (Simpson and Rumak 1981) (Kendrick et al. 1977). One agent, aminorex fumarate, was removed from the European market in the early 1970's after it was implicated in an outbreak involving 32 cases of progressive pulmonary hypertension. A mechanism for this change was never elucidated, but the incidence of the disease so closely followed the sales of the drug that the likelihood of a causal relationship could not be ignored (Follath et al. 1971).

The principal lesion seen in the aminorex fumarate related cases, either at autopsy or biopsy, was medial hypertrophy with widening of the arterial media to occupy more than 10% of the vessel's cross sections. In one-third of the cases there was also evidence of eccentric intimal fibrosis with cushion-like thickening of the arterial intima (Pietra and Rüttner 1987). Such lesions are reminiscent of those produced by Szakacs in his experimental studies of catechol toxicity (Szakacs et al. 1959). Similar medial hypertrophy has also been noted in the small coronary arteries of cocaine users, though the pulmonary vessels have not been studied (Majid et al. 1990).

Fenfluramine is synthetic amphetamine which, unlike amphetamine and methamphetamine, exerts its effects primarily on serotonergic neurons. Its use has been linked to both the occurrence of progressive pulmonary hypertension (Douglas et al. 1981) and to acute respiratory failure (Simpson and McKinaly 1975). In the rat model, respiratory arrest, probably mediated by some central mechanism, precedes terminal cardiac arrhythmias. If fenfluramine's effects are partially blocked with a serotonin antagonist, the animals develop extensive intraalveolar hemorrhages and edema, consistent with the diagnosis of acute pulmonary hypertension (Hunsinger and Wright 1990).

3.1.8.3 Central Nervous System

Some, if not all, of the "designer" amphetamines are toxic to serotonergic neurons (Ricaurte et al. 1985). Otherwise, the neurotoxicity of the phenylisopropylamines is manifest principally as psychosis and stroke. When large doses of methamphetamine (10–15 mg/kg) are given to rats, the brain's serotonergic and dopaminergic systems are quickly altered. Tyrosine hydroxylase activity, the rate-limiting enzyme in the synthesis of dopamine and norepinephrine, decreases in a dose related fashion and so does the brain's content of dopamine and homovanillic acid (Koda and Gibb 1973) (Gibb et al. 1990). These decreases are not uniform. For instance, some studies have shown that while dopamine levels in the caudate nucleus are decreased, levels in the nucleus accumbens actually go up at the same time (Swerdlow et al. 1991).

These alterations persist for months after the initial treatment but, in the case of methamphetamine, have never been linked with any demonstrable CNS lesions, either in humans or experimental animals. In 1986 all of the same chemical alterations, except for decreased levels of tyrosine hydroxylase, were demonstrated in animals treated both with MDA (3,4-Methylenedioxyamphetamine) and MDMA (3,4 methylenedi-oxymethylamphetamine) (Stone et al. 1986). More importantly, both MDA and MDMA were shown to cause CNS lesions in experimental animals. Similar lesions have not been demonstrated in humans (Yeh and Desouza 1991).

Amphetamine-related psychotic reactions were recognized very early on. The first paper on the subject appeared in 1938 (Young and Scoville 1938). A paper published in 1958 reviewed 36 cases from the world's literature and commented on the similarities between the symptoms of amphetamine-induced psychosis and schizophrenia (Connell 1958). It transpired that large numbers of amphetamine abusers were being admitted to mental hospitals with the mistaken diagnosis of schizophrenia! Cultural determinants may have some bearing on the psychiatric manifestations of amphetamine abuse. Methamphetamine psychosis has been responsible for large numbers of psychiatric hospita-lizations in Japan, but disease on a similar scale has never been seen in the United States.

Even without developing psychosis, amphetamine users may be restless, tense and fearful. Some develop delusions of persecution and ideas of reference. They may have auditory, tactile, and visual hallucina-tions. Strangely, most are not disoriented and will act appropriately, given their paranoid state. The frequency with which hallucinations are visual, and the relative preservation of orientation in amphetamine users, is thought by some to differentiate amphetamine psychosis from true schizophrenia (Kalant 1966). Amphetamine toxicity in animals is associated with stereotyped, compulsive behavior such as grooming and pacing. Similar stereotypical behavior may be apparent in intoxicated humans. Generally, all of these symptoms disappear within a day or two of stopping the drug, though depression can be marked for some time afterwards. The syndrome of agitated delirium, known to occur in conjunction with cocaine use, has not been reported in amphetamine abusers. In animals, at least, the behavioral abnormalities can be prevented by prior treatments which deplete dopamine.

Hemorrhagic and ischemic stroke occur in association with smoking (Rothrock et al. 1988), oral ingestion (Poteliakhoff and Roughton 1956) (Delaney and Estes 1980) (Yu et al. 1983), and intravenous injection of methamphetamine (Lukes 1983) (Bostwick 1981) (Caplan et al. 1982) (Imanse and Vanneste 1990) (Delaney and Estes 1980) (D'Sousa and Shraberg 1981) (Lessing and Hyman 1989), though there are still fewer than 25 cases in the world literature. In some of these cases vasculitis has been present (Yu et al. 1983) (Shibata, 1991), while in others there was bleeding from a preexisting arteriovenous malformation (Lukes 1983). Most of the other phenylisopropylamines have also been implicated, and there are nearly as many reports of phenylpropanolamine related stroke as there are cases related to methamphetamine use (Glick et al. 1987) (Forman et al. 1989). Propylhexedrine (Benzedrex™) causes brainstem dysfunction when used intravenously (Fornazzai et al. 1986), and intracranial hemorrhage has been described in conjunction with pseudoephedrine overdose (Loizou et al. 1982).

The mechanism for stroke in these patients is not always clear. There have been no experimental histologic studies and only a handful of reported autopsies (Bostwick 1981). Amphetamine-related bleeds are more often intracerebral or simultaneously intracerebral and subarachnoid, than pure subarachnoid. Hemorrhage is most often confined to the frontal lobes, though it occasionally involves the basal ganglia. This distribution is in contrast with the pattern seen in hypertensive hemorrhages, which usually involve the basal ganglia and hypothalamus. The pattern is, however, almost exactly the same as that seen in cocaine abuse where the frontal lobes are most often involved.

About one quarter of the patients with intracranial hemorrhage secondary to amphetamine or methamphetamine had subarachnoid bleeds, and the appearance of "beading" considered to be angiographic evidence for arterial spasm. Beading has also been observed in association with phenylpropanolamine and norepinephrine-related strokes. This finding has been interpreted as evidence for arterial spasm, but caution is warranted, since beading is a relatively nonspecific finding and can result from subarachnoid hemorrhage itself (Weingarten 1988).

Necrotizing vasculitis as a consequence of amphetamine and polydrug abuse was first described by Citron in 1970 (Citron et al. 1970). The histological appearance in the cases described was identical to that seen in polyarteritis nodosa. Lesions included fibrinoid necrosis of the intima and media with mixed cellular infiltrates. With longer periods of survival there was intimal proliferation and marked luminal narrowing, especially at the bifurcation of vessels. Characteristically, giant cells were absent and the veins spared. Other reports described involvement of smaller (Stafford et al. 1975), and larger (Bostwick 1981) (Shibata, 1991), vessels. In the case described by Shibata the smaller vessels were spared, but virtually all of the major vessels were necrotic with destruction of the smooth muscle layer, but with scarring of the elastic layer. No leukocytic infiltration of the vessels was seen. During the last 10 years similar reports have been uncommon. A possible explanation for the apparent decline in the number of cases is that the process may have been the result of some contaminants or adulterants introduced during the manufacture of methamphetamine.

3.1.8.4 Renal Disease

The first report linking amphetamine ingestion and reversible renal failure was published in 1970 (Ginsberg et al. 1970). Even though cocaine abuse leads to rhabdomyolysis with some frequency, amphetamine-induced myoglobinuric renal failure is rare, with only a dozen cases in the world literature. A host of unrelated insults can lead to rhabdomyolysis, including heat, alcoholism, drug toxicity, hypokalemia, and muscle ischemia. When rhabdomyolysis occurs, myoglobin, potassium and phosphorus are released into the plasma. The presence of these substances in the plasma sets in train a series of metabolic derangements and fluid shifts. The resultant damage to the kidneys can be indirect, resulting from hypotension and renal ischemia, or direct. Direct toxic effects occur when myoglobin or decomposition products such as ferrihemate cause tubular obstruction. Much of the damage may be mediated by free radical formation (Odeh 1991).

What is not known about amphetamines is just which amphetamine mediated effect causes the syndrome to occur. The first patient described had a consumptive coagulopathy and hyperpyrexia. Several other patients had been hypotensive and comatose, suggesting that prolonged immobilization played a role (Terada et al. 1988) (Scandling and Spital 1982). Other intravenous users had septic shock and disseminated intravascular coagulation (Kendrick et al. 1977). Even without presuming any direct drug toxicity, hyperthermia could account for a number of the cases. Hyperthermia in amphetamine users has multiple causes. Increased motor activity, even without seizures can raise body temperature, especially when heat loss from the skin is inhibited because of catechol induced vasoconstriction. Altered thermoregulation may also be the result of amphetamines' direct actions on the hypothalamic temperature center. The really interesting question is why the syndrome is so much more common in cocaine users than in amphetamine abusers, and there are no ready answers.

3.1.8.5 Hepatic disease

Two of the synthetic analogs, Pemoline™ (2-1-amino-5-phenyl-4--oxazolidinone) and Ritalin™ (methylphenidate) can cause hepatic damage (Tolman et al. 1973) (Patterson 1984) (Goodman 1972), but this complication is rare. Most reported cases have occurred as a result of legitimate drug treatment. In one review of 100 alleged cases of Pemoline-associated hepatotoxicity, there was sufficient data to analyze in only 43. Based on the results of enzyme measurements, and the findings in one autopsy, the injury pattern is said to be hepatocellular in nature, probably due to an idiosyncratic metabolic reaction (Nehara et al. 1990). In another case an 11-year old, taking the medication for an attention deficit disorder, developed frank liver failure. Open-liver biopsy demonstrated submassive hepatic necrosis with extensive fibrovascular replacement (Pratt and Dubois 1990).

Ritalin-associated hepatocellular injuries, unlike those that have been described in pemoline users, have occurred in intravenous abusers (Mehta et al. 1984) (Lundquest et al. 1987). In one instance, liver biopsy demonstrated portal inflammation and hepatocellular disarray in an intravenous abuser who survived a bout of liver failure (Mehta et al. 1984). In a second case, the autopsy findings in a polydrug user who died of amniotic fluid embolus included biventricular hypertrophy and multiple granulomas in the liver and lungs (Lundquest et al. 1987). The autopsy findings in a third polydrug abuser, who injected Ritalin™ and Dilaudid™, are consistent with the sequence of events occurring when tablets meant for oral ingestion are repeatedly injected. Pulmonary hypertension is the ultimate outcome, but, because this particular individual had a patent foramen ovale, the elevated pulmonary pressure caused a right-to-left shunt. Talc granulomas were found throughout the body, including the brain and kidneys (Riddick 1987).

References

Allcott, J, R Barnhart and L Mooney (1987). Acute lead poisoning in two users of illicit methamphetamine. JAMA 258 (4):510-511.

Anderson, E and W Scott (1936). Cardiovascular effects of benzedrine. Lancet 2:1461-1462.

Anderson, R, H Garza, J Garriott and V DiMaio (1979). Intravenous propylhexedrine (Benzedrex) abuse and sudden death. Am J Med 67:15-20.

Änggård, E, L Gunne, L Jönsson, and F Niklasson (1970). Pharmacokinetic and clinical studies on amphetamine-dependent subjects. Eur J Clin Pharmacol 3:3-11.

Anon. (1990). Method disputed as NIDA lab incurs false positives. Clin Chem News. 16:1.

Arnett, E, W Battle, J Russo et al. (1976). Intravenous injection of talc-containing drugs intended for oral use - a cause of pulmonary granulomatosis and pulmonary hypertension. Am J Med 60:711-718.

Baselt, R. and Cravey, B. (1989). The disposition of toxic drugs and chemicals in man. Year Book Medical Publishers, Chicago, London.

Beckett, A. and M Rowland (1965). Urinary excretion kinetics of methylamphetamine in man. J Pharm Pharmac 17:109S-114S.

Bett, W. (1946). Benzedrine sulphate in clinical medicine: a survey of the literature. Postgrad Med J 22:205.

Bost, R., P. Kemp and V. Hnilica (1989). Tissue distribution of methamphetamine and amphetamine in premature infants. J Analyt Toxicol 13:300–302.

Bostwick, D. (1981). Amphetamine induced cerebral vasculitis. Hum Pathol 12:1031–1033.

Burchfield, D., V. Lucas, R. Abrams et al (1991). Disposition and pharmacodynamics of methamphetamine in pregnant sheep. JAMA 265:1968–1973.

Byers, J., J. Soin, R. Fisher and G. Hutchins (1975). Acute pulmonary alveolitis in narcotics abuse. Arch Pathol 99:273–277.

Caldwell, J., L. Dring and R. WIlliams (1972). Metabolism of (C-14) methamphetamine in man, the guinea pig, and the rat. Biochem J 120:11–22.

Call, T., J. Hartneck, W. Dickinson et al. (1982). Acute cardiomyopathy secondary to intravenous amphetamine abuse. Ann Intern Med 97:559–560.

Caplan, L., D. Hier and G. Banks (1982). Current concepts of cerebrovascular disease-stroke: stroke and drug abuse. Stroke 13: 869–872.

Carson, P., K. Oldroyd and K. Phadke (1987). Myocardial infarction due to amphetamine. Br Med J 294:1525–1526.

Cho, A. and J. Wright (1978). Minireview: pathways of metabolism of amphetamine and related compounds. Life Sci 22:363–372.

Cho, A. (1990). Ice: a new dosage form of an old drug. Science 249 (4969):631–634.

Chokshi, S., R. Moore, N. Pandian and J. Isner (1989). Reversible cardiomyopathy associated with cocaine intoxication. Ann Intern Med 111: 1039–1040.

Citron, B., M. Halpern, M. McCarron et al., (1970). Necrotizing angiitis associated with drug abuse. N Engl J Med 283:1003–1011.

Connell, P. (1958). Amphetamine psychosis. 1st ed., London: Chapman and Hall.

Cravey, R. and D. Reed (1970). Intravenous amphetamine poisoning. Report of three cases. J Forensic Sci Soc 10:109–112.

Croft, C., B. Firth and L. Hillia (1982). Propylhexedrine-induced left ventricular dysfunction. Ann Intern Med 97:560–561.

D'Sousa, T. and D. Shraberg (1981). Intracranial hemorrhage with amphetamine use. Neurology 31:922–923.

Dayton, P., J. Read and V. Ong (1970). Physiological disposition of methylphenidate-C^{14} in man. Fed Proc 29:345 (abstract).

Delaney, P. and M. Estes (1980). Intracranial hemorrhage with amphetamine abuse. Neurology 30:1125–1128.

DHHS/NIDA. (1990) Notice to DHHS/NIDA certified laboratories. December 19. Department of Health and Human Services.

Douglas, J., J. Munro, A. Kitchin et al. (1981). Pulmonary hypertension and fenfluramine. Br Med J 283:881–883.

Driscoll, R., F. Barr, B. Gragg and G. Moore (1971). Determination of therapeutic blood levels of methamphetamine and pentobarbital by GC. J Pharm Sci 60:1492–1495.

Evrard, P, A. Allaz and P. Urban (1990). Myocardial infarction associated with the use of dextrofenfluramine. Br Med J 301:(6747)345.

Fahlen, M., H. Bergman, G. Helder et al. (1973). Phenformin and pulmonary hypertension. Br Heart J 35:824–828.

Follath, F., F. Burkart and W. Schweitzer (1971). Drug-induced pulmonary hypertension? Br Med J 1:265–266.

Forman, H., S. Levin, B. Stewart et al. (1989). Cerebral vasculitis and hemorrhage in an adolescent taking diet pills containing phenylpropanolamine: case report and review of literature. Pediatrics 83 (5):737–741.

Fornazzari, L., P. Carlen and B. Kapur (1986). Intravenous abuse of propylhexedrine (Benzedrex™) and the risk of brainstem dysfunction in young adults. Can J Neurol Sci 13:337–339.

Fukunaga, T., Y. Mizoi and J. Adachi (1987). Methamphetamine-induced changes of peripheral catecholamines: an animal experiment to elucidate the cause of sudden death after methamphetamine abuse. Jpn J Legal Med 41 (4a):335–341.

Fukunaga, T., Y. Mizoi, J. Adachi and Y. Tatsuno (1987). Methamphetamine concentrations in blood, urine and organs of fatal cases after abuse. Jpn J Legal Med 41 (4b):328–334.

Furst, S., S. Fallon, G. Reznik and P. Shah (1990). Myocardial infarction after inhalation of methamphetamine. N Engl J Med 323 (16):1147.

Garriott, J. and F. Spruill. 1973. Detection of methamphetamine in a newborn infant. J Forensic Sci 18:434–436.

Gaul, G., G. Blazek, E. Deutsch and H. Heeger (1982). Ein Fall von chronischer pulmonaler Hypertonie nach Fenfluramineinnahme. Wein Klin Wochenschr 94:618–622. (English abstract)

Gibb, J., M. Johnson and G. Hanson (1990). Neurochemical basis of neurotoxicity. Neurotoxicology 11 (2):317–322.

Gillogley, K., A. Evans, R. Hansen et al. (1990). The Perinatal impact of cocaine, amphetamine, and opiate use detected by universal intrapartum screening. Am J Obstet Gynecol 163 (5):1535–1542.

Ginsberg, M., M. Hertzman and W. Schmidt-Nowara (1970). Amphetamine intoxication with coagulopathy, hyperthermia, and reversible renal failure. A syndrome resembling heatstroke. Ann Intern Med 73:81–85.

Glick, R., J. Hoying, L. Cerullo and S. Perlman (1987). Phenylpropanolamine: an over-the-counter drug causing central nervous system vasculitis and intracerebral hemorrhage. Neurosurgery 20 (6):969–974.

Goodman, C.. (1972). Hepatotoxicity due to methylphenidate hydrochloride. NY State J Med 72:2339–2340.

Groth, D., G. Mackay, J. Crable and T. Cochran (1972). Intravenous injection of talc in a narcotics addict. Arch Pathol 94:171–178.

Gualtieri, C., R. Hicks, K. Patrick et al. (1984). Clinical correlates of methylphenidate blood levels. Ther Drug Monit 6 (4):379–392.

Hahn, H., A. Schweid and H. Beaty (1969). Complications of injecting dissolved methylphenidate tablets. Arch Intern Med 123:656–659.

Henzlova, M., S. Smith, V. Prchal, and F. Helmcke (1991). Apparent reversibility of cocaine-induced congestive cardiomyopathy. Am Heart J 122 (2): 577–579.

Hong, R., E. Matsuyama and K. Nur (1991). Cardiomyopathy associated with the smoking of crystal methamphetamine. JAMA 265 (9):1152–1154.

Hotchkiss, A. and J. Gibb (1980). Long-term effects of multiple doses of methamphetamine on tryptophan hydroxylase activity in rat brain. J Pharmacol Exp Ther 214:257–262.

Hunsinger, R. and D. Wright (1990). A characterization of the acute cardiopulmonary toxicity of fenfluramine in the rat. Pharm Res 22 (3):371–378.

Imanse, J. and J. Vanneste (1990). Intraventricular hemorrhage following amphetamine abuse. Neurology 40:1318–1319.

Jacobs, L. (1989). Reversible dilated cardiomyopathy induced by methamphetamine. Clin Cardiol 12:725–727.

Kalant, Oriana Josseau (1966). The amphetamines: toxicity and addiction. Vol. No 5. Brookside Monographs, ed. PJ Griffen and RE Popham. Toronto: Charles C. Thomas.

Kendrick, W., A. Hull and J. Knopchel (1977). Rhabdomyolysis and shock after intravenous amphetamine administration. Ann Int Med 86:381–387.

Koda, L. and J. Gibb (1973). Adrenal and striatal tyrosine hydroxylase activity after methamphetamine. J Pharmacol Exp Ther 185:42–48.

Kojima, T., I. Une and M. Yashiki (1984). CI-mas fragmentographic analysis of methamphetamine and amphetamine in human autopsy tissues after acute amphetamine poisoning. Forensic Sci Int 21:253–258.

Kojima, T., I. Une, M. Yashiki et al. (1984). A fatal methamphetamine poisoning associated with hyperpyrexia. Forensic Sci Int 24:87–93.

Kringsholm, B. and P. Christoffersen (1987). Lung and heart pathology in fatal drug addiction. A consecutive autopsy study. Forensic Sci Int 34:39–51.

Lam, D. and N. Goldschlager (1988). Myocardial injury associated with polysubstance abuse. Am Heart J 115 (3):675–680.

Lebish, P., B. Finkle and J. Brackett (1970). Determination of amphetamine, methamphetamine, and related amines in blood and urine by gas chromatography with hydrogen-flame ionization detector. Clin Chem 16:195–200.

Lessing, M. and N. Hyman (1989). Intracranial hemorrhage caused by amphetamine abuse. J Roy Soc Med 82 (12):766–767.

Levine, B., Y. Caplan and G. Kauffman (1986). Fatality resulting from methylphenidate overdose. J Analyt Toxicol 10 (5):209–210.

Lewman, L. (1972). Fatal pulmonary hypertension from intravenous injection of methylphenidate (Ritalin) tablets. Hum Pathol 3:67–70.

Loizou, L., J. Hamilton and S. Tsementzis (1982). Intracranial hemorrhage in association with pseudoephedrine overdose. J Neurol Neurosurg and Psychiat 45:471–472.

Lukes, S. (1983). Intracerebral hemorrhage from an arteriovenous malformation after amphetamine injection. Arch Neurol 40:60–61.

Lundquest, D., W. Young and J. Edland (1987). Maternal death associated with intravenous methylphenidate (Ritalin™) and pentazocine (Talwin™) abuse. J Forensic Sci 32 (3):798–801.

Majid, P., B. Patel, H. Kim et al. (1990). An angiographic and histologic study of cocaine-induced chest pain. Am J Cardiol 65 (11):812–814.

Marsden, P. and J. Sheldon (1972). Acute poisoning by propylhexedrine. Br Med J i:730.

Matoba, R., S. Onishi and I. Shikata. Cardiac lesions in cases of sudden death in methamphetamine abusers. Heart and Vessels 1 (Suppl 1 1985):298–300.

McMurray, J., P. Bloomfield and H. Miller (1986). Irreversible pulmonary hypertension after treatment with fenfluramine. Br Med J 292:239–240.

Mehta, H., B. Murray and T. Loludice (1984). Hepatic dysfunction due to intravenous abuse of methylphenidate hydrochloride." J Clin Gastroenterol 6:149–151.

Monroe, R. and H. Drell (1947). Oral use of stimulants obtained from inhalers. JAMA 135 (14):909–915.

National Institute on Drug Abuse (1990a). Annual Emergency Room Data. Data from the Drug Abuse Warning Network. Statistical Series, Number 10-A. Rockville, Maryland, U.S. Department of Health and Human Services.

National Institute on Drug Abuse (1990b). Annual Medical Examiner Data. Data from the Drug Abuse Warning Network. Statistical Series, Number 10-B. Rockville, Maryland, U.S. Department of Health and Human Services.

Nehra, A., F. Mullick, K. Ishak and H. Zimmerman (1990). Pemoline-associated hepatic injury. Gastroenterology 99:1517–1519.

Odeh, M. (1991). The role of reperfusion-induced injury in the pathogenesis of the crush syndrome. N Engl J Med 324 (20):1417–1422.

Olsen, K., Gulliksen, M. and Christophersen, A. (1992). Metabolites of chloropromazine and brompheniramine may cause false-positive urine amphetamine results with monoclonal EMIT dau immunoassay. Clin Chem 38:611–612.

Orrenius, S. and A. Maehly (1970). Lethal amphetamine intoxication - a report of three cases. Z Rechtsmed, 67:184–189.

Packe, G., M. Garton and K. Jennings. Acute myocardial infarction caused by intravenous amphetamine abuse. Br Heart J 64 (1):23–24.

Paré, J., Citem G. and R. Fraser (1990). Long-term follow-up of drug abusers with intravenous talcosis. Am Rev Respir Dis 139 (1989):233–241.

Parran, T. and D. Jasinski (1991). Intravenous methylphenidate abuse - prototype for prescription drug abuse. Arch Intern Med 151 (4):781–783.

Patterson, J. (1984). Hepatitis associated with pemoline. South Med J 77 (7):938.

Pentel, P., J. Jentzen and J. Sievert (1987). Myocardial necrosis due to intraperitoneal administration of phenylpropanolamine in rats. Fundam Appl Toxicol 9:167–172.

Pentel, P., F. Mikell and S. Zavoral (1982). Myocardial injury after phenylpropanolamine ingestion. Br Heart J 47:51–54.

Pietra, G., W. Edwards, J. Kay et al. (1989). Histopathology of primary pulmonary hypertension. A qualitative and quantitative study of pulmonary blood vessels from 58 patients in the National Heart, Lung, and Blood Institute, Primary Pulmonary Hypertension Registry. Circulation 80:1198–1206.

Pietra, G. and J. Rüttner (1987). Specificity of pulmonary vascular lesions in primary pulmonary hypertension. Respiration 52 :81–85.

Poteliakhoff, A. and B. Roughton (1956). Two cases of amphetamine poisoning. Br Med J January 7:26–27.

Pouwels, H., J. Smeets, E. Cheriex and E. Wouters. Pulmonary hypertension and fenfluramine. Eur Respir J 3 (5 1990):606–607.

Pratt, D. and R. Dubois (1990). Hepatotoxicity due to pemoline (Cylert): a report of two cases. J Ped Gastro and Nutr 10:239–241.

Rajs, J., T. Härm and K. Ormstad (1984). Postmortem findings of pulmonary lesions of older datum in intravenous drug addicts. Virchows Arch 402: 405–414.

Ricaurte, G., G. Bryan, L. Strauss et al. (1985). Hallucinogenic amphetamines selectively destroy brain serotonin nerve terminals. Science 229:986–988.

Richards, H. and A. Stephens (1973). Sudden death associated with the taking of amphetamines by an asthmatic. Medicine, Science, and the Law 13 (1):35–38.

Riddick, L. (1987). Disseminated granulomatosis through a patent foramen ovale in an intravenous drug user with pulmonary hypertension. Am J Forensic Med and Pathol 8 (4):326–333.

Rona, G. (1985). Catecholamine cardiotoxicity.J Mol Cell Cardiol 17:291–306.

Rothrock, J., R. Rubenstein and P. Lyden (1988). Ischemic stroke associated with methamphetamine inhalation. Neurology 38:589–592.

Scandling, J. and A. Spital (1982). Amphetamine-associated myoglobinuric renal failure. South Med J 75 (2):237–240.

Schmidt, R., R. Glenny, J. Godwin et al. (1991). Panlobular emphysema in young intravenous Ritalin™ abusers. Am Rev Respir Dis 143:649–656.

Sekine, H. and Y. Nakahara (1987). Abuse of smoking methamphetamine mixed with tobacco: I. Inhalation efficiency and pyrolysis products of methamphetamine. J Forens Sci 32 (5):1271–1280.

Sherman, C., L. Hudson and D. Pierson (1987). Severe precocious emphysema in intravenous methylphenidate (Ritalin) abusers. Chest 92 (6): 1085–1087.

Shibata, S., Mori, K., Sekine, I. and Suyama, H. (1991). Subarachnoid and intra-cerebral hemorrhage associated with necrotizing angiitis due to meth-amphetamine abuse, an autopsy case. Neurol Med Chir 31 (Tokyo): 49–52.

Simpson, D. and B. Rumak (1981). Methylenedioxyamphetamine: clinical des-cription of overdose, death and review of pharmacology. Arch Intern Med 141:1507–1509.

Simpson, H. and I. McKinaly (1975). Poisoning with slow-release fenfluramine. Br Med J 4:462–463.

Smith, H., A. Roche, M. Jagusch and P. Herdson (1976). Cardiomyopathy associated with amphetamine administration. Am Heart J 91:792–797.

Smith, L. (1939). Collapse with death following the use of amphetamine sulfate. JAMA 113:1022–1023.

Soine, W. (1986). Clandestine drug synthesis. Med Res Rev 6:41-74

Soine, W. Contamination of clandestinely prepared drugs with synthetic by--products. In Proceedings of the 50th Annual Scientific Meeting, The Committee on Problems of Drug Dependence, in NIDA Research Monograph 95, Louis S. Harris (ed), National Institute on Drug Abuse, 1989, pg 44–50.

Stafford, C., B. Bogdanoff, L. Green and H. Spector (1975). Mononeuropathy multiplex as a complication of amphetamine angiitis. Neurology 25: 570–572.

Stecyk, O., T. Loludice, S. Demeter and J. Jacobs (1985). Multiple organ failure resulting from intravenous abuse of methylphenidate hydrochloride. Ann Emerg Med 14 (6):597–599.

Steiner, E., Envill, T., Hallberg, M., Rane, A. (1984). Amphetamine secretion in breast milk. Euro J Clin Pharm, 27:123–124.

Stone, D., D. Stahl, G. Hanson and J. Gibb (1986). The effects of 3,4-methylene-dioxymethamphetamine(MDMA)and3,4-methylenedioxyamphetamine (MDA) on monoaminergic systems in the rat brain. Eur J Pharmacol 128:41–48.

Swerdlow, N., R. Hauger, M. Irwin et al. (1991). Endocrine, immune, and neurochemical changes in rats during withdrawal from chronic amphetamine intoxication. Neuropsychopharmacology 5 (1):23–31.

Szakacs, J. and Cannon A. (1958). l-Norepinephrine myocarditis.Am J Clin Pathol 30:425–434.

Szakacs, J., R. Dimmette and E. Cowart (1959). Pathologic implications of the catecholamines: epinephrine and norepinephrine. US Armed Forces Med J 10:908–925.

Tazelaar, H., S. Karch, M. Billingham, and BS Stephens (1987). Cocaine and the heart. Hum Pathol 18:195–199.

Terada, Y., S. Shinohara, N. Matui and T. Ida (1988). Amphetamine-induced myoglobinuric acute renal failure. Jpn J Med 27:305–308.

Tolman, K., J. Freston, M. Berenson and J. Sannella (1973). Hepatotoxicity due to pemoline: report of two cases. Digestion 9:532–539.

Tomashefski, J. and C. Hirsch (1980). The pulmonary vascular lesions of intravenous drug abuse. Human Pathol 11:133–145.

Tomashefski, J., C. Hirsch and P. Jolly (1981). Microcrystalline cellulose pulmonary embolism and granulomatosis. Arch Pathol & Lab Med 105: 89–93.

Van der Ark, A., A. Verweij and A. Sinnema (1978). Weakly basic impurities in illicit amphetamine. J Forensic Sci 23:693–700.

Vevaina, J., F. Civantos, M. Viamonte and W. Avery (1974). Emphysema associated with talcum granulomatosis in a drug addict. South Med J 67: 113–116.

Von Hoof, F., A. Heyndrickx and J. Timperman (1974). Report of a human fatality due to amphetamine. Arch Toxicol 32:307–312.

Wagner, G., Ricaurte, G., Johanson, C. et al. (1980). Amphetamine induces depletion of dopamine and loss of dopamine uptake sites in caudate. Neurology 20:547–550.

Waller, B., W. Brownlee and R. Roberts (1980). Self-induced pulmonary granulomatosis. Chest 78:90–94.

Wan, S., S. Matin and D. Azarnoff (1978). Kinetics, salivary excretion of amphetamine isomers, and effect of urinary pH. Clin Pharmacol Ther 23: 585–590.

Wargin, W., K. Patrick, C. Kilts et al. (1983). Pharmacokinetics of methylphenidate in man, rat, and monkey. J Pharmacol Exp Ther 226 (2):382–386.

Weingarten, K. (1988). Cerebral vasculitis associated with cocaine abuse or subarachnoid hemorrhage? JAMA 259:1648–1649.

Wu, A., Wong, S., Johnson, K. et al. (1992). The conversion of ephedrine to methamphetamine-like compounds during and prior to gas chromatographic/mass spectrometric analysis of CB and HFB derivatives. Biol Mass Spect 21:278–284.

Yamamoto, K., Watanabe, H., Ukita, K., et al. (1992). 3 Tödesfalle nach gemein-
schaftlichem Konsum von Methaphetamin. Archive Kriminologie, 188:
72–76.

Yeh, S.Y. and E.B. De Souza (1991). Lack of neurochemical evidence for neurotoxic effects of repeated cocaine administration in rats on brain monoamine neurons. Drug Alcohol Depend 27 (1):51–61.

Young, D. and W. Scoville (1938). Paranoid psychosis in narcolepsy and the
possible danger of Benzedrine treatment. Med Clin N Amer 22 (3):637.

Yu, Y., D. Cooper, D. Wellenstein et al. (1983). Cerebral angiitis and intracerebral hemorrhage associated with methamphetamine abuse. J Neurosurg
58:109–111.

Zalis, E., C. Lundberg and R. Knutson (1967). The pathophysiology of acute
amphetamine poisoning with pathologic correlation. J Pharmacol Exp
Ther 158 (1):115–127.

Zalis, E. and L. Parmley (1963). Fatal amphetamine poisoning. Arch Intern Med
112:822–826.

3.2. PHENYLPROPANOLAMINE

3.2.1 HISTORICAL ASPECTS

Structurally and functionally, phenylpropanolamine (PPA) is similar to ephedrine and amphetamine. Like the amphetamines, PPA causes the increased release of norepinephrine from nerve terminals. Like ephedrine, it also is a directly acting alpha and, to a lesser degree, beta agonist (Pentel 1984) (Schmidt and Fleming 1962). PPA alone, or in combination with other drugs, was responsible for less than 2% of all drug related emergency room visits reported in the 1990 DAWN survey. During that same period 19 PPA related deaths were reported (National Institute on Drug Abuse, 1992).

PPA is the fifth most consumed medicinal chemical used in the United States. It is the major ingredient in numerous over-the-counter preparations. According to industry surveys, more than 6 billion doses are consumed annually at a cost of well over $200 million (Morgan 1990). PPA is a component in over 100 different products sold in the United States. Most of the drug is used to make cough and cold products, but since 1979, when the FDA published a monograph declaring that PPA was safe and effective when used as an anorectic, increasing amounts have been used to produce over-the-counter diet pills. During the early 1980's additional amounts were funneled into the making of "look-alike" stimulants. In 1981 and 1982 nearly half the confiscated samples of amphetamine contained PPA, along with caffeine and ephedrine (Morgan et. al. 1987).

During the mid 1970's an enterprising truck driver named Edward Seay began merchandising caffeine tablets that had been designed to look exactly like prescription amphetamine (Morgan et al. 1987). Sales through truck stops and mail-order catalogs amounted to millions of tablets per month. The Seay Drug Company, of Union City, Georgia sold imitations of virtually all the Schedule III and IV amphetamines and stimulants. In 1977 Seay began advertising in magazines such as *Penthouse, Hustler and High Times*, as well as in women's beauty magazines. At about that same time Seay, and other similar manufactures, began adding caffeine and ephedrine to their pills. Almost immediately, reports of toxicity began to appear. There is some debate as to whether these products really have stimulant or euphorogenic properties when used at recommended levels (Lake et al. 1990), but there is no question that phenylpropanolamine use can be associated with stroke, infarction, and myocardial necrosis. The fact that fewer cases are being reported may have to do with a decrease in the popularity of the "look-alike" drugs.

The toxicity of PPA itself remains an extremely controversial topic. Given the millions of doses that have been consumed, the reported the number of ADRs (adverse drug reports) is quite low. Nonetheless, there are a sizable number of case reports documenting exactly the same sorts of disorders are seen in association with amphetamine abuse (Winick, 1990) (Miller, 1990).

TABLE 3.2.1
**PEAK PPA BLOOD LEVELS IN FIVE VOLUNTEERS
AFTER DIFFERENT ORAL DOSES**

Dosage	Range of Peak Blood Levels
25 mg	67 – 185.3 ng/mL
50 mg	147.7 – 190.1 ng/mL
100 mg	290.6 – 480.6 ng/mL

Except for modest increases in systolic blood pressure with 50 and 100 mg doses, these individuals were otherwise asymptomatic (*from Dowse et al.*)

3.2.2 CHEMISTRY

Phenylpropanolamine is alpha-(1-Aminoethyl)benzenemethanol hydrochloride. Its formula is $C_9H_{14}CLNO$, with a molecular weight of 187.67. It is composed of 57.6% carbon, 7.5% hydrogen, 18.9% chloride, 7.5% nitrogen, and 8.5 % oxygen. Crystals composed of racemic forms have a melting point of 199°–194°C.

3.2.3 METABOLISM

Phenylpropanolamine, also called norephedrine, has very nearly the same half-life as ephedrine, attains nearly the same blood levels, and produces nearly the same effects as ephedrine. Peak levels occur between 0.67 and 2.5 hours after oral dosing. Regardless of the dose taken, the half-life is on the order of 1.5 hours, though in some individuals it may be much shorter. Almost all of a given dose is excreted unchanged in the urine (Heimlich et al. 1961). The table below shows the peak concentrations produced after different dosing regimens (Dowse et al. 1990)

Toxic blood and tissue levels are poorly characterized (Pentel et al. 1987). Postmortem blood from a woman who expired of an apparent cardiac arrest, after taking an unspecified number of cold pills, had a concentration of 2 mg/L (Baselt and Cravey 1989). A 20-year old suicide described as taking a "large overdose" had a postmortem blood level of 48 mg/L and hepatic levels that were 10 times higher than the blood level. The concentration in the brain was twice that in the blood (Baselt and Cravey 1989). Because this level is hundreds of times higher than therapeutic levels, or even previously reported toxic levels, its relevance is open to some question. Blood levels in 12 pediatric deaths reported to the National Association of Medical Examiners Pediatric Toxicology Registry ranged from as low as 0.04 mg/L to as high as 0.84 mg/L (Hanzlick and Davis 1992).

PPA is mainly an alpha adrenergic agonist, but it also possesses some ß activity, and as a result, toxic (as opposed to fatal) reactions appear to be not uncommon. The standard PPA dose of 50–75 mg is not associated with significant increases in levels of circulating cate-cholamines (Lake et al. 1990), but doses of 85–100 mg have been implica-ted as the cause of severe hypertensive reactions (Pentel 1984).

PPA increases plasma caffeine levels, and when the two agents are taken at the same time, the resultant blood pressure increases are greater than those observed when either drug is taken alone. When test subjects were given 400 mg of caffeine and 75 mg of PPA at the same time, the peak plasma caffeine concentration was 8.0 ± 2.2 μg/mL, nearly 4 times higher than the result when the same amount of caffeine is given alone (Lake et al. 1990). This interaction may explain why there is an increased incidence of adverse reactions when PPA is taken together with caffeine and/or ephedrine.

Case reports have described patients with arrhythmias, chest pain and even electrocardiographic changes (Pentel et al. 1982). Arrhyth-mic sudden death also occurs (Bernstein, 1973) (Dietz 1981) (Pentel 1984), but no autopsy findings have been reported. In experimental animals PPA produces exactly the same constellation of lesions that are associated with classic catecholamine toxicity. Rats given varying doses of intraperitoneal PPA displayed dose-related myocardial necrosis with contraction bands, eosinophilia and occasional infiltrates (Pentel et al. 1987). Myocardial fibrosis was not observed in this model because the animals were sacrificed before it could develop (Karch and Billingham 1986). However, the lesions which were observed are known to heal by fibrosis and the presence of microfocal fibrosis could well account for the arrhythmias which have been described in PPA users. Based on the number of published case reports, PPA seems to be more toxic to the cerebral than the coronary vasculature. The difference is unexplained, but likely has to do with receptor distribution and regulation.

3.2.4 TOXICITY BY ORGAN SYSTEM

3.2.4.1 Neurologic Disease

The most commonly encountered complications of PPA use are neurologic. Frank psychotic episodes have occurred after using therapeutic doses of PPA containing decongestants (Traynealis and Brick 1986) (Kane and Green 1966) (Wharton 1970) (Norvenious et al. 1979) (Lake, 1991). Seizures also have been described (Cornelius et al. 1984) (Muller 1983). Stroke has been reported with some frequency (Johnson et al. 1983) (Kizer 1984) (Mesnard and Ginn 1984) (Fallis and Fisher 1985) (Traynealis and Brick 1986) (Maher 1987) (Maertens et al. 1987) (Le Coz et al. 1988) (King 1979) (Bernstein and Diskant 1982) (Kase et al. 1987) (Kita et al. 1985) (Forman et al. 1989) (McDowell and LeBlanc 1985) (Bale et al. 1984) (Stoessl et al. 1985) (Glick et al. 1987) (Lake 1991). When angiograms were done, these patients usually, but not always, were found to have changes consistent with vasospasm or angiitis. Many of these patients are normotensive when they are first seen, and almost all are women. In other cases, hypertension has been a factor. Doses much over 50 mg are associated with significant blood pressure increases (Lake, 1991). As is the case with cocaine and amphetamine, most of the PPA-associated stroke patients are quite young, usually in their late 20's or early 30's.

The mechanism for stroke in PPA users has not been explained. Animal studies have shown that very high doses of PPA (200 mg/kg) produce slight decrease in formal cortex dopamine levels but no other effects on the monoamine systems (Woolverton 1986). Biopsy findings are available from only one case, and there have been no autopsy studies. The biopsy was from a 35-year old woman with an intracerebral hemorrhage (Glick et al. 1987). Arteriography showed diffuse segmental narrowing. When the hemorrhage was evacuated, multiple specimens of tissue were obtained. There was necrotizing vasculitis of the small arteries and veins which were infiltrated with polymorphonuclear leukocytes. There was lumenal narrowing and even vessel occlusion. As in intravenous methamphetamine abuse, there was fragmentation of the elastic lamina and occasional microaneurysm formation, but no granulomas and no giant cells. In general the findings are consistent with a drug-induced vasculitis and contrast markedly with the findings in primary or idiopathic cerebral vasculitis where granulomas and giant cells are always seen.

3.2.4.2 Cardiac Disease

EKG changes, arrhythmias and chest pain have all been described (Pentel et al. 1982), (Chouinard et al. 1978) (Conway 1989). Typical catechol lesions can easily be produced in rats treated with PPA, but only at dosages that produce blood levels 4–6 times as high as seen with normal clinical regimens (Pentel et al. 1987).

3.2.4.3 Pulmonary Disease

Autopsy information is sparse. In one case a 15-year old who died 32 hours after taking 400 mg of PPA, was found to have changes consistent with the diagnosis of acute respiratory distress syndrome (ARDS) (Logie and Scott 1984). In a second case, death resulted from a 600-mg overdose and multiple pulmonary emboli were found in addition to changes consistent with ARDS (Patterson 1980). Blood and tissue levels were not reported for either case.

3.2.4.4 Renal Disease

Like the other amphetamines, PPA can cause acute myoglobin-uria renal failure (Swenson et al. 1982), and there is one report of biopsy-proven interstitial nephritis (Bennett 1979). The incidence of both complications seems to be quite low.

References

Bale, J., M. Fountain and R. Shaddy (1984). Phenylpropanolamine associated CNS complications in children and adolescents. Am J Dis Child 138:683–685.

Baselt, R. and R. Cravey (1989). Disposition of toxic drugs and chemicals in man. 3rd ed., Chicago, London: Year Book Medical Publishers.

Bennett, W. (1979). Hazards of appetite suppressant phenylpropanolamine. Lancet 2:42–43.

Bernstein, E. and B. Diskant (1982). Phenylpropanolamine: a potentially hazardous drug. Ann Emerg Med 11:311–315.

Chouinard, G., A. Ghadirian, B. Jones (1978). Death attributed to ventricular arrhythmia induced by thiordiazine in combination with a single Contac C capsule. Can Med Assoc J 119:729–731.

Conway Jr, E., C. Walsh, A. Palomba (1989). Supraventricular tachycardia following the administration of phenylpropanolamine in an infant. Pediatr Emerg Care 5 (3):173–174.

Cornelius, J., P. Soloff and C. Reynolds (1984). Paranoia, homicidal behavior, and seizures associated with phenylpropanolamine. Am J Psychiat 141:120–121.

Dietz, A. (1981). Amphetamine-like reactions to phenylpropanolamine. JAMA 245:601–602.

Dowse, R., Scherzinger, S., Kanfer, I. (1990). Serum concentrations of phenyl-propanolamine and associated effects on blood pressure in normotensive subjects: a pilot study. Int J Clin Pharmacol Ther Toxicol 28 (5): 205–210.

Fallis, R. and M. Fisher (1985). Cerebral vasculitis and hemorrhage associated with phenylpropanolamine. Neurology 35:405–407.

Forman, H., S. Levin, B. Stewart et al. (1989). Cerebral vasculitis and hemorrhage in an adolescent taking diet pills containing phenylpropanolamine: case report and review of literature. Pediatrics 83 (5):737–741.

Glick, R., J. Hoying, L. Cerullo and S. Perlman (1987). Phenylpropanolamine: an over-the-counter drug causing central nervous system vasculitis and intracerebral hemorrhage. Neurosurgery 20 (6):969–974.

Hanzlick, R. and Davis G. (1992). National Association of Medical Examiners Pediatric Toxicology Registry. Report 1: phenylpropanolamine. Am J Forensic Med and Pathol 13 (1):37–41.

Heimlich, K., D. MacDonnell, T. Flanagan and P. O'Brien (1961). Evaluation of a sustained release from of phenylpropanolamine hydrochloride by urinary excretion studies. J Pharm Sci 50:232–237.

Johnson, D., H. Etter and D. Reeves (1983). Stroke and phenylpropanolamine use. Lancet 2:970.

Kane, F. and B. Green (1966). Psychotic episodes associated with the use of common proprietary decongestants. Am J Psychiat 123 (4):484–487.

Karch, S. and Billingham M. (1986). Myocardial contraction bands revisited. Hum Pathol 17:9–13.

Kase, C., T. Foster, J. Reed et al. (1987). Intracerebral hemorrhage and phenylpropanolamine use. Neurology 37:399–404.

King, J. (1979). Hypertension and cerebral hemorrhage after timolets ingestion. Med J Aust 2 (5):258.

Kikta, D., M. Devereaux and K. Chandar (1985). Intracranial hemorrhages due to phenylpropanolamine. Stroke 16:510–512.

Kizer, K. (1984). Intracranial hemorrhage associated with overdose of decongestant containing phenylpropanolamine. Am J Emerg Med 2:180–181.

Lake, C., Rosenberg, D. and Quirk R. (1990). Phenylpropanolamine use among diet patients. Int J Obesity 14:575–582.

Lake, C., D. Rosenberg, S. Gallant et al. (1990). Phenylpropanolamine increases plasma caffeine levels. Clin Pharmacol Ther 47:675–685.

Lake, C., S. Gallant, E. Masson, P. Miller (1990). Adverse drug effects attributed to phenylpropanolamine: a review of 142 case reports. Am J Med 89: 195–208.

Lake, C. (1991). Manic psychosis after coffee and phenylpropanolamine. Biol Psychiatry 30:401–404.

Le Coz, P., F. Woimant, D. Rougemont et al. (1988). Angiopathies cerebrales benignes et phenylpropanolamine. Rev Neurol (Paris) 144:295–300.

Logie A., Scott C. (1984). Fatal overdosage of phenylpropanolamine. Br Med J 289:591.

Maertens, P., G. Lum, J. Williams et al. (1987). Intracranial hemorrhage and cerebral angiopathic changes in a suicidal phenylpropanolamine poisoning. South Med J 80:1584–1586.

Maher, LM. (1987). Postpartum intracranial hemorrhage and phenylpropanolamine use. Neurology 37:1686.

McDowell, J. and H. LeBlanc (1985). Phenylpropanolamine and cerebral hemorrhage. West J Med 142:688–691.

Mesnard, B. and D. Ginn (1984). Excessive phenylpropanolamine ingestion followed by subarachnoid hemorrhage. South Med J 77:939.

Miller, L. (1991). Phenylpropanolamine: the saga continues. J Clin Psychopharm 11:82–83.

Morgan, J. (1990). Cardiovascular toxicity of cocaine. J Appl Cardiol 5:321–322.

Morgan, J., D. Wesson, K. Puder and D. Smith (1987). Duplicitous drugs: the history and recent status of look-alike drugs. J Psychoactive Drugs 19:21–23.

Muller, S. (1983). Phenylpropanolamine, a nonprescription drug with potentially fatal side effects. N Engl J Med 308:653.

Nagata, T., Kimura, K., Hara, K. and Kudo, K. (1990). Methamphetamine and amphetamine concentrations in postmortem rabbit tissues. Forensic Sci Int 48:39–47.

National Institute on Drug Abuse. (1990a). Annual Emergency Room Data. Data from the Drug Abuse Warning Network. Statistical Series, Number 10-A. Rockville, Maryland, U.S. Department of Health and Human Services.

National Institute on Drug Abuse. (1990b). Annual Medical Examiner Data. Data from the Drug Abuse Warning Network. Statistical Series, Number 10-B. Rockville, Maryland, U.S. Department of Health and Human Services.

Neelakantan, L. and H. Kostenbauder (1976). Electron-capture GLC determination of phenylpropanolamine as a pentafluorophenyloxazolidine derivative. J Pharm Sci 65:740–742.

Norvenious, G., E. Widerlov and G. Lonnerhom (1979). Phenylpropanolamine and mental disturbances. Lancet 2:1367–1368.

Patterson F. (1980). Delayed fatal outcome after possible Rutuss overdose. J Forensic Sci 25:349–352.

Pentel, P. (1984). Toxicity of over-the-counter stimulants. JAMA 252:1898–1903.

Pentel, P., J. Jentzen and J. Sievert (1987). Myocardial necrosis due to intraperitoneal administration of phenylpropanolamine in rats. Fundam Appl Toxicol 9 (1):167–172.

Pentel, P., F. Mikell and S. Zavoral (1982). Myocardial injury after phenylpropanolamine ingestion. Br Heart J 47:51–54.

Stoessl, A., G. Young and T. Feasby (1985). Intracerebral hemorrhage and angiographic beading following ingestion of catecholaminergics. Stroke 16: 734–736.

Swenson, R., T. Golper and W. Bennet (1982). Acute renal failure and rhabdomyolysis after ingestion of phenylpropanolamine-containing diet pills. JAMA 248:1216.

Traynealis, V. and J. Brick (1986). Phenylpropanolamine and vasospasm. Neurology 36:593.

Wharton, B. (1970). Nasal decongestants and paranoid psychosis. Br J Psych 117:429–440.

Winick, C. (1991). Phenylpropanolamine: toward resolution of a controversy. J Clin Psychopharm 11:79–81.

Woolverton, W., Johanson, C., de la Garza, R. et al. (1986). Behavioral and neurochemical evaluation of phenylpropanolamine. J Pharmacol Exp Ther 237 (3):926–930.

3.3 FENFLURAMINE

3.3.1 HISTORICAL ASPECTS

Fenfluramine (Ponderax, Pondimin) was first synthesized in 1963 for use as an anorectic. Fenfluramine is still primarily used as an appetite suppressant, though it has been suggested as a treatment for autism. Fenfluramine causes anorexia by stimulating satiety centers located in the ventromedial hypothalamic nuclei (Teitelbaum 1970). This action seems to be a result of fenfluramine's ability to cause the release of serotonin (5-HT) and its added ability to interfere with the 5-HT uptake carrier (Fuller et al. 1988). In experimental animals, fenfluramine treatment causes large, rapid decreases in brain serotonin and 5-hydroxyindoleacetic acid (5-HIAA) (Garattini 1980). Tryptophan hydroxylase activity is decreased as well (Steranka and Sanders-Bush 1979). Rats given one dose of fenfluramine still have decreased serotonin levels 30 days later (Harvey and McMaster 1975). Fenfluramine hydrochloride is not truly a drug of abuse, but it is an amphetamine derivative with significant pulmonary and neurologic toxicity. A closely related compound, Aminorex fumarate, widely prescribed during the early 1960's as an appetite suppressant, was withdrawn from the market when it became apparent that users were developing pulmonary hypertension (Follath et al. 1971).

3.3.2 DRUG CONSTANTS

Fenfluramine is N-Ethyl-alpha-methyl-3 (trifluromethyl) benzene-ethanamine. Its formula is $C_{12}H_{16}F_3N$, with a molecular weight of 231.27. It is composed of 62.3% carbon, 7% hydrogen, 24.7% fluorine, and 6.1% nitrogen. Crystals of the racemic mixture have a melting point of 108–112°C. Commercial fenfluramine is supplied as a racemic mixture.

3.3.3 METABOLISM

Following a single oral dose of 60 mg, peak plasma concentrations are 0.05 to 0.07 mg/L at 3 hours. This drug has a very long half life (13 to 30 hours), and patients tend to maintain consistent steady-state concentrations (average of 0.16 mg/L) when therapeutic doses are regularly taken (Campbell 1970). In stabilized patients, levels of its principal metabolite, norfenfluramine, are about half as high (Innes et al. 1977). Like the other amphetamines, fenfluramine's excretion depends on the urinary pH. About 20% is excreted unchanged in the urine, and another 20% as the N-dealkylation product norfenfluramine (Beckett and Brookes 1967).

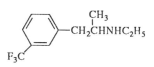

Figure 3.3 Fenfluramine molecule

3.3.4 Blood and tissue levels

One adult surviving a 1,600-mg overdose had peak concentrations of 0.85 mg/L in the plasma (Richards 1969) and a 2-year old who ingested 440 mg had a peak level of 0.78 mg/L with 0.17 mg/L of norfenfluramine (Campbell and Moore 1969). Overdose-related deaths have been reported, though not very frequently. Fenfluramine blood levels in three different children who died after ingesting up to 1,200 mg ranged from 6.5 to 16 mg/L. Hepatic concentrations in these same children were 4 to 9 times higher (24–136 mg/Kg) (Gold et al. 1969) (Simpson and McKinaly 1975). Similar levels were seen in a teenager who died 3.5 hours after taking 2 grams of fenfluramine. Both liver and brain had fenfluramine concentrations 9 times that found in the blood (6.5 mg/L) (Fleisher and Campbell 1969). Low CNS concentrations were seen in the patient reported by Kintz and Mangin. They described the case of a 36-year old woman who died after ingesting an unknown amount of fenfluramine. The blood level was 7.46 mg/L but the brain level was only 0.48 mg/L, while the concentration in the liver was over 155 mg/L. Fenfluramine levels in the hair were 14.1 ng/mg (Kintz & Mangin, 1992).

3.3.5 Toxicity by Organ System

3.3.5.1 Cardiopulmonary

Two patients with fenfluramine-associated pulmonary hypertension came to notice in 1981. Both patients were women who had been taking the medication for over 8 months. In both cases a thorough evaluation disclosed that pulmonary hypertension was due to greatly increased vascular resistance that cleared when the drug was discontinued (Douglas et al. 1981). There are no autopsy reports, but some animal studies are relevant, because pulmonary toxicity has been simulated in an animal model. Dogs infused with fenfluramine have increased pulmonary diastolic pressure. In the rat, massive overdose (130 mg/kg) causes respiratory depression and cardiac ischemia. Electrocardiographic changes in this model include ischemia and conduction delays with widening of the QRS and PR prolongation.

Animals given smaller doses still develop respiratory distress and extensive alveolar and interstitial pulmonary hemorrhages after 24 hours. The changes are worse when animals are pretreated with a serotonin antagonist (Hunsinger and Wright 1990).

3.3.5.2 Neurological

Neurotoxicity has been demonstrated in several animal models. In the rat, structural damage to the serotonergic (5-HT) neurons is evident 36 hours after injecting a single 10 mg/kg dose. Immunochemical studies showed 5-HT axons that were markedly swollen while the cell body remained intact (Molliver and Molliver 1990). Other studies have demonstrated the presence of intralysosomal lamellar bodies in the endothelial cells, pericytes and perivascular astrocytic process of rats given 5 mg/kg doses of fenfluramine, suggesting an inability to metabolize a yet to be identified fenfluramine-phospholipid reaction product. Human studies are nonexistent (Thakkar et al, 1990).

References

Campbell, D. (1970). Gas chromatographic measurement of levels of fenfluramine and norfenfluramine in human plasma, red cells and urine following therapeutic doses. J Chrom 49:442–447.

Campbell, D. and B. Moore (1969). Fenfluramine overdosage. Lancet 2:1306.

Douglas, J., J. Munro, A. Kitchin et al. (1981). Pulmonary hypertension and fenfluramine. Br Med J 283:881–883.

Fleisher, M. and D. Campbell (1969). Fenfluramine overdosage. Lancet 2:1306.

Follath, F., F. Buckart and W. Schweitzer (1971). Drug-induced pulmonary hypertension? Br Med J i:265–266.

Fuller, R., H. Snoddy and D. Robertson (1988). Mechanisms of effects of d-fenfluramine on brain serotonin metabolism in rats: uptake inhibition versus release. Pharmacol, Biochem. Behav 30:715–721.

Garattini, S. (1980). Recent studies on anorectic agents. Trends Pharmaceut Sci 1 :354–356.

Gold, R., H. Gordon, R. DaCoasta et al. (1969). Fenfluramine overdosage. Lancet 2:1306.

Harvey, J. and S. McMaster (1975). Fenfluramine: evidence for a neurotoxic action on midbrain and a long-term depletion of serotonin. Psychopharmacol Commun 1:217–228.

Hunsinger, R. and D. Wright (1990). A characterization of the acute cardiopulmonary toxicity of fenfluramine in the rat. Pharm Res 22 (3):371–378.

Innes, J., M. Watson, M. Ford et al. (1977). Plasma fenfluramine levels, weight loss, and side effects. Br Med J 2:1322–1325.

Kintz, P. and Mangin, P. (1992). Toxicological findings after fatal fenfluramine self-poisoning. Hum & Exp Tox, 11:51–52.

Molliver, D. and M. Molliver (1990). Anatomic evidence for a neurotoxic effect of (+/-)- fenfluramine upon serotonergic projections in the rat. Brain Res 511:165–168.

Richards, A. Fenfluramine overdosage. Lancet 2 (1969):1367.

Schmidt, J. and W. Fleming (1962). The structure of sympathomimetics as related to reserpine induced sensitivity changes in the rabbit ileum. J Pharmacol Exp Ther 139:230–237.

Simpson, H. and I. McKinaly (1975). Poisoning with slow-release fenfluramine. Br Med J 4:462–463.

Steranka, L. and E. Sanders-Bush (1979). Long-term effects of fenfluramine on central serotonergic mechanisms. Neuropharmacology 18:895–903.

Teitelbaum, P. (1970). The biology of drive. In The Neurosciences, ed. GC Guarton, T Melnechuck, and FO Schmitt. 557. New York:The Rockefeller University Press.

Thakkar, B., D. Dastur and D. Manghani (1990). Neuropathology & pathogenesis of experimental fenfluramine toxicity in young rodents. Ind J Med Res B92:54–65.

3.4 MESCALINE ANALOGS ("DESIGNER DRUGS")

"Designer" is a not very satisfactory term for a group of drug analogs that are manufactured illegally. The term has been used to describe such disparate agents as fentanyl, meperidine, amphetamine analogs, and mescaline along with its analogs. Amphetamines share some common mechanisms of toxicity and, for that reason, are considered separately from other psychoactive drugs such as the indole alkylamines (LSD and psilocybin) and the piperidines (phencyclidine).

Compared to the amphetamines, little clinical information is available about any of the "designer drugs", and even less is known about the pathology of the other agents. Often referred to as hallucinogens, they certainly cause changes in how reality is perceived. But whether smaller, recreational doses, actually induce true hallucinosis is difficult to say. More often than not, individuals under the influence of these drugs can distinguish their visions from reality. On the other hand, judgment certainly is impaired. Occasionally it may be so impaired that fatal accidents can result. Mescaline abuse is rare, but abuse of the methyoxylated amphetamines, particularly MDMA, is increasingly popular.

3.4.1 MESCALINE

3.4.1.1 Historical Aspects

Mescaline comes from the cactus referred to as either as *Lophora williamsii* or *Anhalonium Lewinii*. Lewin was one of the first to systematically study this group of plants and their active principle, mescaline. This small cactus can be found growing in dry places and rocky slopes throughout the southwestern United States. It grows singly or in clusters. It is an inconspicuous plant that can be hard to find. Unless it is in flower, it tends to look like a small rock. The dried tops of the plants, know as peyote buttons, have been used by Indian shamans for

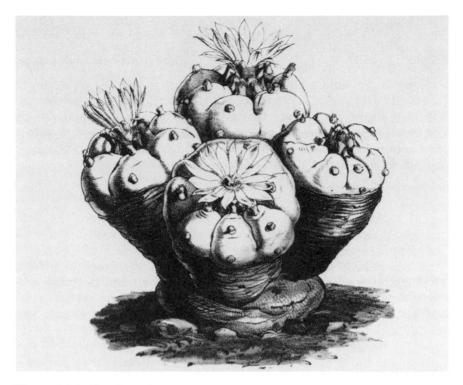

Figure 3.4.1 Peyote cactus
Even though it grows wild throughout the American Southwest, it can be very hard to find. Except when it is in bloom, it tends to resemble a small rock.

centuries. During the early 1800's the Apaches, Kiowas, and Commanches of the Great Plains also began to chew the buttons and incorporated them into their religious rites. The practice quickly spread among the plains Indians who combined its use with elements of Christianity. Their ceremonies still begin with the chewing of peyote buttons, followed by nights of prayers and singing. The sect is now known as the Native American Church and has more than 200,000 members (Barron et al. 1964). Mescaline, or 3,4,5-trimethoxy -ß-phenethylamine, is the active principle found in peyote cactus. The average mescaline content is 6%. No mescaline-related deaths or emergency room visits were reported in the 1990 DAWN survey (National Institute on Drug Abuse, 1992).

The first systematic chemical and pharmacologic studies were reported by Lewin and Henning in 1888 (Lewin and Henning 1888). Lewin's work attracted the attention of the famous American neurologist, S. Weir Mitchell (Prentiss and Morgan 1895). Mitchell, who was a prolific writer and a pioneer in the study of peripheral nerve injuries, was also interested in toxicology and psychiatry (Metzer 1989). He obtained some peyote buttons and took them himself, then published an account of his experiences in the *British Medical Journal* (Mitchell 1896).

He thought that the plant might be of great value in the study of psychological disorders, but he also warned of the abuse potential. The famous sexologist Havelock Ellis also dabbled with mescaline, and described the many benefits to be derived from its use (Anon 1898). Neither the benefits nor the epidemic of abuse ever really materialized. The active principal alkaloid was isolated in 1896, but it structure wasn't elucidated until 1919. Since that time, structural modifications of the mescaline molecule have been used to create a host of other psychoactive compounds. Some have been mostly laboratory curiosities, but others, such as MDMA, are widely used.

3.4.1.2 Drug Constants and Drug Preparation

Mescaline is 3,4,5-Trimethoxybenzeneethanamine or 3,4,5, trimethoxyphenethylamine. Its formula is $C_{11}H_{17}NO_3$, with a molecular weight of 211.23. It is composed of 62.5% carbon, 8.1% hydrogen, 6.6% nitrogen and 22.7% oxygen. Mescaline crystals have a melting point of 35–36°C. Pure mescaline will combine with carbon dioxide in the air to from crystalline carbonates. The hydrochloride form of mescaline, $C_{11}H_{18}CLNO_3$, forms colorless, needle-like crystals, with a melting point of 181°C.

Mescaline is extracted from the cactus by first drying and then grinding the tops of the plants. The ground material is then soaked in methanol for a day, filtered and acidified. After evaporating off the alcohol the solution is neutralized and the mescaline extracted with chloroform. Less sophisticated chemists cook the cactus in a pressure cooker until they end up with a tarry material that can be formed into small pills. Some clandestine producers will even apply an enteric coating, or place the tarry material in gelatin capsules, the idea being to reduce the nausea that often accompanies mescaline use.

3.4.1.3 Metabolism and Tissue Levels

There have been no autopsy reports, and there are only limited metabolic studies. The latter studies were published nearly 30 years ago and were done with techniques that are now considered antiquated. The hallucinogenic dose is thought to be on the order of 200 to 500 mg. Tracer studies in healthy volunteers showed levels of 3.88 mg/L two hours after a 500-mg dose. A 350-mg dose given intravenously produced a peak blood level of 14.8 mg/L at 15 minutes, declining to 2.1 mg/L at 2 hours. The half-life of mescaline is on the order of 6 hours. Most of a given dose is excreted in the urine. About 60% will be excreted unchanged, and about 30% as 3,4,5-trimethoxyphenylacetic acid. Smaller amounts of other inactive metabolites also appear (Charalampous et al. 1966) (Charlampous et al. 1964) (Mokrasch and Stevenson 1959). Generalizing from animal studies is difficult because mescaline is metabolized differently by different species.

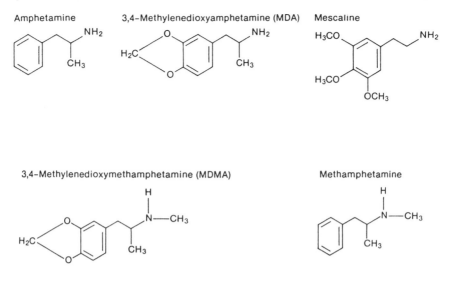

Figure 3.4.1.2 Mescaline and the "designer" amphetamines
Whether small recreational doses of these drugs are hallucinogenic is hard to say, but all of these agents can impair judgment and their use occasionally leads to fatal accidents.

When dogs are injected subcutaneously with mescaline, the highest concentrations are found in the liver and kidneys. Concentrations in the liver, spleen and kidneys are 3 to 6 times the concentration found in the blood stream. Brain levels tend to parallel the blood levels (Kapadia, 1970). Tissue levels have been measured at autopsy in only one case. A mescaline user who died of a head injury had a blood level of 9.7 mg/L with a concentration 8 times as high in the liver (Reynolds 1985).

3.4.1.4 Clinical syndromes

Half a milligram of mescaline given to healthy volunteers produces an artificial psychosis that is indistinguishable from acute schizophrenia. Neuropsychologic measurements made during mescaline intoxication suggest that the behavioral changes are due to right hemispheric striato-limbic hyperactivity, with associated left hemispheric dysfunction (Oepen et al. 1989). The results of PET scanning studies would be of considerable interest, but they are yet to be done. Otherwise, the symptoms associated with mescaline abuse are mostly those of sympathetic stimulation. Transient rises in pulse, blood pressure, and temperature all occur (Kapadia 1970). Laboratory studies on mescaline's cardiovascular effects have yielded inconsistent results.

3.4.1.5 Pathologic findings

Lethal overdoses of mescaline have never been reported, nor have there been any reports of medical complications associated with its use. The deaths that have been reported have been accidental, usually as a result of drug-induced confusion (Reynolds and Jindrich 1985).

References

Anon (1898). Paradise or inferno. Br Med J, 1:390.

Barron, F., M. Jarvik and S. Bunnell. (1964) The hallucinogenic drugs. Sci Am, 210:29–37.

Charalampous, K., A. Orengo, K. Walker and J. Kinross-Wright (1964). Metabolic fate of ß (3,4,5-trimethoxyphenyl)-ethylamine (mescaline) in humans: isolation and identification of 3,4,5-trimethoxyphenylacetic acid. J Pharm Exp Ther, 145:242–246.

Charalampous, K., K. Walker and J. Kinross-Wright (1966) Metabolic fate of mescaline in man. Psychopharmacologia, 9:48–63.

Kapadia, G., Fayez, M. (1970) Peyote constituents: chemistry, biogenesis, and biological effects. J Pharm Sci, 59:1699–1727.

Lewin, T., and Henning (1888). Anhalonium Lewinii. Therapeutic gazette 231–237.

Metzer, W. (1989) The experimentation of S. Weir Mitchell with mescal. Neurology, 39:303–304.

Mitchell, S. (1896) Remarks on the effects of *Anhalonium lewinii* (the mescal button). Br Med J, 2:1625–1629.

Mokrasch, L. and I. Stevenson. (1959) The metabolism of mescaline with a note on correlations between metabolism and psychological effects. J Nerve Ment Dis, 129:177–183.

National Institute on Drug Abuse. (1990a). Annual Emergency Room Data. Data from the Drug Abuse Warning Network. Statistical Series, Number 10-A. Rockville, Maryland, U.S. Department of Health and Human Services.

National Institute on Drug Abuse. (1990b). Annual Medical Examiner Data. Data from the Drug Abuse Warning Network. Statistical Series, Number 10-B. Rockville, Maryland, U.S. Department of Health and Human Services.

Oepen, G., M. Fuenfgeld, A. Harrington et al. (1989). Right hemisphere involvement in mescaline-induced psychosis. Psychiatry Research 29 (3): 335–336.

Prentiss, D. and F. Morgan. (1893) *Anhalonium lewinii* (mescal buttons): study of the drug with special reference to its physiological action upon man, with report of experiments. Ther Gazette, 11:577–585.

Reynolds, P. and E. Jindrich. (1985) A mescaline associated fatality. J Analyt Toxicol 9 (4):183–184.

3.4.2 METHYOXYLATED AMPHETAMINES

Since 1947, when researchers produced the first psychoactive mescaline analog (TMA), structural modifications of the mescaline molecule have been used to produce a succession of psychoactive derivatives. Very little information is available about these agents. As a group, their toxicity is quite low, accounting for the lack of autopsy studies. In most cases, even meaningful animal experiments are lacking. Thus the toxicity of MDMA, which is, at the moment, a widely abused drug, remains poorly characterized.

3.4.2.1 TMA (2,4,5-Trimethoxyamphetamine)

This drug has twice the psychoactive potency of mescaline (Shulgin 1973). It was first synthesized in 1933, but it was never used as a psychedelic until 1962. It produces all the same effects as mescaline, but is said to have a lower therapeutic index. The amount required to cause hallucinatory or psychedelic experiences is not very different from the amount needed to produce toxicity (Chesher 1990).

3.4.2.2 DOM (Methyl-2,5-dimethoxyamphetamine)

This drug was first synthesized in 1963 shortly after TMA (Shulgin 1977). The first reports of abuse appeared in 1967. It was also referred to as "STP" ("serenity, tranquility and peace"). It is a white solid, soluble in most organic solvents and has a melting point 60-61°C. The melting point for the hydrochloride salt is 190-191°C. In doses of less than 3 mg, DOM's effects are said to be like those of mescaline. Higher doses cause hallucinations and unpleasant side effects that may last for as long as 8 hours (Snyder et al 1967).

DOM rapidly developed a rather bad reputation on the streets, probably because it was being used in excessively high doses (Snyder et al. 1967) (Shulgin 1977). Regardless of the dose, about 20% will appear unchanged in the urine with peak excretion occurring at between 3 and 6 hours, the period when intoxication is most intense. Hallucinations produced by higher doses are associated with nausea, diaphoresis and tremor. Moderate elevations in pulse and systolic, but not diastolic pressure occur. Blood and tissue levels have never been determined and the pathologic changes associated with its use, if any, are unknown.

3.4.2.3 PMA (paramethoxyamphetamine)

This interesting compound is a potent hallucinogen that also has sympathomimetic effects. Animal studies done in the early 1960's suggested that PMA's hallucinogenic potency was nearly as great as LSD's (Smythies et al. 1967), though the effects were not quite so marked in man. In limited human studies, occasional instances of marked hypertension were observed. The first PMA fatalities were reported in 1974 (Cimbura 1974). All of the dead were males, between 17 and 30 years of age. Clinical observations on those who died are rather sparse, but they all suffered from the same constellation of symptoms: agitation, seizures, and hyperthermia. Autopsy findings were not described. PMA was rapidly classified as a restricted drug and there have been no further reports of abuse or fatalities.

3.4.2.4 DOB (4-bromo-2,5-dimethoxyamphetamine, also called Bromo-DMA)

This is also an agent with potent hallucinogenic and sympathomimetic properties. It is fairly long acting. Symptoms begin 3–4 hours after ingestion and may take 24 hours to resolve. Because of its high potency it can be sold impregnated in blotter paper, and sometimes has been passed off for LSD (Shulgin 1981). DOB was especially popular in Australia where it was often falsely represented as LSD. After synthesis DOB was impregnated onto sheets of colored paper, usually embossed with some sort of logo or animal sketch. The impregnated sheets were then cut up an sold as 1-cm squares. The problem with this method of distribution is that during preparation the drug may migrate to the corners or bottom of the sheet. Users who bought squares from the center often received less than they paid for, while those who bought squares from the margins of the sheet often got more than they bargained for, which may explain why so many bad experiences were associated with use of the drug (Delliou 1980). This agent is associated with more morbidity than the others. (Bohn 1981) (Buhrich et al. 1983) (Wineck et al. 1981). Diffuse vascular spasm, identical to the classic picture of ergotism, has been reported after DOB use (Bowen et al. 1983). This syndrome has not been reported in conjunction with other "designer" amphetamines, but it is a well known complication of LSD use. Scant autopsy information is available. In one reported case, a 21-year old woman was found dead at the wheel of her parked car. Gross autopsy findings included cerebral edema with uncal herniation. The lungs were minimally congested. Microscopic findings were not reported. Blood and tissue concentrations were as below:

Table 3.4.2.4.1
BLOOD LEVELS IN CASE OF FATAL DOB INTOXICATION

Blood	Bile	Vitreous	Brain	Liver	Kidney
0.9 mg/L	0.64 mg/L	0.51 mg/L	0.25 mg/L	9.0 mg/L	1.1 mg/L

3.4.2.5 MDA (3,4-Methylenedioxyamphetamine, "The Love Drug")

MDA was first synthesized by two Merck chemists, Mannich and Jacobsohn, in 1910 (Mannich and Jacobsohn 1910). It was recognized early on that MDA had marked sympathomimetic effects, including tachycardia and hypertension (Gunn et al. 1939). Gordon Alles tried it on himself in a series of experiments which were described in Hoffer and Osmond's text on the hallucinogenic drugs (Hoffer and Osmond 1967). MDA was patented both as an anorectic agent and as an antitussive (Lukaszewski 1979), but never saw commercial distribution.

Like the other members of this group, MDA exhibits both amphetamine and hallucinogenic properties. The amphetamine-like actions are more pronounced with the (L)-isomer and the hallucinogenic effects with the (D)- isomer. The (D)-isomer, at least in rats, is extremely arrhythmogenic and even moderate doses can provoke ventricular tachycardia. This may explain some reported cases of MDA-associated sudden death. Illicitly manufactured MDA is always a racemic mixture (Marquardt et al. 1978), but the proportions of each isomer present may vary. Some batches may be more toxic than others, even if they contain pure MDA. Amphetamine-associated effects include vasoconstriction, tachycardia,and pupillary dilatation. There may also be convulsions and hyperthermia. MDA first appeared on the illicit market in the early 1960's and was responsible for a number of deaths. Its share of the illicit market rapidly faded when MDMA was introduced, but it still remains available on the black market. The last death to be reported was in 1990 (Nichols et al. 1990). Other than that one case, there were no mentions in the 1990 DAWN survey.

The principal oil in nutmeg, safrole, can be used as a precursor to synthesize MDA by amination, and this process has been utilized in some clandestine laboratories. Illicitly produced MDA is sold in powder or liquid form, almost always as the hydrochloride salt (Ratcliffe 1974). It is generally taken orally, but can be snorted or injected, and fatalities have been associated with each route. Clinical studies with MDA are limited. The effects of a 150-mg dose will peak at 1.5 hours, but can last for as long as 8 hours. MDA is said to produce feelings of well-being and heightened tactile sensations. Detection of this drug is likely to be serendipitous. Both MDA and MDMA cross-react with the screening agents used to detect amphetamine and methamphetamine (Ramos et al. 1988). Blood and tissue levels have been reported in several fatal cases; reported levels have been remarkably similar in all cases.

Dogs treated with large doses of MDA die from hyperthermia and acidosis (Davis et al. 1987). Human autopsy findings in the case reported by Poklis, other than visceral congestion, included epicardial, subendocardial, gastric and subpleural petechiae (Poklis et al. 1979). In the five cases described by Cimbura, agitation, hallucinations and delirium were prominent features, but autopsy findings were not mentioned. Compared to other amphetamines, blood levels in these five individuals were quite high, ranging from 6 to 26 mg per liter. In two of the cases hepatic concentrations were lower than blood levels, in one case they were higher (Cimbura 1972). The case described by Reed had visceral congestion with pulmonary edema and there were petichae on the surface of the heart (Reed et al. 1972). The latter is probably not of great significance since the patient had undergone resuscitative measures which can cause such petichae (Karch 1987). The last reported case was that of a 26-year old whose clinical history suggested arrhythmia. At autopsy fresh thrombosis was found in a severely obstructed (75%) left main coronary artery. Microscopic features were not described (Nichols et al. 1990).

3.4.2.6 MDMA (3,4-methylenedioxymethamphetamine; other names include XTC, Adam, MDM)

The free base is white and musty smelling. Salts are readily soluble in water. The empiric formula is $C_{11}H_{15}NO_2$. Such a wide range of melting points have been reported for the different salts as to make them of little value. Merck was issued a patent for MDMA in 1914, but the toxicology of this compound wasn't studied systematically until the early 1950's when the U.S. Army contracted with a group at the University of Michigan to study MDMA's toxicity. The results of the Michigan studies, which were finally declassified and published in 1973, showed that MDMA was somewhat less toxic than MDA, but more toxic than mescaline (Hardman et al. 1973). Prior to its classification as a schedule I drug in 1985, MDMA enjoyed some popularity in the psychiatric community, and arguments were (Shulgin 1986), and continue to be (Grob et al., 1992) made for its therapeutic value. It has been suggested that the use of MDMA, in a controlled, therapeutic setting, promotes trust and confidence between patients and therapists. MDMA's reputation as an empathy-enhancing compound (Eisner 1989), or "empathogen", is fairly well established.

The illicit production of this drug is fairly straightforward. Safrole, the active ingredient in nutmeg, is used to prepare the starting ketone (3,4-(methylenedioxy)phenylpropanone) by oxidization with hydrogen peroxide in an acid medium. The resulting compound is then combined with methylamine in alcohol. Aluminum powder, freshly treated with mercuric chloride in ethanol, is added to the mixture which is then boiled for several hours. MDMA can then be distilled off under pressure (Verweij, 1990).

MDA is a known breakdown product of MDMA, but how much is metabolized via this pathway is hard to say, because illicitly manufactured MDMA usually also contains small amounts of MDA. Very little is known about the pharmacology of MDMA in humans. Its half-life is on the order of 8 hours, but levels in intoxicated patients are poorly characterized, and the clinical pharmacology has been studied in only one patient. In Army experiments the LD_{50} in dogs was found to be 8–23 mg/kg when the drug was injected intravenously. In rhesus monkeys the range was 17–28 mg/kg. After ingesting 50 mg orally, a 74-kg man had a peak level of 105 ng/mL at 2 hours. Blood levels declined to 5.1 ng/mL at 24 hours. Over the course of three days, 72% of the dose was

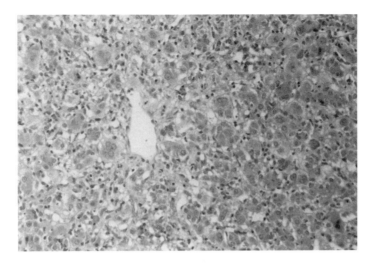

Figure 3.4.2.6 MDMA hepatitis
Florid hepatitis with inflammatory cell infiltrates and lobular disarray. The infiltrate is predominantly mononuclear, but a number of eosinophils and neutrophils are present in the portal tracts. It is not clear whether these changes represent a reaction to MDMA or to some contaminant in the drug. Courtesy of Dr. N. G. Ryley, John Radclyffe Hospital, Oxford.

excreted unchanged in the urine (Verebey et al. 1988). Blood levels in intoxicated drivers have ranged from 0.11 to 0.59 mg/L (Bost 1988). There is one case report of a 13-month old child who ingested a capsule of MDMA, containing anywhere from 50 to 150 mg of drug. The child developed a typical hyperadrenergic syndrome with fever, tachycardia, hypertension and convulsions. Serum MDMA measured roughly 90 minutes after ingestion was 700 ng with 100 ng of MDA detected at the same time (Russell, Schwartz, Dawling 1992).

There appears to be tremendous overlap between recreational and toxic levels. In seven patients who died of MDMA toxicity, blood levels ranged from 110 ng/mL to 1260 ng/mL. Levels in five patients who survived serious bouts of toxicity were from 200 to 970 ng, while levels in five car-accident victims were from 50 to 340 ng/mL (Henry, Jeffreys, Dawling 1992). Reports from England have described patients with severe hepatitis. Liver damage seems to have been the result of an idiosyncratic reaction to MDMA or to some contaminant ingested along with it. In the cases that have been reported to date, all of the standards tests for hepatitis have been negative. A liver biopsy in one case showed florid changes with both portal and lobular necrosis. There was an inflammatory infiltrate containing mostly monocytes and there were substantial numbers of eosinophils. Liver biopsy in another case showed extensive necrosis concentrated in the periportal areas. The infiltrate was comprised of plasma cells and lymphocytes with only an occasional eosinophil. In both the biopsied cases, recovery was uneventful.

Rat liver and brain microsomes both metabolize MDA, via demethylation, to dihydroxyamphetamine and MDMA to dihydroxymethamphetamine. In both locations the conversion is cytochrome P450 dependent. Both of the metabolites can be further oxidized to form quinone or semiquinones that can react with sulfhydryl groups. The presence of these latter compounds could account for the known toxic effects of MDMA on serotonergic neurons (Hiramatsu et al. 1990) (Lin et al., 1992).

MDMA shares the same properties as the other members of this group, affecting both the heart and the central nervous system. Neurotoxicity in animals is manifested by damage to serotonergic neurons. In the rat model even one dose results in degeneration of serotonin-containing neurons. Animals treated with massive and repeated doses, while showing initial damage, do eventually recover and at one year after treatment have no apparent lesions (Battaglia et al. 1987). There is considerable interspecies variation in the response to MDMA. The monkey is much more sensitive to the MDMA's serotonin depleting effects than is the rat (Ricaurte et al. 1985) (Barnes 1988).

No brain lesions have been demonstrated in humans, but chronic paranoid psychosis has been reported in MDMA abusers (McGuire, 1991). Clinically, there is no evidence that humans ever develop typical symptoms of serotonin depletion (disorders of sleep, mood, appetite). On the other hand, at least one preliminary study found that humans previously exposed to MDMA have lower concentrations of 5-HIAA in their spinal fluid than non drug using controls. When compared to normals, MDMA users had 26% less 5-HIAA, and since the 5-HIAA content of the spinal fluid is thought to reflect the activity of central serotonergic neurons, the results suggest the presence of at least impaired function, if not morphologic changes. The situation is analogous to the problems with fenfluramine. It is a definite neurotoxin in animals, but no pathology has been reported in the 50 million plus users who have taken it for diet control (Grob et al. 1990).

In spite of very wide-spread use, reports of adverse effects in the United States have been rare. However, a number of fatalities have been described in the British literature, and from the data that has been presented, it appears that the increased toxicity seen in the U.K. is a function of how the drug is used (Chadwick et al. 1991) (Campkin & Davies, 1992) (Screaton et al., 1992) (Fahal et al., 1992) (Henry, 1992). Almost all of the case reports from England involve young people who develop hyperthermia, rhabdomyolysis, renal failure and disseminated intravascular coagulation. Common to almost all the cases is the fact that, after taking the drug, the victims danced for many hours in hot, poorly ventilated clubs. That such cases are rarely encountered in the United States probably has to do with the fact that American users tend to take the drug while they are alone, or at small gatherings, and that they don't do anything to generate more heat over and above that generated by MDMA's disruption of serotonin metabolism. The situation is likely to change in the near future, as "rave" parties, where participants use MDMA and dance all night, have become increasingly popular in the United States.

Autopsy information about MDMA-related deaths is very spotty. Some of the deaths appear to have been secondary to malignant rhythm disturbances. Dowling described a case with high-grade multivessel disease who collapsed and died at the wheel of his car. His blood level was 0.95 mg/L, and autopsy was otherwise unremarkable (Dowling et al. 1987). Suarez described a 34-year old with Wolf-Parkinson-White syndrome and an MDMA blood level of 0.2 mg%, who died of a cardiac arrhythmia. Findings at autopsy were unremarkable except for the heart which had areas of patchy fibrosis (Suarez and Riemersma 1988). Other deaths manifested fairly classic amphetamine/catechol toxicity with hyperadrenergic symptoms, including fever, tachycardia and hypertension, as well as rhabdomyolysis, renal failure and disseminated intravascular coagulation (Chadwick, Curry, Linsely et al., 1991) (Campkin & Davies, 1992). One such patient died after taking an undetermined amount of MDMA (only a qualitative toxicology screen was done). No microscopic findings were reported, and the general autopsy disclosed diffuse pulmonary and cerebral edema with "evidence of a generalized hemorrhagic diathesis" (Simpson and Rumak 1981). Another individual survived in spite of developing fever, tachycardia and pulmonary edema, apparently brought on by only 150 mg (twice a normal dose) (Brown et al. 1987). MDMA can precipitate death by misadventure. One intoxicated individual electrocuted himself (Dowling et al. 1987). Of course the presence of the drug might also be just an accidental finding. Dowling described one asthmatic with a blood MDMA of 1.1 mg/L and autopsy findings of severe chronic lung disease.

3.4.2.7   MDEA (3,4-methylenedioxyethamphetamine, Eve)

This agent appeared on the market shortly after MDMA. It is a close relative of MDMA, with essentially the same actions. It was banned in 1985 along with MDMA. Neither the clinical pharmacology nor toxicology of this compound have been studied. There is one reported fatality in an individual with an enlarged heart and some non-specific histologic changes. His blood contained 2.0 mg/L of MDEA.

3.4.2.8   4-MAX (U4Euh,EU4EA,U4EA,4-Methylaminorex,Aminorex)

4-MAX and 4-Methylaminorex belongs to a group of compounds know as oxazolines. Aminorex was sold in Europe by McNeil Laboratories during the 1960's under the brand names Menocil™ and Apiquel™. It was promoted for appetite suppression and weight reduction, but had to be withdrawn from the market when its use was linked with the development of fatal pulmonary hypertension. The first reports of 4-Methylaminorex abuse were from Florida during the mid-1980's, but since then sporadic seizures have occurred across the country. On the street it is sometimes called "Ice" or "Blue Ice". Instead of being sold under its own name it is often misrepresented as methamphetamine. Because it is relatively simple to synthesize, it has the potential to become a low-cost substitute for cocaine or methamphetamine (World Health Organization, 1991). 4-methylaminorex was classified as a Schedule I substance in April 1989. No deaths or emergency room visits were attributed to 4MAX in the 1990 DAWN report.

The cis -(+)isomer is the form found in most clandestine drug laboratories. It is synthesized in a one-step reaction by condensing phenylpropanolamine with cyanogen bromide. It could also be produced starting with norpseudoephedrine. Both phenylpropanolamine and norpseudoephedrine are unrestricted and easily available. In laboratory experiments 4-MAX produces the same effects as the other amphetamines, causing substantial increases in brain dopamine release and decreases in tryptophan hydroxylase activity (Hanson, Bunker, Johnson et al.1992). When it was discovered that aminorex had lethal side effects, all work with it and related compounds stopped, and current clinical research is all but nonexistent. In animal trials, 4-MAX seems to be more epileptogenic than the other compounds in this class (Hanson et al. 1991), but otherwise it would be logical to suppose that 4-methylaminorex shares common mechanisms of toxicity with the rest of the amphetamines.

Pharmacokinetic studies of Aminorex were done before sophisticated methods became available, and the pharmacokinetics of 4MAX have been studied hardly at all. Aminorex absorption is relatively rapid. A single 15-mg oral dose produces peak plasma concentration of 40 μg/mL at two hours. Concentrations decline slowly after that, dropping to 5 μg/mL at 24 hours. The reported half-life for aminorex in humans is 7.7 hours. Studies have not been done on 4MAX, but the similarities to Aminorex are so great that it should behave in much the same way. Most of a given dose is eliminated unchanged in the urine (World Health Organization, 1991).

Detecting 4-MAX in blood or body fluids is problematic, because neither aminorex nor 4-MAX are detectable with the routinely used screening tests. None of the currently available radioimmunoassays (RIA), fluorescence polarization assays (TDX) or enzyme multiplied immunoassays (EMIT) for amphetamines cross-react with the oxazolines. Detection with chromatographic or spectrophotometric techniques is not a problem, but since most medical examiners and all workplace testing programs screen with immunoassays, the presence of the oxazolines is likely to go undetected. Blood and urine levels have been measured in one fatality. The 4MAX concentration in the blood was 21.3μg/Ml in the

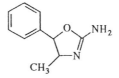

Figure 3.4.2.8 Aminorex molecule
4-Methylaminorex differs from MDMA and other ring-substituted amphetamines. It is classified as an oxazoline and has a side chain substitution that resembles pemoline, a potent stimulant.

blood and 12.3 μg/mL in the urine (World Health Organization, 1991).

3.4.2.9 Ephedrone
(2-methylamino-1-phenylpropan-1-one, "Jeff")

This agent has been in use in the former USSR for several years, and there are sporadic reports from elsewhere in Europe. It is synthesized directly from ephedrine by oxidation with potassium permanganate. Of course in the United States the preferred route is reduction to form methamphetamine. The popularity of this form in the former USSR may have to do with the availability of raw materials. A number of deaths have been attributed to "Jeff" overdoses, but nothing is known of the pathology or clinical pharmacology of this agent (Zhingel et al. 1991).

References

Barnes, D. (1988). New data intensify the agony over Ecstasy. Science 239: 864–866.

Battaglia, G., S. Yeh and E. DeSouza (1988). MDMA-induced neurotoxicity: parameters of degeneration and recovery of brain serotonin neurons. Pharmacol Biochem Behav 29:269–274.

Bedford, A., Schwartz, R., Dawling, S. (1992). Accidental ingestion of "Ecstasy" (3,4-methylenedioxymethylamphetamine). Arch Dis Child, 67: 1114–1115.

Bohn, G. (1981). Illegally manufactured 2,5-dimethoxy-4-bromoamphetamine in connection with a fatal intoxication. Toxichemistry 14 (1981):140–141.

Bost, R. (1988). 3,4-Methylenedioxymethamphetamine (MDMA) and other amphetamine derivatives. J Foren Sci 33 (2):576–587.

Bowen, J., G. Davis, T. Kearney and J. Bardin (1983). Diffuse vascular spasm associated with 4-bromo-2,5-dimethoxyamphetamine ingestion. JAMA 249:1477–1479.

Brown, C., J. Osterloh (1987). Multiple severe complications from recreational ingestion of MDMA ('Ecstasy'). JAMA 258 (6):780–781.

Buhrich, N., G. Morris and G. Cook (1983). Bromo-DMA: the Australian hallucinogen? Australia and New Zeland J Psych 17 (3):275–279.

Campkin, T., U. Davies. (1992). Another death from Ecstasy. J R Soc Med, 85(1):61.

Chadwick, I., Curry, P., Linsley, A. et al. (1991). Ecstasy, 3-4 Methylenedioxy-methamphetamine (MDMA), a fatality associated with coagulopathy and hyperthermia. J R Soc Med, 84(6):371.

Chesher, G. (1990). Designer drugs - The "whats and the whys." Med J Aust 153 (3):157–161.

Cimbura, G. (1972). 3,4-Methylenedioxyamphetamine (MDA): Analytical and forensic aspects of fatal poisoning. J Forensic Sci 17:329–333.

Cimbura, G. (1974). PMA deaths in Ontario. Can Med Assoc J 110:1263–1267.

Davis, W., H. Hatoum and I. Waters (1987). Toxicity of MDA (3,4-methylene-dioxyamphetamine) considered for relevance to hazards of MDMA (Ecstasy) abuse. Alcohol and Drug Res 7:123–134.

Delliou, D. (1980) Bromo-DMA: new hallucinogenic drug. Med J Aust:83.

Dowling, G., E. McDonough and R. Bost (1987). "Eve" and "Ecstasy": a report of five deaths associated with the use of MDEA and MDMA. JAMA 257:1615–1617.

Eisner, B. (1989). Ecstasy, the MDMA story. Berkeley: Ronin Publishing.

Fahal, I., D. Sallomi, M. Yaqoob & G. Bell. (1992). Acute renal failure after ecstasy. Br Med J 305:29.

Grob, C., G. Bravo and R. Walsh (1990). Second thoughts on 3,4-Methylenedi-oxymethamphetamine (MDMA) neurotoxicity. Arch Gen Psychiatry 47: 288.

Grob, C., Bravo, G., Walsh, R. and Liester, M. (1992). The MDMA-neurotoxicity controversy: implications for clinical research with novel psychoactive drugs. J Nerve Ment Dis, 180:355–356.

Gunn, J., M. Gurd and I. Sachs (1939). The action of some amines related to adrenaline: methoxy-phenylisopropylamines. J Physiol 95:485–500.

Hanson, G., Bunker, C., Johnson, M. et al. (1992). Response of monoaminergic and neuropeptide systems to 4-methylaminorex: a new stimulant of abuse. Euro J Pharm, 218:287–293.

Hanson, G., Johnson, M., Bush, L. et al. (1991). Behavioral and neurochemical responses to 4-methylaminorex: a new stimulant of abuse. In L. Harris, (ed.) In Committee for problems of drug dependency, Annual Conference. Published in National Institute on Drug Abuse Monograph Series, in press.

Hardman, H., C. Haavik and M. Seevers (1973). Relationship of the structure of mescaline and seven analogs to toxicity and behavior in five species of laboratory animals. Toxicol and Appl Pharmacol 25 (2):299–309.

Henry, J., Jeffreys, K. and Dawling, S. (1992). Toxicity and deaths from 3,4-methylenedioxymethamphetamine ("ecstasy"). Lancet, 340:384–387.

Henry, J. (1992). Ecstasy and the dance of death: severe reactions are unpredictable. Br Med J 305:5–6.

Hiramatsu, M., Kumagai, Y., Unger, S. and Cho, A. (1990). Metabolism of methylenedioxymethamphetamine:formation of dihydroxymethamphe-tamine and a quinone identified as its glutathione adduct. J Pharmacol Exp Ther, 254:521–527.

Hoffer, A. and H. Osmond (eds.) 1967. The Hallucinogens, New York: Academic Press.

Karch, S. (1987). Resuscitation-induced myocardial necrosis. Am J Forensic Med and Path 8 (1):3-8.

Lin, L., Kumagai, Y. and Cho, A. (1992). Enzymatic and chemical demethylenation of (Methylenedioxy) amphetamine and (Methylenedioxy)methamphetamine by rat brain microsomes. Chem Res Toxicol, 5:401-406.

Lukaszewski, T. (1979). 3,4-Methylenedioxyamphetamine overdose. Clin Toxicol 15:405-409.

Mannich, C. and W. Jacobsohn (1910). Hydroxy phenyalkylamines and dihydroxyphenalkylamines. Berichte 43:189.

Marquardt, G., V. DiStefano and L. Ling (1978). Pharmacological and toxicological effects of ß-3,4-methylenedioxyamphetamine isomers. Toxicol Appl Pharmacol 45 (1978):675-683.

Nichols, G., G. Davis, C. Corrigan and J. Ransdell (1990). Death associated with abuse of a "designer drug". Kentucky Med Assn J 88 (November): 600-603.

Poklis, A., M. Mackell and W. Drake (1979). Fatal intoxication from 3,4-methylenedioxyamphetamine. J Forensic Sci 24:70-75.

Ramos, J., R. Fitzgerald and A. Poklis (1988). MDMA and MDA cross reactivity observed with Abott TDx amphetamine/ methamphetamine reagents. Clin Chem 34 (5):991.

Ratcliffe, B. (1974) Editorial: MDA. Clin Toxicol 7 (4):409-411.

Reed, D., R. Cravey and P. Sedgwick (1972). A fatal case involving methylenedioxyamphetamine. Clin Toxicol 5:3-6.

Ricaurte, G., G. Bryan, L. Strauss et al. (1985). Hallucinogenic amphetamine selectively destroys brain serotonin nerve terminals. Science 229: 986-988.

Screaton, G., H. Cairns, M. Sarner et al. (1992). Hyperpyrexia and rhabdomyolysis after MDMA ("ecstasy") abuse. Lancet 33:677-678.

Shulgin, A., Sargent, T., Naranjo, C. (1973). Animal pharmacology and human psychopharmacologyofß-methoxy-4,5-methylenedioxyphenylisopropylamine (MMDA). Pharmacology 10:12-18.

Shulgin, A. (1977). Profiles of psychedelic drugs: STP. J Psychedelic Drugs 9:171-172.

Shulgin, A. (1981). Profiles of psychedelic drugs:DOB. J Psychedelic Drugs 13:99.

Shulgin, A. (1986). The background and chemistry of MDMA. J Psychoact Drugs 18:291-304.

Simpson, D. and B. Rumak (1981). Methylenedioxyamphetamine: Clinical description of overdose, death and review of pharmacology. Arch Intern Med 141:1507-1509.

Smythies, J., V. Johnston, R. Bradley et al. (1967) Some new behaviour-disrupting amphetamines and their significance. Nature 216 (October 14): 128-129.

Snyder, S., L. Failace and L. Hollister (1967). 2,5-dimethoxy-4-methyl-amphetamine (STP): a new hallucinogenic drug. Science 158 (1967):669-670.

Suarez, R. and R. Riemersma (1988). "Ecstasy" and sudden cardiac death. Am J For Med and Pathol 9 (4):339-341.

Verebey, K., J. Alrazi, and J. Jaffe (1988). The complications of 'Ecstasy' (MDMA). JAMA 259 (11):1649-1650.

Verweij, A. (1990) Clandestine manufacture of 3,4 methylenedioxymethylamphetamine (MDMA) by low pressure reductive amination. A mass spectrometric study of some reaction mixtures. Forensic Sci Int 45:91–96.

World Health Organization (1991). Information manual designer drugs. World Health Organization, Vienna, 103–119.

Winek, C., W. Collom and J. Bricker (1981). A death due to 4-bromo-2,5-dimethoxyamphetamine. Clin Toxicol 18:267–271.

Zhingel, K., W. Dovensky, A. Crossman and A. Allen (1991). Ephedrone: 2-methylamino-1-phenylpropan-1-one (Jeff). J Forensic Sci 36 (3):915–920.

4 Indole Alkylamines, Arylhexylamines and Phenylalkylamines

4.1 PSILOCYBIN

4.1.1 HISTORY

Psilocybin-containing mushrooms were probably used by the Aztecs, but until the 1960's they aroused little interest outside of Mexico. The name psilocybin is derived from the Greek roots "psilo" meaning bald and "cybe" meaning head, presumably because of the shape of the mushrooms from which the compounds are derived. The molecule's structure wasn't even established until 1958, when the active principle of these mushrooms was isolated by Albert Hoffman at Sandoz Pharmaceuticals. Hoffman had succeeded in synthesizing LSD only a few years earlier. For some time Sandoz marketed pure psilocybin under the brand name Indocybin™ (Stafford 1982).

Psilocybin can be found in three different genera of mushrooms: *Psilocyba, Panelous, and Concybe.* All three varieties grow naturally in the northwestern and southeastern portions of the United States. Related or identical forms grow wild in Central and South America as well as South East Asia, and India. Large quantities are cultivated for illegal distribution. The most common species is *Psilocybe cubensis,* and it grows wild in the manure of cattle, water buffalo, and other ruminants, including deer, and possibly even kangaroos. In Southeast Asia, farmers collect droppings from these animals and systematically grow the fungi in disused rice paddies (Allen & Merlin, 1992).

All three genera contain the tryptophan derivatives psilocybin (4-phosphoryloxy-N-N-dimethyltryptamine) and psilocin (4-hydroxyl-N, N-dimethyltryptamine. *Psilocybe cubensis* is generally the preferred cultivar, and on average yields 10 mg of psilocybin per gram of fresh mushroom, which is equal to an average dose. Psilocin is 1.5 times more potent than psilocybin, but because the latter oxidizes more slowly than the former, both contribute about equally to the mushroom's effect (Leikin, Krantz et al. 1989). During the early 1980's, growing kits complete with spores were advertised in magazines. They are now illegal (Schwartz and Smith 1988).

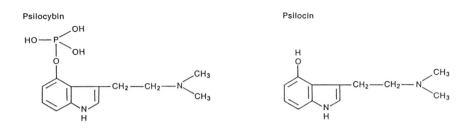

Figure 4.1 Psilocybin and Psilocin molecules

Identifying wild *Psilocyba* is difficult and can be dangerous. Psilocybin-containing mushrooms grow side by side with the poisonous *Galerina autumnalis*. The two can be separated by the fact that Galerina species have rust brown colored spores while the spores of Psilocybe species are gray to lilac. Some, but not all, species of *Psilocybe* mushrooms can be distinguished from poison mushrooms by the fact that, when cut, they will oxidize and turn blue within 30 to 60 minutes. Unfortunately, some poisonous mushrooms can do the same thing. As a result, pathologists are much more likely to encounter cases of mushroom poisoning than they are to encounter psilocybin-associated medical problems!

4.1.2 CHEMICAL CONSTANTS

Psilocybin is 3-[2-(Dimethylamino)ethyl]-1 H-indol-4-ol dihydrogen phosphate ester. Its formula is $C_{12}H_{17}N_2O_4P$ with a molecular weight of 284.27. It is composed of 50.7% carbon, 6% hydrogen, 9.9% nitrogen, 22.5% oxygen and 10.9% phosphorus. The melting point is variable, depending on how it was crystallized. Psilocin, the 4-hydroxy analog of psilocybin, is formed by metabolic dephosphorylation. It is also contained in hallucinogenic mushrooms, but in much smaller amounts. Psilocin is the active form within the central nervous system and, on a weight for weight basis, is much more potent than psilocybin. Its formula is $C_{11}H_{16}N_2O$ with a molecular weight of 204.27. It forms plate-like crystals and has a melting point of 173–176°C (Merck, 1989).

4.1.3 METABOLISM AND TISSUE LEVELS

Controlled human studies are nonexistent. Pharmacokinetic studies in rodents, which may or may not be relevant to man, suggest that 50% of a given dose will be absorbed from the stomach, and that 65% will be excreted in the urine, with another 20% appearing in the bile and stool. Most of the excretion occurs in the first 8 hours but, in the rat at least, labeled drug may appear in the urine for as long as a week (Aboul-Enein 1974). Tissue levels have not been reported in humans.

4.1.4 CLINICAL FINDINGS

Symptoms consistent with sympathetic stimulation have been described. A 30-year old case report describes the death of a 6-year old child who developed hyperthermia and status epilepticus after ingesting an undetermined number of mushrooms (McCawley, Brummett et al. 1962). A review of 27 patients with "magic mushroom" poisoning found that mydriasis and hyperreflexia were as common as disorders of perception, and that all of the individuals recovered uneventfully (Peden, Macaulay et al. 1981). A paper published in 1983 reviewed 318 cases reported to Poison Control Centers and found increasing use, but no serious toxicity (Francis and Murray 1983). Since then no other cases have been reported. It seems probable that any deaths that do occur are likely to be accidental, usually as a result of drug-induced confusion. In times of shortage, dealers may misrepresent LSD or PCP as psilocybin, producing a somewhat puzzling clinical picture.

REFERENCES TO 4.1

Aboul-Enein, H. (1974). Psilocybin: a pharmacological profile. Am J Pharm 146: 91–95.

Allen, J. and M. Merlin (1992). Psychoactive mushroom use in Koh Samui and Koh Pha-Ngan Thailand. J. Ethnopharm 35:205–228.

Francis, J. and V. Murray (1983). Review of enquiries made to the NPIS concerning psilocybe mushroom ingestion, 1978-1981. Hum Toxicol 2:349–352.

Leikin, J., A. Krantz et al. (1989). Clinical features and management of intoxication due to hallucinogenic drugs. Med Toxicol Adverse Drug Exp 4(5):324–350.

McCawley, E., R. Brummett et al. (1962). Convulsions from Psilocybe mushroom poisoning. Proc West Pharmacol Soc 5:27–33.

Peden, N., K. Macaulay et al. (1981). Clinical toxicology of "magic mushroom" ingestion. Postgraduate Med J 57:543–545.

Schwartz, R. and D. Smith (1988). Hallucinogenic mushrooms. Clin Peds 27(2): 70–73.

Stafford, P. (1982). Psychedelics encyclopedia, revised edition. J.P Tarcher, Inc, Los Angeles and Boston.

4.2 LYSERGIC ACID DIETHYLAMINE

4.2.1 HISTORY

Albert Hoffman synthesized LSD in 1938. He had been working as a research chemist at Sandoz Laboratories in Basel, where his chief interest was the chemistry of ergot. He isolated lysergic acid from ergot and then combined it with various amines via peptide linkages. He was

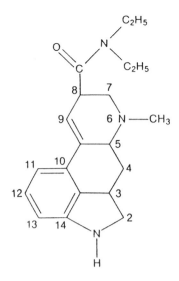

Figure 4.2 LSD-25
LSD-25 was produced by Albert Hoffman at Sandoz Laboratories. He had
isolated lysergic acid from ergot and was trying to make a chemical agent that
would act as a circulatory stimulant. LSD-25 was the 25th compound that he
produced.

trying to produce chemical agents that lacked some of ergot's toxic side
effects, but which might have use as circulatory or respiratory stimulants. In that goal, at least, he was successful. He synthesized Methergi-
ne™, which is still used today to stop uterine bleeding after birth.
During the course of his experiments he created a series of related
compounds. The twenty-fifth substance he produced was d-lysergic acid
diethylamine (LSD-25). When tested on laboratory animals, the results
were disappointing.

For five years Hoffman worked on other projects, but in April
of 1943 he decided to re-evaluate LSD-25. The hallucinogenic experience
which ensued when he accidentally ingested some LSD led to the start
of the modern "psychedelic" age. After further studies, Sandoz eventually marketed LSD as Delysid™, recommending, among other things,
that psychiatrists try it on themselves so that they might find out first-
hand what the subjective experiences of a schizophrenic were like
(Ulrich and Patten 1991).

LSD was never a great commercial success, but its availability
fostered research into the chemical origins of mental illness. None of the
theories proposed during the 50's and 60's proved correct, but these
theories eventually did lead to more modern research into serotonin
metabolism and receptor research. They also led to some rather bizarre
experiments by the Central Intelligence Agency. It was thought that
LSD had great potential for mind control. To verify that theory, the CIA

mounted a special operation called MK-ULTRA. Prostitutes were used to lure business men to brothels where they were secretly dosed with LSD and their behavior observed. The experiments were unsuccessful.

The psychedelic age began in the early 1960's when Timothy Leary undertook his researches with psilocybin at Harvard. In 1961 he tried LSD and was so altered by the experience that he dropped his psilocybin studies and began researching the effects of LSD. He was forced to leave Harvard in 1962, but by that time the media had launched the psychedelic age to the tune of Leary's anthem: "Tune in, Turn on, Drop Out". LSD was finally outlawed by the Federal government in 1965. The outlawing of LSD use, coupled with questionable studies demonstrating chromosomal damage as a consequence of LSD use, led to a rapid decline in popularity (Ulrich, 1991). Sporadic reports from around the country indicate there is renewed interest in LSD use, but the seizure of a clandestine LSD laboratory is a distinctly rare event. Over the past few years here has been some fluctuation in the price of LSD. The average price on the street for one "hit" ranges from $1 to $10. At wholesale (more than 1,000 "hits"), prices range from 35 cents to $3.50 per dose. (US Department of Justice, 1992).

LSD is usually available at the same "rave" parties where MDMA is sold. However the doses used today are only a fraction of what was taken in the 1960's, and that may explain why current reports of toxicity are uncommon.

4.2.2 CHEMICAL CONSTANTS AND DRUG MANUFACTURE

LSD is 9,10-Didehydro-N-diethyl-6-methylergoline-8ß-carboxamide. It is also referred to as LSD25 because it was the 25th derivative of lysergic acid that Hoffman synthesized. Its formula is $C_{20}H_{25}N_3O$, with a molecular weight of 323.42. It is composed of 74.3% carbon, 7.8% hydrogen, 13% nitrogen, and 5% oxygen. When crystallized from benzene it forms pointed prisms with a melting point of 80–85°C.

Clandestine chemists have two options when it comes to producing LSD. Alkaloid related to LSD can be extracted from the seeds of plants such as morning glories, and then further processed to make LSD. The Hawaiian baby woodrose is the preferred seed, since it contains nearly 7 mg of alkaloid per gram of seeds (Smith, 1981). Alternatively, *Claviceps purpurea* can be cultured with yields of egotamine as high as 4 grams per liter. Even if starter fungus can't be purchased commercially, it can be found growing on top of rye grass, just by the seed-bearing area. Growing large quantities of fungus is technically demanding, and probably not done that often.

The result in either case is an assortment of different lysergic acid molecules, each linked to different amide groups. The amide is hydrolyzed off and used as the starting point for the synthesis of LSD. The synthesis utilizes a number of fairly toxic and potentially explosive chemicals, including hydrazine, trifluoroacetic acid and diethylamine. The dangerous nature of the business may account for the infrequency with which LSD labs are discovered.

4.2.3 TISSUE LEVELS AND METABOLISM

The standard street dose is between 100 and 300 μg (Cohen 1984). This small amount of drug can be impregnated in almost any medium, including sugar cubes and chewing gum. A recurring urban myth has it that children may be exposed to the drug by applying temporary (water soluble) tattoos. While in theory such could certainly be the case, in fact this occurrence has never been reported. Smaller quantities of LSD are being used today than in the past. In the early 1980's the standard "street" dose was from 100 to 300 μg (Cohen, 1984). The standard dose today is much lower, typically ranging from 20 to 80 μg (Nelson, Foltz 1992).

Absorption is rapid and almost complete. LSD circulates in the blood mostly bound to protein and has an estimated half-life of 2.5 hours. Human volunteers given 2 μg/kg intravenously had plasma levels of 6–7 ng/ml 30 minutes later. After that, the level gradually declined with an apparent half-life of 175 minutes (Aghajanian and Bing 1964). When a single oral dose of 160 μg was given, the peak blood level was 9 ng/mL, and the calculated half-life was almost identical (180 minutes) to the half-life seen after intravenous administration (Upshall and Wailling 1972). When 50 micrograms were given to a volunteer, LSD was detectable 3 days after ingestion at a cut off level of less than 1 ng (Vu-Duc, 1991). Levels have been measured in emergency room patients with LSD intoxication. Blood samples were obtained anywhere between 2 and 11 hours after ingestion, and levels were found to range from 0.5 to 1.9 ng/mL (McCarron, Walberg et al. 1990). Urine concentrations in the same patients were between 0.2 and 7.7 ng/mL. Serum levels in other cases of severe intoxication have been remarkably similar, ranging between 2 and 4 ng/mL (Baselt and Cravey 1989). Tissue levels have not been measured in humans.

4.2.4 CLINICAL SYNDROMES

LSD usage results in somatic, perceptual and psychic symptoms that seem to follow each other in a fairly predictable order. Physiologic effects are, however, minimal and unpredictable. The clinical changes produced by LSD seem to be indistinguishable from those produced by mescaline. It has been suggested that changes in pulse rate, respiration and blood pressure seen with LSD use are probably just the result of varying anxiety levels (Klepitz and Racy 1973). In the past there were frequent reports of acute panic reactions (Barnett 1972), "flashbacks" (Moskowitz 1971), and homicides while under the influence (Klepitz and

Racy 1973). Lapses of judgment resulting in self-injury can also occur, but the incidence of such events also seems to be decreasing. There have been no reports of fatalities due directly to LSD effects and no reported autopsy studies.

4.2.5 DETECTION

Since the half-life of LSD is relatively short and the amounts ingested quite small, detection is a problem. Urine concentrations reach sub-nanogram levels within a few hours after ingestion, and there are problems with most of the currently used detection techniques. Since LSD is not one of the "NIDA 5", there has been relatively little incentive to develop effective detection techniques. Newer approaches using the combination of gas chromatography and tandem mass spectrometry should allow the detection of LSD and its metabolites in low-pg/mL concentrations in both urine and blood (Nelson, Foltz 1992).

REFERENCES TO 4.2

Aghajanian, G. and O. Bing (1964). Persistence of lysergic acid diethylamide in the plasma of human subjects. Clin Pharm Ther 5:611–614.

Barnett, B. (1972). Diazepam treatment for LSD intoxication. Lancet II(270):

Baselt, R. and RH. Cravey (1989). Disposition of toxic drugs and chemicals in man. Chicago, London, Year Book Medical Publishers, 470–473.

Cohen, S. (1984). The hallucinogens and the inhalants. Psych Clin N Amer 7: 681–688.

Klepfisz, A. and J. Racy (1973). Homicide and LSD. JAMA 223:429–430.

McCarron, M., C. Walberg et al. (1990). Confirmation of LSD intoxication by analysis of serum and urine. J Analyt Toxicol (May/June):165–167.

Moskowitz, D. (1971). Use of haloperidol to reduce LSD flashbacks. Milit Med 136:754–756.

Nelson, C., Foltz, R. (1992). Determination of lysergic acid diethylamide (LSD), iso-LSD, and n-demethyl-LSD in body fluids by gas chromatography/tandem mass spectrometry. Anal Chem, 64:1578–1585.

Smith, M. V. (1981). Psychedelic chemistry. Loompanics Unlimited, Port Townsend, Washington.

Ulrich, R. and B. Patten (1991). The rise, decline and fall of LSD. Persp Biol and Med 34(4):561–578.

Vu-Duc, T, Vernay, A. and Casalanca, A. 1991. Detection of lysergic acid diethylamine in human urine: elimination, screening and analytical confirmation. Schweizerische Medizinische Wochenschrift (French). 121 (50):1887–1890.

4.3 PHENCYCLIDINE

4.3.1 HISTORICAL ASPECTS

Phencyclidine (1-(1-phenylcyclohexyl piperidine, or PCP) was discovered by pharmacologists at Parke-Davis in 1956 (Greifenstein,

Devault et al. 1958). Marketed as an intravenous anesthetic called Sernyl™ (Collins, Gorospe et al. 1960), it had a number of advantages over other surgical anesthetics. In recommended doses it produced neither respiratory nor cardiovascular depression and, at least in animals, it appeared to be devoid of cellular toxicity (Chen and Weston 1960). Unfortunately, human use had to be discontinued because 10 to 20% of patients became delirious and unmanageable for many hours after surgery (Greifenstein, Devault et al. 1958). Even so, it was a good veterinary anesthetic that continued in use until production was discontinued in 1979. Recreational abuse was first reported in California during the late 1960's, and the drug soon developed a reputation for causing antisocial, violent behavior (Fauman, Aldinger et al. 1976). Abuse was prevalent during the 1970's and early 1980's, but during the last 10 years illicit use of PCP has markedly decreased, while the price at wholesale has increased. The DAWN report for 1990 lists only 4,400 PCP-related emergency room visits and no fatalities (National Institute on Drug Abuse 1990a; National Institute on Drug Abuse 1990b).

Phencyclidine's mode of action is probably the most complex of any abused drug. Many of PCP's central nervous system effects are similar to those of methamphetamine. PCP blocks dopamine uptake, and on a weight-per-weight basis, is nearly as potent a reuptake blocker as the amphetamines. PCP also causes the release of stored catecholamines, but in this respect, at least, it is much less potent than methamphetamine (Johnson and Jones 1990) (Yang, Moroji et al. 1991). In addition to its stimulant properties, PCP has depressant, hallucinogenic and analgesic effects (Peterson, Stillman, 1978). PCP abusers report experiencing heightened sensitivity to stimuli, along with mood elevation, and feelings typical of inebriation (Siegel 1978).

PCP has become the subject of intense interest in the scientific community. There is strong evidence that PCP, and other related compounds, protect against the effects of cerebral ischemia (Olney, Price et al. 1987). PCP binds with high affinity to membrane receptors located in the NMDA receptor (N-methyl-D-aspartate) complex (Su 1991). The fact that PCP competitively binds at the NMDA receptor complex is of interest, because it is stimulation of this complex that mediates the neurotoxic events responsible for tissue damage in stroke (Nuglisch, Rischke et al. 1991). Some PCP derivatives, such as MK-801, show even more neuroprotective activity than PCP. Binding in the NMDA complex probably does not explain the behavioral effects of PCP, because PCP also binds the sigma receptor. Sigma receptors are found not just in the central nervous system, but also on membranes from endocrine, immune and peripheral tissues (Su, 1991). Their stimulation is thought to be responsible for many of the unpleasant side effects associated with opiate use. In addition to PCP, cocaine, pentazocine, and even anabolic steroids all bind sigma receptors, which may explain certain similarities in the behavioral effects of all these drugs.

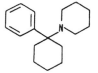

Figure 4.3.3 Phencyclidine molecule
The preferred route in clandestine labs starts with condensation of 1-phenyl-cyclopentylamine with pentamethylene dibromide. The ethyl ether and other volatile solvents used in the process give off a dinstinctive odor that often gives away the location of the laboratory.

Whatever the mechanism for PCP's behavioral and psychological effects, death appears to be a consequence of respiratory and cardiac depression. In the dog model of extreme PCP intoxication, death results when convulsions are followed by respiratory failure and cardiac failure that is secondary to hypoxia, hyperpyrexia and acidosis. If the animals are paralyzed, convulsions and hyperthermia are prevented, but respiratory and cardiac depression still occur. At the highest doses, death seems to be entirely due to myocardial depression (Davis, Hackett et al. 1991). These results can be extrapolated to humans only with great caution, because reports of massive overdose (blood level > 1,800 ng/mL) in humans don't mention myocardial compromise (Jackson, 1989).

4.3.2 PHYSICAL CONSTANTS
Phencyclidine has a molecular weight of 243, and its hydrochloride form has a melting point range of 234 to 236° C. It is water-soluble with a pKa of 8.5. It is a tertiary amine and its most important physical property, at least so far as toxicity is concerned, is its lipid solubility. PCP is extremely lipophilic and is rapidly shifted from the blood stream into adipose tissue and the brain.

4.3.3 CLANDESTINE LABORATORIES
In clandestine labs the preferred route of synthesis involves condensation of 1-phenylcyclopentylamine with pentamethylene dibromide (Kalir, Sadeh et al. 1969). Other routes are possible and many different analogues have been detected in street samples. PCP is sold in bulk either in liquid or powder form. Street drug may be anywhere from 50 to 100% pure. The ethyl ether and other volatile solvents used in the production process give off a distinctive odor that often gives away the location of the laboratory. The fumes are also quite explosive, making illicit PCP production a risky affair. Street prices have risen over the years, but have leveled off recently. In 1976 the price on the street was

1–3 dollars per hit (Lundberg, Gupta et al. 1976). Depending on the part of the country, one gallon of illicit PCP sells for $3,000 to $10,000. The national range for one ounce of powder is $1,000 to $2,000. At the street level, prices are much higher than they were during the 1970's, and PCP soaked cigarettes (which contain 5–10 mg of PCP) sell from 10–20 times more than they did in the 1970's (Department of Justice, 1992).

4.3.4 ROUTES OF ADMINISTRATION

PCP can be smoked, snorted, injected, or swallowed. Cigarettes soaked in PCP were very popular during the 1980's. In some parts of the country, PCP-laced cigarettes are called "Sherms", because the cigarette preferred for soaking purposes was produced by a company called Nat Sherman. Parsley leaves soaked in PCP are an occasionally used alternative. Studies on human volunteers who smoked 100 μg of (^{3}H)-phencyclidine indicate that most of smoked PCP is absorbed. Peak blood levels occur 15 to 20 minutes after smoking, but there is a second peak, suggesting delayed release from the lungs. The maximum concentration achieved in this particular smoking study was 1.5 ng/mL. The mean half-life of the smoked PCP was 24 hours ±7 hours (Cook, Brine et al. 1982a). Oral absorption is nearly as good as intravenous administration. Volunteers given 1 mg orally had average PCP concentrations of 2.7 ng/mL. Plasma concentration after 1 mg given intravenously were 2.9 mg/mL. Peak plasma levels after oral dosing were at 2.5 hours, although levels were near maximal at 1.5 hours. After both oral and intravenous administration there follows a 1–2 hour plateau period, where plasma levels remain relatively stable (Cook, Brine et al. 1982b).

Some skin absorption does occur, and can result in positive urine tests, possibly at levels exceeding NIDA cutoffs. In one study a crime lab chemist was found to have a PCP level of 28 ng/mL (Pitts et al, 1981). Just how relevant all of these measurements are to the problems of clinical intoxication is not entirely clear. The amounts used for the volunteer studies are probably very small when compared to the amounts taken by abusers. When PCP was first introduced as a legal anesthetic, sophisticated techniques for measuring blood levels were not available. Now that such techniques exist, ethical considerations prevent the administration of PCP in quantities that accurately reflect street practices.

4.3.5 METABOLISM

PCP is extensively metabolized and less than 10% is excreted unchanged in the urine (Woodworth, Owens et al. 1985) (Wall, Brine et al. 1981). Recovery of PCP and its metabolites in urine and feces is incomplete. Hydroxylated derivatives accounting for less than 50% of a total dose can be recovered from the urine. At the same time, unchanged PCP can be found in saliva and sweat, suggesting that some elimination may occur by these routes (Cook, Brine et al. 1982b).

Phencyclidine is metabolized by hydroxylation on position 4 of the cyclohexane ring and/or on the piperidine moiety. Both of the resulting metabolites are pharmacologically inactive. The metabolites then undergo glucoronidation, and are excreted in the urine. Since PCP is a weak base, acidification of the urine enhances its excretion. In the past, PCP overdoses were given ammonium chloride or ascorbic acid, in hopes of increasing excretion and minimizing toxicity, but this approach was eventually found to be ineffective. On the other hand, continuous gastric suction has proved a useful treatment because PCP is excreted into the stomach, setting up a pathway for gastroenteric recirculation (Aniline and Pitts 1982) .

The window for detection of PCP in the urine is variable. In experimental animals the half-life for PCP is only 3–5 hours (Woodworth, Owens et al. 1985), but in humans it is much longer. After oral administration the terminal half-life may approach 24 hours, which means that PCP should still be detectable in the blood for 5 days, and for at least as long in the urine. NIDA cutoffs require the presence of at least 25 ng/ml before a measurement may be reported out as positive.

4.3.6 TISSUE LEVELS

PCP levels during clinically apparent intoxication, and at autopsy, have been extensively reported. Intoxication is not apparent with blood levels lower than 3 ng/mL, but otherwise clinical correlations between blood levels and physical findings, except for systolic blood pressure, are generally poor (Bailey, Shaw et al. 1978b). In 70 cases where PCP was deemed a factor in the death, 90% of the cases had blood levels ranging from 10 to 300 ng/mL (Budd and Liu 1982). In a smaller series of 5 PCP-related deaths and 10 cases of intoxication, levels at autopsy ranged from 8–2,100 ng/mL. The 10 individuals with clinical evidence of intoxication had plasma levels ranging from < 10 ng up to 812 ng/mL (Bailey, Shaw et al. 1978a). The PCP blood levels that result from a given dose may vary depending on what other drugs are being used at the same time. In a dog model of PCP intoxication, concurrent administration of PCP with marijuana results in higher blood and brain levels of PCP than when PCP is used alone. Alcohol, on the other hand, does not exert this effect (Godley 1991). This synergy may explain why PCP and marijuana are frequently detected in the same urine specimens.

Table 4.3.6.1
BLOOD AND TISSUE LEVELS IN 70 FATAL CASES OF PCP INTOXICATION.

Blood	Urine	Liver	Bile	Brain	Kidney
100–2,400	100–7,600	100–7,820	100–1,690	30–710	400–900

Concentrations are in ng/mL. *Adapted from Budd and Liu.*

4.3.7 INTERPRETING BLOOD AND TISSUE LEVELS

PCP blood and urine measurements are of historical interest only. They prove that the individual in question did, at one time, take PCP. The clinical and forensic importance of isolated blood and urine levels is impossible to determine. PCP is rapidly extracted from the blood by brain and fatty tissues which then slowly release PCP back into the circulation. In one animal study, PCP levels in adipose tissue were 13 times higher than brain levels and 20 times higher than blood levels (James and Schnoll 1976). Continued slow release from these depots can occur over an extended period of time. PCP also makes its way back into the circulation after being reabsorbed from the gastric contents entering the small bowel. Measurable levels may persist for months (Aniline and Pitts 1982). NIDA guidelines call for screening and confirmation tests with a 25 ng/mL cutoff, thereby significantly reducing the time frame for detectability. If the cutoff were reduced by one half, the period during which PCP could be detected might be lengthened by a period of weeks! Controlled studies on the limits of detection have not been published, but in one case report a police chemist who had daily contact with PCP still had a blood level of 70 ng/mL 6 months after leaving the laboratory to go back to school (Pitts et al. 1981). PCP remains stable in stored urine specimens for long periods of time. There is almost no change in PCP concentration after 3 months of cold storage, and half of the initial concentration of PCP will still be present after 6 months (Hughes, Hughes et al. 1991). Since PCP is no longer marketed, either as a human or veterinary anesthetic, its presence can only be explained by illicit use.

Episodes of fatal PCP intoxication, as opposed to homicides and trauma deaths where PCP is an incidental finding, are uncommon (Noguchi and Nakamura 1978) (Poklis, Graham et al. 1990). Tolerance to PCP is seen in animals, and almost certainly in man. It has been argued that tolerance in humans is proven by the fact that blood levels in patients dying directly from PCP's effects overlap with the blood levels seen in individuals with accidental deaths (Poklis, Graham et al. 1990) (Bailey 1979). This same phenomenon can be seen in cocaine-related deaths, and probably in all other stimulant related fatalities.

A case report from 1989 is of some interest. A man swallowed two balloons full of PCP and promptly lapsed into a coma, however the particulars of his history were unknown to his physicians until he passed the two balloons, one ruptured, while he was still comatose on day 11. His maximum blood level on the third hospital day was 1,879 ng/mL. His blood level at the time he passed the two balloons was not recorded, but the level in his cerebrospinal fluid was 245 ng/mL, and the blood level the day before was nearly 1,000 ng/mL (Jackson 1989). Maternal/fetal relationships have not been studied in depth, but the limited number of studies that have been published have shown not only that PCP crosses the placenta with ease, but also that the fetus concentrates the drug and usually has higher levels than the mother (Aniline and Pitts 1982).

4.3.8 TOXICITY BY ORGAN SYSTEM

4.3.8.1 Neurologic disorders

The limited number of autopsy studies that have been reported make no mention of neuropathologic changes. Whether this reflects a lack of toxicity or just limited numbers of observations remains to be seen. All of the arylhexylalkyamines that have been tested, including MK-801, ketamine, and tiletamine produce acute changes in rat brains. Vacuolization of neurons in the posterior cingulate and retrosplenial cortices can be seen within 4 hours of subcutaneously injecting 1 mg/kg of PCP. There is some evidence that the changes resolve and that tolerance to the effects develops with repeated usage (Olney and al 1989). It is conceivable that these transient changes could account for behavioral disorders that are seen in human PCP users, but there is no proof one way or the other. Fatal status epilepticus has been reported (McCarron, 1981) (Kessler, Demers et al. 1974), but these cases are difficult to interpret, because PCP, and related compounds such as MK-801, have anticonvulsant properties (Balster 1987)!

4.3.8.2 Renal Disorders

In one series of 1,000 PCP intoxicated patients, 2.2% had rhabdomyolysis, and three of these patients had renal failure requiring dialysis (McCarron, 1981). Most instances of renal failure appear to be in deeply comatose patients who also were suffering from drug-induced seizures (Hoogwerf, Kern et al. 1979) (Fallis, Aniline et al. 1982)(Cogen, Rigg et al. 1978) (Cho, Hiramatsu et al. 199)

REFERENCES TO 4.3

Aniline, O. and F. Pitts (1982). Phencyclidine (PCP): a review and perspectives. CRC Crit Rev Toxicol. 10:145-177.

Bailey, D. (1979). Phencyclidine abuse: clinical findings and concentrations in biological fluids after nonfatal intoxication. Am J Clin Path. 72:796-799.

Bailey, D., R. Shaw and J. Guba (1978a). Phencyclidine abuse: plasma levels and clinical findings in casual users and in phencyclidine-related deaths. J Analyt Toxicol. 2:233–237.

Bailey, D., R. Shaw and J. Guba (1978b). Phencyclidine abuse: plasma levels and clinical findings in phencyclidine-related deaths. J Analyt Tox. 2: 233–237.

Balster, R. (1987). The behavioral pharmacology of phencyclidine. Psychopharmacology: The third generation of progress. New York, Raven Press.

Budd, R. and Y. Liu (1982). Phencyclidine concentrations in postmortem body fluids and tissues. J Toxicol Clin Toxicol. 19(8):843–850.

Chen, G. and J. Weston (1960). The analgesic and anesthetic effect of 1-(1-phenylcyclohexyl)piperidine HCL on the monkey. Anesth Analg. 39:132–137.

Cho, A., M. Hiramatsu, R. Pechnick and E. Di Stefano (1989). Pharmacokinetic and pharmacodynamic evaluation of phencyclidine and its decadeutero variant. J Pharm & Exp Ther. 250:210–215.

Cogen, F., Z. Rigg, J. Simmons and E. Domino (1978). Phencyclidine associated acute rhabdomyolysis. Ann Intern Med. 88:210–212.

Collins, V., C. Gorospe and E. Rovenstine (1960). Intravenous nonbarbiturate, nonnarcotic analgesics: preliminary studies. I. Cyclohexylamines. Anesth Analg. 39:302–306.

Cook, C., B. Brine, B. Quin et al. (1982a). Phencyclidine and phenylcyclohexene disposition after smoking phencyclidine. Clin Pharmacol Ther. 31(5):635–641.

Cook, C., D. Brine, R. Jeffcoat et al. (1982b). Phencyclidine disposition after intravenous and oral doses. Clin Pharm Ther. 31(5):625–634.

Davis, W., R. Hackett, K. Obrosky, and I. Waters (1991). Factors in the lethality of IV phencyclidine in conscious dogs. Gen Pharmacol, 22(4):723–728.

Fallis, R., O. Aniline, F. Pitts Jr. and L. Weiner (1982). Massive phencyclidine intoxication. Arch Neurol. 39:316.

Fauman, B., G. Aldinger, M. Fauman and P. Rosen (1976). Psychiatric sequelae of phencyclidine abuse. Clin Toxicol. 9:529–537.

Godley, P., Moore, E., Woodworth, J. and J. Fineg (1991). Effects of ethanol and delta-9-tethrahydrocannabinol on phencyclidine disposition in dogs. Biopharmaceutics and Drug Disp, 12:189–199.

Greifenstein, F., M. Devault, J. Yoshitake and J. Gajewski (1958). A study of 1-arylchclohexamine for anesthesia. Anesth Analg. 37:283–294.

Hoogwerf, B., J. Kern, M. Bullock and C. Comty (1979). Phencyclidine-induced rhabdomyolysis and acute renal failure. Clin Toxicol. 14:47–53.

Hughes, R., Hughes, A., Levine, B, and M Smith (1991). Stability of phencyclidine and amphetamines in urine specimens. Clin Chem, 37 (12): 2141–2142.

Jackson, J. (1989). Phencyclidine pharmacokinetics after a massive overdose. Ann Intern Med. 111:613–615.

James, S. and S. Schnoll (1976). Phencyclidine: tissue distribution in the rat. Clin Toxicol. 2:573–582.

Johnson, K. and S. Jones (1990). Neuropharmacology of phencyclidine: basic mechanisms and therapeutic potential. Am Rev Pharmacol Toxicol. 30: 707–750.

Kalir, A., S. Sadeh, H. Karoly et al. (1969). 1-Phenylcycloalkylamine derivatives, II. J Med Chem. 12:473.

Kessler, G., L. Demers, C. Berlin et al. (1974). Phencyclidine and fatal status epilepticus. N Engl J Med. 291:979.

Lundberg, G., R. Gupta and S. Montgomery (1976). Phencyclidine: patterns seen in street drug analysis. Clin Toxicol. 9:503–511.

McCarron, MM, Schuylze, B, Thompson, GA et al. (1981). Acute phencyclidine intoxication: clinical patterns, complications and treatments. Ann Emerg Med, 10:290–297.

National Institute on Drug Abuse (1990a). Annual Emergency Room Data. Data from the Drug Abuse Warning Network. Statistical Series, Number 10-A. Rockville, Maryland, U.S. Department of Health and Human Services.

National Institute on Drug Abuse (1990b). Annual Medical Examiner Data. Data from the Drug Abuse Warning Network. Statistical Series, Number 10-B. Rockville, Maryland, U.S. Department of Health and Human Services.

Noguchi, T. and G. Nakamura (1976). Phencyclidine-related deaths in Los Angeles County, 1976. J Forensic Sci. 23:503–507.

Nuglisch, J., R. Rischke and J. Krieglstein (1991). Preischemic administration of flunarizine or phencyclidine reduces local cerebral glucose utilization in rat hippocampus seven days after ischemia. Pharmacology. 42(6): 333–339.

Olney, J., Labruyere, J. and M. Price (1989). Neurotoxic effects of phencyclidine. Science. 244:1360–1362.

Olney, J., M. Price, K. Salles et al. (1987). MK-801 powerfully protects against N-methyl aspartate neurotoxicity. Eur J Pharmacol. 141:357–361.

Petersen, R., and Stillman, R. (1978). Phencyclidine: an overview. In Phencyclidine (PCP) Abuse: an appraisal. NIDA Research Monograph 21. Petersen R, and Stillman, R eds, pg 1-17, National Institute on Drug Abuse, Rockville, MD.

Pitts, F., Allen, R., Aniline, O, and L. Yago (1981). Occupational intoxication and long-term persistence of phencyclidine (PCP) in law enforcement personnel. Clin Toxicol, 18 (9) 1015–1020.

Poklis, A., M. Graham and D. Maginn (1990). Phencyclidine and violent deaths in St. Louis Missouri: a survey of Medical Examiners' cases from 1977 to 1986. Am J Drug Alcohol Abuse. 16(3&4):265–274.

Siegel, R. (1978). Phencyclidine and ketamine intoxication: a study of four populations of recreational users,. Phencyclidine (PCP) abuse: an appraisal. NIDA Research Monograph 21. Washington, DC, National Institute on Drug Abuse.

Su, T-P. (1991). Review. Sigma receptors, putative links between nervous, endocrine and immune systems. Eur J Biochem, 200:633–642

Wall, M., D. Brine, A. Jeffcoat et al. (1981). Phencyclidine metabolism and disposition in man following a 100 μg intravenous dose. Res Comm in Substance Abuse. 2:161–172.

Woodworth, J., S. Owens and M. Mayersohn (1985). Phencyclidine (PCP) disposition kinetics in dogs as a function of dose and route of administration. J Pharm Exp Ther. 234:654–661.

Yang, Q., T. Moroji, Y. Takamatsu, Y. Hagino and M. Okuwa (1991). The effects of intraperitoneally administered phencyclidine on the central

nervous system - behavioral and neurochemical studies. Neuropep-
tides. 19(2):77–90.

5 Narcotics

5.1 INTRODUCTION

5.1.1 PREVALENCE OF OPIATE RELATED MORBIDITY

Medical examiners participating in the Federally sponsored DAWN (Drug Abuse Warning Network) program reported 5,830 drug related deaths in 1990. Heroin toxicity accounted for approximately one third of the cases (National Institute on Drug Abuse 1990), and opiates, as a group, for two thirds. Toxicity from the other opiates was much less frequent than with heroin. Table 5.1.1 lists the other agents that were encountered in the United States during that same time period.

TABLE 5.1.1
DEATHS FROM NARCOTIC ANALGESICS IN 1990 (DAWN REPORT).

DRUG	Number of Mentions	Percentage of Mentions
Heroin/Morphine	1976	34
Codeine	682	12
Methadone	421	7
D-Propoxyphene	258	4
Hydrocodone	45	0.7
Meperidine	35	0.6
Oxycodone	25	0.4
Hydromorphone	14	0.2
Oxymorphones	12	0.2

As a group, the narcotic analgesics accounted for slightly more than 50% of all drug related deaths compared to 43% attributable to cocaine.

5.1.2 CLASSIFICATIONS OF NARCOTIC AGENTS

Opiate-related toxicity may be due to (1) direct effects of the drug or its metabolites (2) direct effects of adulterants or expients injected along with the drug, or (3) infectious, mechanical, or lifestyle complications associated with the practices of drug abuse. Earlier schemes classified opiates on the basis of their source, as either naturally occurring (morphine or codeine), semisynthetic, morphine-based (heroin or hydromorphone), semisynthetic thebane based (oxymorphone or oxycodone), or purely synthetic (meperidine or pentazocine) (Inturrisi 1982). This classification, while possibly of some interest to forensic chemists, does little to explain mechanisms of toxicity. A much more useful way to classify these drugs is by the receptors to which they bind.

The body produces endogenous pain-relieving substances that have molecular structures similar to that of morphine. These substances, called endorphins or enkephalins, along with exogenous opiates such as morphine, bind to opioid receptors located in the brain, and throughout the body. Depending on which receptor is activated, the result may be, among other things, analgesia, dysphoria, or respiratory depression. At least 5 different types of opiate receptors are thought to exist. The receptors have been given Greek names based on the type of drugs that bind to them. The Mu receptor is so named because morphine binds to it. Other molecules that bind at this same site are called mu agonists, not only because they bind to the same receptor, but also because they cause the same effects as morphine. The effects associated with mu receptor activation are supraspinal analgesia, euphoria, moderate sedation, and respiratory depression. Table 5.1.2 lists the principal receptor types and the effects that can be anticipated when they are stimulated (Lipman 1990).

TABLE 5.1.2
OPIATE RECEPTOR TYPES

Receptor Type	Result of Stimulation
Mu_1	supraspinal analgesia
Mu_2	respiratory depression, sedation, bradycardia
Kappa	spinal analgesia, sedation
Sigma	dysphoria, psychomotor stimulation, tachycardia

Morphine also binds to sigma receptors. Activation of these receptors produces most of the undesirable effects associated with the clinical use of morphine: dysphoria, psychomotor stimulation, and hallucinations. With a few notable exceptions (such as propoxyphene, which, in addition to being a mu agonist, is also a potent local anesthetic), direct opiate toxicity is due to mu receptor activation. While there may be some important clinical differences between mu agonists, there is little to distinguish the direct toxic effects of one from another. For that reason, the pathologic changes attributable to opiate abuse are considered here as a group. Pharmacokinetic and toxicologic data is supplied for the 10 agents cited most frequently in the DAWN reports. Toxicity from the other opiates is too rare to be characterized.

REFERENCES

Inturrisi, C. (1982). Narcotic drugs. Med Clin North Am. 66:1061–1071.
Lipman, A. (1990). Clinically relevant differences among the opioid analgesics. Am J Hosp Pharm. 47(Suppl 1):S7–S13.
National Institute on Drug Abuse (1990). Annual Medical Examiner Data. Data from the Drug Abuse Warning Network. Statistical Series, Number 10-B. Rockville, Maryland, U.S. Department of Health and Human Services.

5.2. HISTORY OF OPIATE ABUSE

5.2.1 ORIGINS IN ANTIQUITY

Opium poppies can be seen on coins and in drawings that antedate written mentions in the Greek literature by at least 1,000 years (Kritikos and Papadaki 1967). Homer and Hesiod discussed the medicinal merits of poppies, and writings from the classical period of ancient Greece frequently mentioned the same subject. In Greek the poppy was referred to as *opion*. The term was derived from the word for juice (*opos*). Translated into Latin, *opion* becomes *opium*. For the ancients, the poppy symbolized sleep, occasionally everlasting. The cup given to Socrates contained the standard solution used at the time for purposes of euthanasia and suicide: a mixture of hemlock and opium. Opium was known, but used sparingly in Europe during the Middle Ages, possibly because medieval surgeons seemed to have been largely indifferent to the suffering of their patients (Kramer 1979).

5.2.2 INTRODUCTION TO EUROPE AND ASIA

During the Renaissance opium's popularity increased. This was partially due to the efforts of Philippus Aureolus Theophrastus Bombast von Hohenheim, a.k.a. Paracelsus (1490-1540). Paracelsus recognized that, no matter what the cause of a disease, sleep and pain relief were part of the cure. And so Paracelsus medicated his patients with formulas that contained opium. He prescribed opium in a host of different formulations. He called one of the formulations "laudanum" (from the Latin, "something to be praised."). It was comprised of one fourth opium, to which was added henbane juice, crushed pearls and coral, "bone of the heart of a stag, bozar stone, amber, musk, and essential oils." An alternative preparation used opium in combination with orange and lemon juice, frogs' sperm, cinnamon, cloves, ambergris and saffron (Macht 1915). Somewhat more streamlined versions of laudanum were used

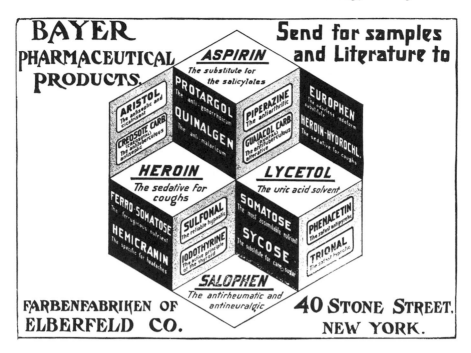

Figure 5.2.1 Heroin
First marketed as a cough suppressant, it was especially recommended for the treatment of tuberculosis. Bayer began selling heroin in 1898. The name derives from the German for "great" or "heroic". Courtesy of the National Library of Medicine.

well into the nineteenth century (Lewin 1931). In much the same way that Freud later enthusiastically recommended the use of cocaine as a panacea (Freud 1884), Sydenham (1624-1689) argued that opium was the drug of choice for a range of conditions, not all of them painful (Sydenham 1848). Thomas Dover, a ship's doctor and one of Sydenham's students, earned his place in history for two contributions: he rescued the real Robinson Crusoe, and he created a powdered opium formulation that became an immensely popular home remedy. Dover's Powder was still being used in the early 1900's.

Medical writers began to discuss opiate toxicity as early as 1700. Terry quotes an English physician who claimed to have successfully separated opium's "noxious Quality" from its "palliative" and "curative" actions, thereby avoiding the complications associated with excessive opium use. That physicians over-relied on opium should not be surprising: opium worked. It improved the conditions it was prescribed for. It relieved pain, calmed stomachs, and suppressed coughs. Until the 20th century, such efficacy could be claimed for few other drugs. Because opium was widely available and widely used, it was inevitable that many would became addicted (Haller 1989) .

In 1803 Sertürner began his experiments with opium, trying to separate its components. In 1805 he published a report announcing that he had isolated an alkaline base in opium called *morphium*. He continued his researches on *morphium* for many years, frequently using himself as a subject; at one point he nearly died of an overdose. His discovery of morphine was certainly important clinically, but his discovery also marked a sea change in the way chemists thought about the chemicals contained in plants. Prior to the discovery of morphine, it was universally held that plants could only produce products that were acid or, at most, neutral. It was believed that only metallic compounds could be alkaline. When Sertürner successfully crystallized morphine, it completely changed the way chemists thought about plant products. In relatively rapid succession, hundreds of other potent plant alkaloids, including quinine and cocaine, were isolated (Macht 1915). Commercial morphine production began not long after morphine's isolation. The founder of England's Royal Pharmaceutical Society, Thomas Morson, started refining and selling morphine in 1821. Merck of Darmstad began wholesale production at about the same time (Berridge 1987).

Addiction and abuse were major problems by the dawn of the nineteenth century, although there is some evidence to suggest that morphine addiction (as opposed to opium eating), may not have been all that wide-spread (Kramer 1979). Patent medications, such as Dover's Powder, and other "cordials", "carminatives", or "soothing syrups" were nothing more than tincture of opium combined with flavorings. Case reports describing "morphia" toxicity were being published with some regularity by the late 1830's. The best known addict of that period was De Quincey. He first used opium to treat a gastrointestinal upset, but he rapidly developed a formidable habit. At one point he was consuming more than 20 grams (not grains) per day (De Quincey 1822).

Opium and Islam were introduced into China by Arab traders during the Tang Dynasty (618–907 A.D). At first, the Chinese used opium only for medicinal purposes. The *Pen Tsao Kang Mu*, a materia medica published in 1590, nearly 1,000 years after opium was first introduced into China, makes absolutely no mention of addiction or abuse (Way 1982). Opium was only taken orally, and then only for treatment of pain and diarrhea. Opium smoking, which probably originated in Java, began nearly a millennium later. The first mentions of opium smoking in China are from the 16th century, at just about the same time the Portuguese were introducing the Chinese to tobacco smoking. Opium and tobacco were often smoked together.

By the beginning of the 18th century, opium smoking had become as big a problem for the Chinese as opium "eating" was in Europe. In 1729 an Imperial edict was issued prohibiting the sale of opium. It imposed fines for trafficking, but the edict was ignored and

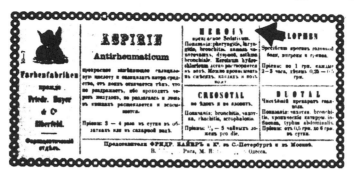

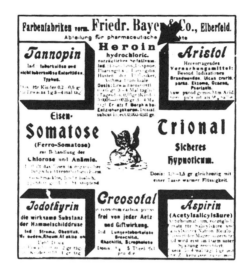

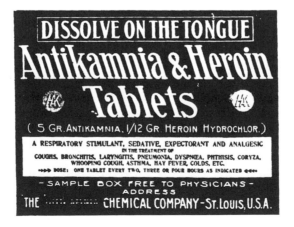

Figure 5.2.2 Heroin
Because of its effectiveness, heroin and heroin-containing products weren't all that difficult to market. Many different formulations were sold in Europe and in the United States.

opium smoking steadily increased. In 1880, for reasons having more to do with an increasing balance of trade deficit than concerns with abuse, Emperor Chin Ching banned opium importation. The East India Company ignored the ban and continued to smuggle large amounts of opium into China. In 1839, when the Chinese government finally decided to take active measures against opium importation, England declared war and China lost. Customs figures from 1881 show that opium imports into China were in excess of 6 million kilograms per year, enough to supply one million smokers. In spite of numerous conventions and treaties, addiction remained a major problem in China until the habit was suppressed by Mao Tse-tung in the early 1960's.

There are some striking historical parallels in the evolution of opium and cocaine abuse. Thousands of years of coca leaf chewing caused few social, and no detectable medical problems, for the Incas. However, as soon as purified cocaine became widely available in Europe, there were huge increases in the amount of cocaine used. As the amount used increased, so did toxicity (Karch 1989). Taking small amounts of opium orally was medically effective and, at worst, a benign indulgence. Much of orally administered opium is inactivated on its first pass through the liver, so this route of ingestion has some built in safeguards. Smoking opium is another mater entirely. When smoked, much more morphine gets into the body, blood levels rise more quickly, and there is no "first pass" effect. The net result is that when opium is smoked, the dosage is effectively multiplied. Not surprisingly, serious toxicity and addiction resulted.

Chinese laborers are said to have introduced opium smoking into the United States, but opium was already popular in America long before the Chinese immigration. In 1844 the New York City coroner held six inquests regarding opium-related deaths and 23 inquests on deaths related to laudanum (Woodman and Tidy 1877). According to U.S. Government figures, over 5 million tons of opium were imported into the United States from 1850 to 1877. This figure does not take into account opium which was smuggled in to avoid taxation, and opium which was cultivated domestically. Opium was produced in California, Arizona, and the New England states (Brecher 1972). Like their European counterparts, American physicians couldn't have practiced without opium. A survey done in Boston in 1888 disclosed that of 10,000 prescriptions dispensed by 35 pharmacies, 15% contained opium and 78% contained opiates! (Way 1982). Whatever the problems associated with opium abuse, they very likely would have been manageable had not for the hypodermic syringe become available in the 1870's, and then heroin at the turn of the century.

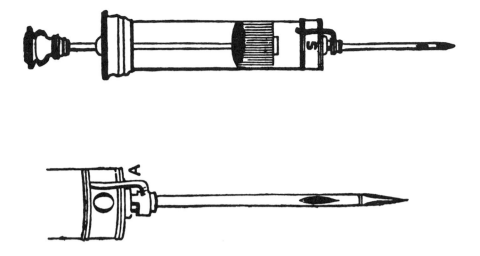

Figure 5.2.3 Hypodermic syringes
Commercial production of syringes began just before the Civil War. Initially, opiates were injected only subcutaneously. The intravenous injection of morphine and heroin did not become common practice until the 1920's.

5.2.3 INVENTION OF THE HYPODERMIC SYRINGE

In 1855 a Scottish physician, Alexander Wood, published an account of his experiments injecting large numbers of people with opium (Wood 1855). He injected tincture of opium and, although his original intent was to achieve something akin to a nerve block, he quickly realized that injected morphine was being carried throughout the body. In the course of his experiments, Wood managed to addict his wife to intramuscular morphine, and she probably was the first woman to die of an injected narcotic overdose (Terry and Pellens 1928).

Wood may have gotten most of the credit, but the idea of injecting people with narcotics had been around for hundreds of years before Wood was born. Christopher Wren, the famous architect and professor of astronomy at Gresham College, Oxford, was also a physician. According to the history of the Royal Society, Wren injected dogs with intravenous opium in 1656. Using a quill attached to a small bladder he injected lean animals with easily visible veins. There were no fatalities. Wren was so encouraged by his preliminary studies that the following year he tried the same experiment on a man. An ambassador to the Court of St. James volunteered the services of a "delinquent servant". The volunteer was injected with an emetic which made him faint. Other experiments were even less successful, and this area of research was ignored for nearly one hundred years (Terry and Pellens 1928).

Wood's publication prompted others to experiment with the parenteral injection of many different drugs, but narcotics attracted the most interest, and injection of narcotics soon became standard practice. Hypodermic syringes were said to have been in great demand and short supply during the U.S. Civil War (Billings 1905), although the shortage couldn't have been all that severe, since many of the veterans became addicts. Addiction, as a problem in America, was slower to evolve than in Europe, but by the 1870's, "morphism" was rampant in both the old and new world. The lag time may have been partially due to the fact that hypodermic injection didn't catch on as quickly in the United States as in Europe.

Even though addiction was common, neither the mechanism of opiate action, nor the process of addiction were even remotely understood. It was widely thought, for instance, that using morphine injections, as opposed to "eating opium", minimized the probability of addiction (Anstie 1868) (Howard-Jones 1972). Accordingly, treatment modalities for addiction were simplistic to the extreme. Freud's *Über coca*, published in 1884 (Freud 1884), reflects the thinking of many during that period. Because cocaine's effects seemed to be so opposite to morphine's, Freud concluded that cocaine would be a logical treatment for "morphinism". Some prominent physicians, including Erlenmeyer (Erlenmeyer 1885), disagreed, but Freud's notions were widely accepted and a large group of patients became addicted simultaneously to cocaine and morphine. It is only quite recently, since the discovery of opiate receptors and neurotransmitters, that rational approaches to narcotics addiction have been formulated.

5.2.4 SYNTHESIS OF HEROIN

The other key development in the history of narcotics addiction was the synthesis of heroin. In 1874, C.R.Wright, of St. Mary's Hospital in London, boiled anhydrous morphine with acetic anhydride and produced a series of acetylated morphine derivatives (Eddy 1953). One of the derivatives was diacetyl morphine (although the nomenclature was different at the time). He sent samples to an associate at Owens College, London, who assayed the substance for biological activity. The ability of the drug to decrease respiratory rate and blood pressure was quickly noted. For reasons that are not clear, the discovery created very little interest. In 1898 Strube published a paper outlining his favorable results using heroin to treat patients with tuberculosis. He found that the drug effectively relieved severe coughs and allowed patients to sleep, and he observed no ill effects (Strube 1898). The Bayer Company in Eberfeld Germany, began commercial production in 1898.

Whatever the medical profession thought about heroin, it was warmly received by the underground. By 1920 heroin addiction was such a problem that the AMA House of Delegates voted to prohibit its importation, manufacture and sale. Legitimate heroin production in the United States ceased after 1924, though low levels of illegal imports persisted. Interestingly, it seems that no one thought to inject heroin intravenously until the early 1920's. The dating is suggested by the fact that the first report describing typical track marks wasn't published until 1929 (Biggam 1929). The outlawing of production, along with international treaties and conventions, but most especially the advent of World War II, led to sharp reductions in clandestine imports. In 1950 there were fewer than 40 heroin seizures within the United States.

Interest in heroin resurfaced with the advent of the Viet Nam War but was temporarily eclipsed by a general disinterest in sedative hypnotics, and a superimposed a cocaine pandemic. Heroin use, at least when judged by the amount of illicit heroin now being confiscated, is again increasing. During 1990, the most recent year for which statistics are available, narcotic analgesics accounted for 57% of all drug related deaths, with 1,976 of the deaths directly attributable to heroin abuse. By comparison, cocaine was responsible for 43% of the drug related deaths reported to the Federal government (National Institute on Drug Abuse 1990).

5.2.5 THE FIRST PATHOLOGY STUDIES

The first autopsy describing both cerebral and pulmonary congestion was that of a New Yorker who died of laudanum overdose. It was reported by a Dr. Lee in 1852 (Woodman and Tidy 1877). Autopsy findings in a second narcotic overdose were published in 1862. A young woman drank "gin mixed with a shilling's worth of laudanum." She quickly became comatose and intense meiosis was noted. Autopsy disclosed cerebral congestion, however the lungs were unremarkable (Slater 1862). In 1861 a report in *Lancet* blamed the death of a child on opiate intoxication from his mother's milk (Anon 1861). A forensics text from 1877 mentions that "congestion of the lungs and of the vessels of the brain" are typically seen in opiate-related deaths, but cautioned that the findings at autopsy were "neither certain nor characteristic," (Woodman and Tidy 1877). Understanding of the problem advanced very little until Helpern and Rho published their paper, "Deaths from Narcotism-Incidence, Circumstances, and Post-mortem findings" in 1966 (Helpern and Rho 1966). In addition to carefully describing the epidemiology of the disease, the authors systematically described all of the signs that have come to be classically associated with narcotism, including pulmonary edema, portal adenopathy, and track marks. Since then opiate receptors have been discovered and other disorders, such as heroin-associated nephropathy (Rao, Nicastri et al. 1974) and leukoencephalopathy (Wolters, Wijngaarden et al. 1982), have been described. None the less, our basic understanding of the pathologic changes produced by narcotic abuse have advanced very little.

References

Anon (1845). Deaths from poisons. Lancet. i:24–25.

Anon (1861). A new theory of poisoning. Lancet. i:93.

Anstie (1868). The hypodermic injection of remedies. Practitioner 1:32–41.

Berridge, V. a. E., G. (1987). Opium and the people. Opiate use in nineteenth-century England. New Haven and London, Yale University Press.

Biggam, A. (1929). Malignant malaria associated with the administration of heroin intravenously. Trans Royal Soc Trop Med and Hyg. 23:147–153.

Billings, J. (1905). Medical reminiscences of the Civil War. Trans Coll Phys Phil. xxvii:115–121.

Brecher, E. (1973). Licit and illicit drugs; the Consumers Union report on narcotics, stimulants, depressants, inhalants, hallucinogens, and marijuana - including caffeine, nicotine, and alcohol. Boston, Little Brown.

Eddy, N. (1953). Heroin (diacetylmorphine): Laboratory and clinical evaluation of its effectiveness and addiction liability. Bull Narcotics. 5:39–44.

Erlenmeyer, A. (1885). Cocaine in the treatment of morphinomania. J Ment Sci. 31: 427–428.

Freud, S. (1884). Über coca. Wien Centralblatt für die ges Therapie. 2:289–314.

Haller, J. (1989). Opium usage in nineteenth century therapeutics. Bull N. Y. Acad. Med. 65(5):591–607.

Helpern, M. and Y. Rho. (1966). Deaths from narcotics in New York City. N.Y. State Med J. 66:2391–2408.

Howard-Jones, N. (1972). The origins of hypodermic medication. Sci Am. 96–102.

Karch, S. (1989). The history of cocaine toxicity. Hum Pathol. 20(11):1037–1039.

Kramer, J. (1979). Opium rampant: medical use, misuse, and abuse in Britain and the West in the 17th and 18th centuries. B J Addict. 74:377–389.

Kritikos, P. and S. Papadaki (1967). The history of the poppy and of opium and their expansion in antiquity in the Eastern Mediterranean area. Bull Narc. 19(4): 5–10.

Lewin, L. (1931). Phantastica: narcotic and stimulating drugs; their use and abuse. New York, E.P. Dutton & Company.

Macht, D. (1915). The history of opium and some of its preparations and alkaloids. JAMA. 64(6):477–481.

Macht, D. (1916). The history of intravenous and subcutaneous administration of drugs. JAMA. 66:856–860.

National Institute on Drug Abuse. (1990). Annual Medical Examiner Data. Data from the Drug Abuse Warning Network. Statistical Series, Number 10-B. Rockville, Maryland, U.S. Department of Health and Human Services.

Quincey, T. D. (1822). Confessions of an English opium eater. London, Taylor and Hessey.

Rao, T., A. Nicastri and E. Friedman (1974). Natural history of heroinassociated nephropathy. N Engl J Med. 290:19–23.

Slayter (1862). Poisoning by opium and gin: fatal result. Lancet 1(March 29):326.

Strube, G. (1898). Mittheilung über therapeutische Versuche mit Heroin. Berl Klinische Wochenschrift. 38:38.

Sydenham, T. (1848). The works of Thomas Sydenham, M.D. Translated from the Latin edition of Dr. Greenhil; with a life of the author by R. G. Latham. London, The Sydenham Society.

Tazelaar, H., S. Karch, M. Billingham and B. Stephens (1987). Cocaine and the heart. Hum Pathol. 18:195–199.

Terry, C. and M. Pellens (1928). The opium problem. New York, Committee on Drug Addictions, Bureau of Social Hygiene, Inc.

Way, E. (1982). History of opiate use in the Orient and the United States. Opioids in mental illness: theories, clinical observations, and treatment possibilities. Ann NY Acad Sci. 398:12–23.

Wolters, E., G. Wijngaarden, F. Stam et al. (1982). Leucoencephalopathy after inhaling "heroin" pyrolysate. Lancet. ii:1233–1237.

Wood, A. (1855). New method of treating neuralgia by the direct application of opiates to painful spots. Edinburgh Med and Surg J. 82:265.

Woodman, W. and C. Tidy (1877). Forensic Medicine and Toxicology. Philadelphia, Lindsay & Blakiston.

5.3 CULTIVATION AND MANUFACTURE

5.3.1 BOTANIC CONSIDERATIONS

There are six genera in the Papaveraceae family, and within the genus there are six distinct species. *Papaver somniferum* is commonly cultivated as the "opium" poppy, but the wild growing *Papaver setigerum* also contains significant amounts of morphine. Over the years, many hybrids have been developed and describing a generic "poppy" is difficult, if not impossible. Flowers may be single or double, with variation in both shape and color. Blossoms may be white, red, pink, purple, crimson, and many shades in between. The capsules, from which the juice is extracted, also vary in shape and alkaloid content. There can be two, three, or more capsules on a plant. Height is also variable, and may range anywhere from 30 to 150 centimeters or more (Anon 1953).

The poppy is an annual plant. It grows in almost any climate, but does best in warm temperate areas and cannot be grown at all in areas that are subject to frost. When grown in humid regions the poppy is vulnerable to infection by a range of fungal and plant parasites. Poppies grow well in average soil, but the soil requires treatment with manure or chemical fertilizers. Plants take two to three weeks to germinate, and two months to fully develop. After a field has been weeded and thinned out, as many as 15 plants can be grown in a square meter. After the plant flowers, and the petals have fallen off, the capsule continues to ripen for about another two weeks, at which time the latex can be harvested. The entire cycle takes less than three months.

Harvesting is a two-step process. First the capsule is incised, allowing the sap to run out and then solidify. Twelve hours after the capsule has been incised the latex is harvested. Incising the capsules is a delicate operation: if the incision is too deep the latex will run down the inside of the plant and be lost to harvest. Farmers prefer to do the incising at sunrise or sunset. That allows the latex to exude and solidify for 8 to 14 hours. The caked latex is then scraped off the capsule using a dull blade. The yield per acre depends on many variables. Historically, the yield in Turkey and the Mediterranean was said to be 10 kg of opium per hectare. Yields in India are said to be higher. Yields in the newer fields being established in South American have yet to be determined.

Well over 20 different alkaloids have been identified in opium, but only three are of any significance: morphine, codeine and thebaine. Thebaine has almost no morphine-like activity of its own, but it can be used to manufacture other narcotic agents. Hundreds of semisynthetic derivatives, referred to as Bentley Compounds, have been synthesized from thebaine, and many of these do have narcotic effects. A few of the derivatives, such as Etorphine, have 1,000 times the activity of morphine. Morphine is the principal alkaloid found in opium. It constitutes between 8 and 19 per cent of air-dried opium. Reported ranges for codeine content are from 1.25 to 3.4% (Anon 1963).

Poppy seeds sold for cooking and baking purposes may contain very substantial amounts of morphine and codeine. In one study the morphine content was found to be anywhere from 7.3 to 60.1 μg per gram of seed, while the codeine content ranged from 6.1 μg to 29.8 μg per gram (Hasegawa, Maseda, Kagawa et al. 1992). It is hardly surprising that the urine of people eating these seeds tests positive on opiate screening tests!

5.3.2 MANUFACTURE

Heroin can be manufactured directly from opium, or from semi-purified morphine. The route utilized depends mostly on the availability of the precursors. Morphine and opium are both sold on the illicit market, and the availability of one or the other depends largely on local conditions.

The clandestine separation of morphine from crude opium involves three separate steps. A kilogram of opium is dissolved in 2 liters of water along with 200 grams of lime, and the resultant solution poured through a coarse filter. Then 250 gm of ammonium chloride is added to the filtrate, causing morphine base to slowly precipitate out. The morphine is collected on a fine cloth filter and then washed with water. The crude morphine is then mixed with charcoal and with either hydrochloric or sulfuric acid. The mixture is filtered and ammonium hydroxide is added to the filtrate, causing purified morphine to precipitate out. The precipitate is collected by filtration and allowed to dry in room air.

In the second phase of production the dried morphine is added to acetic anhydride and the mixture is refluxed at a constant temperature

for five hours. After the mixture has been allowed to cool it is neutralized with sodium carbonate. The crude heroin that precipitates out is
then filtered and washed with water.

In the final stage of production heroin is purified by redissolving
the crude heroin in boiling water that contains citric acid and charcoal.
The mixture is filtered and purified, and heroin is precipitated by the
addition of sodium carbonate. If the lab wants to produce the hydrochloride form instead of heroin base, then the heroin is redissolved in
acetone, and hydrochloric acid is added to the solution.

Depending on market demand, clandestine chemists will sometimes synthesize morphine, instead of opium. Production begins by
dissolving one kilogram of opium in two liters of water and adding 200
grams of slaked lime, 500 mL of alcohol and 500 mL of ether. The
resultant solution is then filtered through a cloth, leaving crude
morphine on the cloth. This material is further purified and decolorized
by refluxing it with 2 liters of dilute sulfuric acid and 250 grams of
charcoal for about half an hour. This solution is then filtered and
ammonium hydroxide added to the filtrate. The off-white colored,
semi-purified morphine that precipitates out is dried in room air.
Hardened dried morphine granules are rubbed against a hard surface to
produce a powder (Anon, 1986) (Narayanaswami 1985).

TABLE 5.3.2.1
**ADULTERANTS FOUND IN HEROIN FROM MEXICO, SOUTHEAST AND
SOUTHWEST ASIA.**

Adulterant	Mexican	S.E. Asian	S.W. Asian
Caffeine	34 %	50 %	4%
Diphenhydramine	16 %	25 %	18 %
Quinine	34 %	25 %	3 %
Procaine	24 %	25 %	1 %
Acetaminophine	10 %	33 %	1 %

Based on data supplied by the Drug Enforcement Administration. Table shows the percentage
of specimen from that area containing a particular adulterant. Acetylcodeine, monacetylmo-
rphine and noscapine are found in all samples, but the amount present in any given
sample is highly variable.

In the past there have been reports of clandestine laboratories
synthesizing methadone, but at present, fentanyl and its analogs are the
only narcotic synthesized clandestinely, and then not very often. The
infrequency of this occurrence probably has to do with the fact that the
synthesis of fentanyl is more difficult than that of other illicit chemicals
such as methamphetamine and phencyclidine. At least three different
synthetic routes are possible. The most popular involves the use of

norfentanyl or 3-methyl-norfentanyl intermediates. These are produced from 1-benzyl-4-poperidone by reductive amination with aniline, then acetylation and hydrogenation to form norfentanyl. Fentanyl and its analogues are then manufactured by alkylating the piperidine nitrogen (World Health Organization, 1990).

5.3.3 SAMPLE ANALYSIS

Even in refined heroin, impurities remain. Substances carried over from the original plant or from opium are referred to as adulterants. Thus the acetylcodeine produced by the acetylation of codeine present in the semipurified morphine can be found in heroin (Lim and Chow 1978). Substances added with the intent of altering the character of the heroin in some way are also called adulterants. Included in this group are compounds such as quinine, caffeine, and diphenhydramine. The term diluent is reserved for those substances, devoid of physiologic effects, that are added to increase the bulk of the final product.

There are, of course, ways to make pure morphine that does not contain other alkaloids, but these methods are not routinely used by clandestine labs. Thus the ratio of heroin to acetylcodeine in illicit heroin is nearly the same as the ratio of morphine to codeine in the illicit morphine that was used to produce the heroin in the first place. Studies have shown that the ratio of heroin to acetylcodeine in an illicit heroin sample may be used to identify that sample's country of origin. The ratio is fairly high for samples emanating from Afghanistan (20.9:1), and quite low for specimens coming from China (6.38:1) (Narayanaswami 1985). However, in the final analysis the ratio of heroin to 6-acetylmorphine and morphine is more an indicator of clandestine lab proficiency than country of origin (Oneil and Pitts 1992).

The origin of particular samples is also suggested by the amount of alkaloid present, and by the type and amount of adulterants and diluents that have been added. "Chinese #4" heroin is almost always more than 80% pure. Samples of semirefined heroin from Pakistan, on the other hand, usually contain less than 50% heroin (Oneil and Pitts 1992). Samples from some areas, particular South West Asia, contain methaqualone, phenobarbitone and caffeine, while specimens from other regions may contain different adulterants.

The average purity of heroin sold on the streets is 24.5%, but, depending on local conditions, there may be extremely wide variation from sample to sample. Heroin sold in the Western states is primarily of Mexican origin, with an average purity of only 13.3 %. Heroin sold on the East coast comes mainly from South East Asia, and has an average purity of 41.6%. Heroin from Southwest Asia (India, Iran, Pakistan) is sold mainly in the East and midwest, and has an average purity of 24 per cent (Drug Enforcement Administration 1992). Table 5.3.2.1 shows the adulterants found in the three principal types of heroin sold in the United States.

The type of material added as diluents varies from region to region, depending on the preferences of the illicit manufacturer. Specimens from Southeast Asia are usually diluted with mannitol or lactose. Mexican specimens often contain lactose, but the addition of mannitol is uncommon. In general these diluents are fairly benign compounds and are unlikely to be responsible for medical complications. Table 5.3.3.1 lists the frequency with which the different diluents are found in samples from the principal growing areas.

TABLE 5.3.3.1
DILUENTS FOUND IN HEROIN FROM MEXICO, SOUTHEAST AND SOUTHWEST ASIA

Diluent	S.E. Asian	S.W. Asian	Mexican
Mannitol	86%	67%	13%
Lactose	40%	50%	35%
Amorphous Material	not present	not present	19%
Dextrose	16%	25%	3%
Starch	14%	17%	6%
Sodium Chloride	2%	8%	3%

Based on data supplied by the Drug Enforcement Administration. The table shows the percentage of specimens from that area containing a particular diluent. Not listed are rarely encountered materials such as citric acid, cellulose and inositol.

References

Anon (1953). The opium poppy. Bull Narc. V (3) (July-September):9–12.

Anon (1963). The opium alkaloids. Bull Narc. V(3) (July-September):13–14.

Drug Enforcement Administration (1992). Domestic Monitor Program. A quarterly report on the source areas, cost, and purity of retail-level heroin, January-March, 1991. DEA #92006.

Hasegawa, M., Maseda, C., Kagawa, M. et al. (1992). Morphine and codeine in poppy seed and poppy seed food. Jpn J Toxicol Environ Health, 38:192–195.

Lim, H. and S. Chow (1978). Heroin abuse and a gas chromatographic method for determining illicit heroin samples in Singapore. J Forensic Sci. 23(2):319–328.

Narayanaswami, K. (1985). Parameters for determining the origin of illicit heroin samples. Bull Narc. 37(1):49–62.

Oneil, P. J. and J. E. Pitts (1992). Illicitly imported heroin products (1984 to 1989) - some physical and chemical features indicative of their origin. J Pharm Pharmacol. 44(1):1-6.

5.4 INDIVIDUAL NARCOTIC AGENTS

5.4.1 MORPHINE

Morphine was isolated from opium by Setürner in 1805. More than one hundred twenty years passed before Sir Robert Richardson characterized morphine's chemical structure in 1927, and total synthesis was only accomplished in 1952. The time lag between morphine's discovery and its chemical characterization is paralleled by the slow evolution in understanding its metabolism and mechanism of action. The principal site of metabolism is the liver, but because the total body clearance of morphine is higher than hepatic flow (Säwe, Kager et al. 1985), questions still remain about extrahepatic metabolism. Other questions remain about the usefulness of blood and tissue levels measured during the 1970's and early 1980's. These measurements were made using radioimmune assays that have since been shown to be unreliable when compared with figures obtained using specific high-performance liquid chromatography (Aherne and Littleton 1985) (Hanks, Hoskin et al. 1988).

5.4.1.1 General considerations

Morphine's elimination is best described as a biphasic process. During an initial phase, lasting only a few minutes, morphine is rapidly distributed throughout the tissues with the highest blood flow. During a second phase, morphine is very quickly converted to its principal metabolite, morphine-3-glucuronide, and somewhat more slowly to smaller amounts of morphine-6-glucuronide. The second phase takes from 1 to 8 hours, with 2 hours as the most widely accepted value (Brunk and Delle 1974) (Dahlstrom, 1979) (Säwe, Dahlstrom et al. 1981) (Murphy and Hug 1981). Conversion of morphine to the 3-glucuronide form is rapid. By 6 minutes after intra-venous injection there is more metabolite than morphine circulating in the blood stream.

The most recent studies in normal volunteers given intravenous morphine showed an initial distribution half-life to be 5 minutes, and the terminal elimination phase 1.7 hours. This means that morphine will be present in measurable quantities in the plasma for between 4 to 6 hours. The fact that M6G is pharmacologically active, and possibly more potent than morphine itself, has only recently been appreciated. The notion that conjugation is the same as detoxification is widely accepted, but not always true. Usually the process of conjugation alters the shape

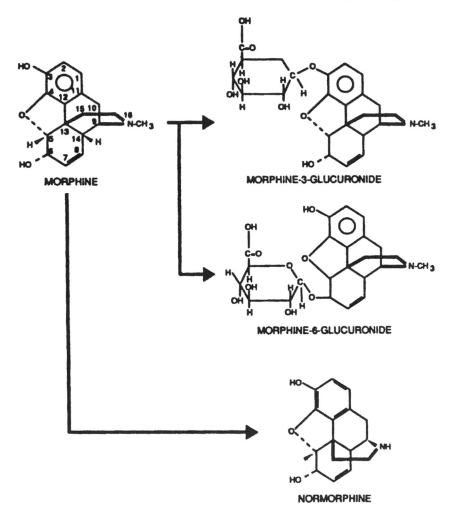

Figure 5.4.1 Basic elements of morphine metabolism.

of the original molecule so that it can't effectively interact with its intended receptor. However, in the case of morphine, glucuronidation at the 6 position increases the affinity of morphine for binding at the μ receptors (Mulder, 1992).

The terminal half-life of M3G is 3.9 ± 1.5 hours, while that of M6G is only 2.6 ± 0.69 hours (Osborne, Joel et al. 1990). The half-life of M6G can, however, rise to over 50 hours in individuals with renal failure. Other morphine metabolites have also been identified, but their importance has yet to be assessed. One metabolite of potential interest is normorphine. Modest amounts are formed after parenteral administration, but when morphine is taken orally, large amounts are produced. This compound is both psychoactive and neurotoxic.

Studies of morphine's metabolism have been hampered by inadequate assay techniques. Until recently, radioimmunoassay was the most widely used method for quantitating morphine in blood and biological fluids. The problem with this approach is that the antibodies used to detect morphine are relatively non-specific, and significantly cross react with morphine metabolites. Plasma morphine measurements made with this technique reflect the presence of two or three different compounds, some of them psychoactive and some not. Measuring plasma half-life, or correlating these levels with specific behavioral effects, toxicity, or lethality is difficult, if not impossible. Recently, the techniques of gas chromatography and high-pressure liquid chromatography with mass spectrometry have been adapted to simultaneously measure morphine and its metabolites.

Once morphine enters the blood stream it is quickly distributed throughout the body to the areas with the highest blood flow. High morphine levels can be measured in lung, kidney, liver, spleen and muscle (Brunk and Delle 1974) (Stanski, Greenblatt et al. 1978). Morphine and its metabolites also quickly cross the blood-brain and placental barriers. One third of a given dose circulates protein bound (Spector and Vessell 1971), so that abnormalities of protein binding, such as would be seen in hepatic failure or malignancies, can alter the degree of protein binding and, indirectly, lead to higher circulating levels of free morphine (Säwe 1986).

Only minimal quantities of morphine are excreted unchanged in the urine. Most morphine is disposed of by glucuronidation. Pathways for ethereal sulfate formation and other oxidative pathways are also known to exist. Most of these biotransformations occur in the liver, but in humans, as much as 38% undergoes glucuronidation elsewhere, probably in the kidney. In animal species, and in the human fetus, the intestinal mucosa may also be an important site of transformation (Laitnen, Kanto et al. 1975) (Iwamato and Klassen 1977) (Pacifici and Rane 1982), but that is not the case in adult human (Mazoit, Sandouk et al. 1990).

Opiate receptor studies have shown that the 3 position in the morphine moiety must remain accessible for a molecule to have opiate activity. Since the 3 carbon position is open in the M6G molecule, it is not surprising that this metabolite has analgesic effects in its own right (Osborne, Joel et al. 1988). Viewed in this light, data from earlier studies distinguishing between free and conjugated morphine levels becomes impossible to interpret, since there are at least two morphine conjugates, and one is psychoactive.

Other controversies about the metabolism and excretion of morphine remain unresolved. One is whether or not morphine is converted to codeine. Whether or not the presence of codeine in a urine specimen can rightly be taken as proof of morphine or heroin abuse is an important issue. The results of earlier studies suggested that, at least in chronic opiate abusers, the conversion occurred (Borner, 1973). The most recent studies, done using gas chromatography/mass spectrometry, indicate that the conversion does not occur (Mitchell, Paul et al. 1991) (Cone, Welch et al. 1991b). The demonstration of codeine in the urine after giving morphine or heroin is probably explained by the presence of codeine impurities present even in pharmaceutical grade morphine (Cone, Welch et al. 1991a). The presence of codeine in a urine or blood specimen is proof only that codeine, and not any other drug, was ingested.

Another controversy concerns the entero-hepatic circulation of morphine. Studies of fecal excretion indicate that this route may account for between 7 and 10% of a given dose in chronic users (Hanks, Hoskin et al. 1988). It had been speculated that chronic users might continue to release unmetabolized morphine into the entero-hepatic circulation. There is evidence for such a route in experimental animals, but the issue has not been resolved in man. Concentrations of unchanged morphine in bile can be extremely high. In one study of narcotic-related deaths the average concentration of morphine in the bile was 312 mg/L (Chan, Chan et al. 1986). In Gottschalk and Cravey's series of 119 cases the median level of morphine in the bile was 33.7 mg/L (Gottschalk and Cravey 1980).

Once morphine has been converted to the glucuronide, excretion is via the kidneys. Less than 10% of a given dose is excreted unchanged in the urine, and elimination of unchanged morphine is not affected by renal failure. On the other hand, elimination of the glucuronides is affected by renal failure, and since M6G is psychoactive, patients with renal failure may become toxic due to the presence of accumulated metabolite (Ball, Moore et al. 1984).

5.4.1.2 Absorption and routes of administration

Almost all of the opiates are well absorbed, no matter the route of administration, but not all opiates are the same. Morphine levels after varying routes of administration have been measured, but only in healthy volunteers, or in cancer patients. Realistic studies, giving large amounts of drug to tolerant addicts, have not been done.

5.4.1.2.1 Intravenous

A 10-mg bolus given to healthy volunteers undergoing elective surgery results in a peak blood level of 200–400 ng/mL five minutes after injection (Berkowitz, Ngai et al. 1975). Whether or not similar situation obtains in addicts is not known.

5.4.1.2.2 Subcutaneous

Absorption via this route, and after intramuscular injection, is almost as rapid as the intravenous route. After either route morphine blood levels peak at 10–20 minutes, somewhat longer than after intravenous injection, but not so much longer as to have much clinical significance. The pharmacokinetics for both routes are nearly the same as after intravenous injection, and plasma levels comparable to those seen after intravenous use can be achieved after subcutaneous injection. That may explain why, in the past, subcutaneous injection (known as "skin popping") enjoyed considerable popularity among some groups of abusers. This practice, and the skin lesions commonly associated with it, seem to be less common today than in the past. It may be that "skin popping" is being replaced by smoking.

5.4.1.2.3 Oral

Morphine is absorbed completely from the small intestine, and peak plasma levels occur after 30–90 minutes, but resultant peak plasma levels are only one tenth as high as after giving the same amount parenterally. Bioavailability is significantly reduced because of first-pass metabolism in the liver. The oral route was popular among the "Opium Eaters" of the 17th and 18th centuries, when distribution was unregulated and prices were low. Today it is an impractical route for abusers because it costs too much. In the case of cancer patients who have access to legally supplied morphine, oral administration is a mainstay in the management (Hoskin, Hanks et al. 1989) (Osborne, Joel et al. 1990) (Gourlay, Cherry et al. 1986).

5.4.1.2.4 Rectal

Plasma levels after rectal administration are somewhat higher than after oral morphine, but are much less than after parenteral (Ellison and Lewis 1984). This route does not seem to be particularly popular among abusers, at least when compared to the rectal use of cocaine, which is a fairly common practice. When 0.6 mg/kg of morphine was given to women undergoing cancer treatment, there was considerable variation between individuals, but peak concentrations of 31–75 ng/mL were reached at between 45 and 120 minutes (Westerling, Lindahl et al. 1982). Fatalities have been reported at levels that were not much higher, and seizures, particularly in neonates, have been reported at levels that were much lower. Morphine-induced seizures have occurred at levels as low as 9 ng/mL (Koren 1983), and one report describes the postoperative death, from cerebral hypoxia, of a child given 4-mg morphine suppositories roughly every 4 hours. Blood levels measured 1.5 hours after death were 94 ng/mL (Gourlay and Boas 1992). Rectal absorption of morphine is variable. Different studies have shown rectal bioavailability to be anywhere from 12 to 61% (Westerling, Lindahl 1982) (Lindahl et al. 1981). Pharmacologic manipulation of the morphine medium can improve absorption and result in levels comparable to oral administration. If the carrier medium is acidified, then the percentage of un-ionized drug increases, as does absorption.

5.4.1.2.5 Intranasal

Heroin and morphine can both be used intranasally, but the practice is not cost effective because transnasal absorption, of morphine at least, is poor when compared with other agents such as cocaine. There are no published studies on absorption by this route. At the turn of the century, probably up to the mid 1920's, nasal insufflation of heroin was at least as popular as injection, and today's abusers seem to have rediscovered this effective route.

5.4.1.2.6 Skin

Morphine is not sufficiently fat-soluble to be absorbed though the skin in quantities sufficient to produce psychological effects. Other opioids, particularly fentanyl and sulfentanyl, but also meperidine, are well absorbed via this route. Since these other agents are also much more potent than morphine or heroin, transdermal application is quite practical. Time-release patches containing fentanyl are now for sale, and are even beginning to appear on the black market (Calis, Kohler et al. 1992).

5.4.1.2.7 Maternal/fetal

It has been recognized for more than a century that mothers can transfer morphine to their children in breast milk (Anon 1861). Depending on the degree of lipid solubility, narcotic agents passively diffuse across the placenta. Fetal uptake after maternal dosing with heroin has been studied in the Rhesus monkey using ^{11}C-heroin and positron tomography. Peak levels in the placenta are reached within a few minutes of administration. Peak maternal levels were twice the fetal level, but by one hour fetal blood levels were higher than maternal levels. Concentrations of labeled morphine in the liver quickly rise and quickly fall (Hartvig, Lindberg et al. 1989). Once the narcotic agents are taken up by the fetus they are metabolized and excreted. They may be detected in the amniotic fluid (Rurak, Wright et al. 1991), or in specimens of hair or meconium (Graham, Koren et al. 1989) (Little, Snell et al. 1989).

5.4.1.3 Tissue disposition

Morphine is rapidly distributed throughout the body, and resultant tissue concentrations reflect the relative blood flow. The time it takes morphine to redistribute, and the resultant tissue concentrations, are altered in older individuals (Chan, Kendall et al. 1975). Concentrations in skeletal muscle never reach those of the blood or other tissues, but muscle is an important storage site for opiates, just by virtue of its sheer bulk. Morphine is not as highly lipophilic as some agents, such as fentanyl, so it tends not to accumulate in fat. Morphine crosses the blood-brain barrier, but not so freely as compounds like heroin and codeine, that possess an aromatic hydroxyl group at the C3 position. Measurements of tissue concentrations from both heroin and morphine overdose are reported together. Since heroin is rapidly converted to 6-acetyl morphine and then to morphine, such extrapolation seems permissible.

5.4.1.3.1 Blood

Blood levels of morphine in six different autopsy series have ranged from 10 (Richards, Reed et al. 1976) to 2,800 ng/mL (Felby, Christensen et al. 1974). Various ranges have been reported for free morphine levels, and in some cases values as high as 2,000 ng/mL have been observed (Reed, Spiehler et al. 1977) (Gottschalk and Cravey 1980) (Sawyer, Waterhouse et al. 1988) (Chan, Chan et al. 1986) (Steentoft, Worm et al. 1988) (Steentoft, Kaa, Worm, 1989) (Kintz, Mangin et al. 1989) (Hine, Wright et al. 1982). Generalizing from these results is extremely difficult for at least three reasons. Firstly, all of the observations were made before it became apparent that M6G was metabolically active. Secondly, many of the measurements were made using immunoassays that cross-react with metabolites. Thirdly, there is the problem of tolerance. Opiate abusers become extremely tolerant to opiate-induced respiratory depression, but this tolerance is rapidly lost (Harding-Pink and Fryc 1988). Even the presence of track marks and other stigmata is not proof that the deceased was tolerant at the time of death, since these signs do not rapidly regress when the drug is discontinued. Except for confirming that the decedent was in fact abusing opiates, quantitation of blood levels helps very little in determining the cause of death (see below). Spiehler analyzed multiple variables common to 200 morphine-induced fatalities, using an artificial intelligence program. The results of her study suggested that the most useful parameters for diagnosis of overdose deaths were blood unconjugated morphine levels, blood total morphine and liver total morphine. Spiehler found that the most reliable predictor for overdose death was the presence of unconjugated morphine levels that were greater than 240 ng/mL (Spiehler 1989) (Spiehler and Brown 1987).

5.4.1.3.2 Brain

Only a handful of measurements have been reported. In the three heroin users described by Kintz the blood brain ratios were 13, 0.24, 1.5, with tissue concentrations ranging from 0.005 mg/Kg to 0.089 mg/Kg of wet brain (Kintz, Mangin et al. 1989). Since heroin crosses the blood-brain barrier much more rapidly than morphine and is then converted to morphine in the brain, it probably is not valid to extrapolate brain morphine concentration from the values that have been observed in heroin-related deaths.

5.4.1.3.3 Liver

Morphine concentrations have been measured in several series. In the ten cases analyzed by Felby the mean was 3.0 mg/kg and the range was from 0.4 to 18 mg/kg (Felby, Christensen et al. 1974). The two cases reported by Chan had levels of 7.0 and 2.9 mg/kg in the liver. The corresponding biliary concentrations in these last two cases were nearly 30 times higher than the blood levels (312 mg/L and 248 mg/L respectively) (Chan, Chan et al. 1986). In other series the differential has not been quite so striking. Kintz found bile levels of 0.087–0.363 mg/L in the bile while concentrations were 0.067–1.424 in the liver. The differences have to do partly with the amount taken before death, and partly with the chronicity of use (Kintz, Mangin et al. 1989).

5.4.1.3.4 Lymph nodes

One of the classic autopsy findings in narcotics addicts is the presence of enlarged hepatic lymph nodes. Whether or not the enlargement is the result of some toxic effect exerted by morphine itself, or the contaminants injected with it, is not known. Nonetheless, lymph nodes concentrate morphine and, in some cases, nodes taken at autopsy may have higher concentrations of morphine than either blood or bile. In the only systematic study published, levels ranged from 0.03 to 0.87 mg/100 grams of tissue (Nakamura and Choi 1983).

5.4.1.3.5 Other Biofluids

Measurements of opiate levels in the vitreous have not been reported. Simultaneous measurement of morphine in saliva, plasma and urine showed that urine concentrations of morphine were 100 times greater than the levels measured in saliva, and 16 times higher than levels in the plasma (Cone 1990). Following an oral dose of 30 mg of codeine, saliva levels were 120 ng/mL three hours later (Sharp 1983). Saliva/plasma ratios for the naturally occurring opiates have not been determined with any accuracy, but similar levels are measured in both fluids (Schramm 1992). On the other hand, the correlations between saliva and plasma levels appear to be excellent in the case of methadone (saliva/plasma ratio is about 0.5), and probably for other synthetic opiates as well. One hour after administration, the saliva hydromorphone concentration is the same as that in plasma (Ritschel 1987).

Morphine levels in spinal fluid have been studied under controlled conditions, but not in addicts or in drug related deaths. CSF levels peak 3 hours after a dose of morphine is given intramuscularly, and at equilibrium the ratio of CSF to plasma is very nearly 1. The elimination half-life of morphine from CSF is the same as the elimination half-life of morphine from the blood (Nordberg 1984).

5.4.1.3.6 Urine

Most of a given dose of morphine is excreted in the urine after it has been converted to glucuronide. In previously reported autopsy studies, urine concentration of conjugated morphine have ranged from 100 ng/mL to 120,000 ng/mL (Säwe 1986). The observed concentration depends largely on the volume of urine that is allowed to collect between measurements (Cone 1990).

5.4.1.4 Excretion and detectability

Since the half-life of morphine is under two hours, measurable levels are unlikely to be detected after 12 hours have passed. The half-lives of the glucuronides are nearly twice that of morphine. The excretion of morphine and its glucuronides is predominantly renal. Over 85% of a given dose can be recovered in the urine within 24 hours of administration. Less than 10% of the excreted material will be unchanged morphine, 50–60% will be morphine-3-glucuronide, and 15% will be in the form of other metabolites such as morphine-6-glucuronide and normorphine. Given current levels of sensitivity, morphine or its metabolites should be detectable for at least 48 hours after administration. Since morphine also undergoes enterohepatic circulation and can reach high concentrations in the gallbladder with chronic use, it would not be surprising if very small amounts, certainly well below the NIDA cut offs, could be excreted for days after the drug was last used.

5.4.2 HEROIN

Heroin is a synthetic morphine derivative, first marketed by Bayer in 1898. It is produced by the acetylation of morphine's two hydroxyl groups. Once in the body, heroin is very rapidly converted, by deacetylation, to 6-acetylmorphine, and thence to morphine. Conversion to 6-acetylmorphine is completed within ten to fifteen minutes. The second step deacetylation is completed within a few hours, resulting in the complete conversion of heroin to morphine.

5.4.2.1 Routes of administration

Heroin and morphine levels after smoking opium, or heroin, have not been measured. Measurements after administration by rectal and nasal routes have not been reported either, though these routes are certainly used. This is unfortunate, because one result of the HIV pandemic is that intravenous heroin abusers are, in increasing numbers, smoking heroin in order to avoid sharing needles. Heroin can be heated on a piece of folded tinfoil and the fumes inhaled, or it can be inhaled into the nose, sometimes through a straw. In Hong Kong, heroin used for this purpose was often dyed red, and as the fumes rise from the foil they can be imagined to have the undulating shape of a dragon's tail, explaining why the practice is called "chasing the dragon". Alternatively, the lighted end of a cigarette can be dipped in powdered heroin and then smoked. In order to keep the heroin from falling off the end of the cigarette, the smoker has to hold his head tilted backwards. The heroin can also be mixed into the contents of a cigarette. None of these routes is particularly effective. Studies have been done in addicts that compared urinary excretion after heroin was administered by injection, volatilization, and by smoking it in a cigarette. The mean percentage of morphine recovered after injection was 68%, after volatilization it was 26%, and after cigarette smoking it was only 14% (Pui-nin 1966).

TABLE 5.4.2.2.1
TISSUE LEVELS FROM 5 CASES OF ACUTELY FATAL HEROIN OVERDOSE

Tissue	Range
Blood	0.06–0.90
Urine	0.21–6.60
Bile	0.09–1.25
Stomach contents	0.01–0.03
Lung	0.09–0.18
Liver	0.07–0.29
Kidney	0.01–1.18
Heart	0.09–0.10
Spleen	0.11–0.95
Brain	0.01–0.10
Vitreous humor	0.03–0.35
Testicle	0.03–0.09
Muscle	0.01–0.04

Values are in mg/L or mg/Kg. Urine and bile specimens were hydrolyzed to free morphine from its conjugate. *Adapted from Kintz et al., 1989.*

5.4.2.2 Tissue distribution

Even though 6-acetylmorphine is a unique heroin metabolite, it has a very short half-life and usually is not quantitated. Toxicologic investigations of opiate-related deaths have traditionally been centered about measurements of morphine concentrations in blood, liver, urine and bile (Steentoft, Worm et al. 1988) (Felby, Christensen et al. 1974) (Reed, Spiehler et al. 1977) (Sawyer, Waterhouse et al. 1988). Separate measurements of morphine-6-glucuronide in drug-related deaths have not been made, because it has only recently become apparent that M6G exerts opiate effects in its own right. Only one study of heroin-related deaths has made simultaneous measurements of morphine levels in multiple organs, and these values are reported in Table 5.4.2.2.

5.4.2.3 Excretion and detectability

Since the conversion of heroin to morphine is so rapid, the probability of detecting heroin in either blood or urine is quite small. Once the conversion to morphine is complete, the limits of detection are the same as for morphine itself (see above).

Testing for opiates in urine is a problem. Poppy seeds are widely eaten and they contain morphine and codeine. On the other hand, poppies do not contain heroin. Thus an individual who eats poppy seeds may well be found to have codeine or morphine in their urine. Poppy seed eaters will not have detectable levels of 6-acetylmorphine (6-MAM). The latter compound is seen only in the blood or urine of individuals who have taken heroin. Small amounts of 6-MAM may also be ingested directly as contaminants present in heroin, introduced during the clandestine refining process (Oneil and Pitts 1992).

The presence or absence of 6-MAM cannot be used to reliably separate innocent poppy seed ingestion from heroin abuse, because 6-MAM is only detectable for a few hours. If it is absent from a suspect specimen, that may only mean that heroin use occurred more than 3 or 4 hours earlier. In the absence of 6-MAM, separating innocent poppy ingestion from heroin abuse can be difficult, and is a real problem for medical review officers. In the past they have had to rely on detecting confirmatory evidence of drug abuse, such as track marks. Recently it has been shown that 6MAM is deposited within the hair matrix, where it is stable for many months. It has been suggested that the demonstration of 6MAM in hair might be another conclusive way to prove than an individual had been using heroin (Cone, Welch et al. 1991b). Heroin samples can also contain 6MAM. That means that the presence of 6-MAM, like the presence of heroin itself, might be the result of external contamination (as in a customs officer who confiscates a large quantity of heroin).

5.4.3 CODEINE

5.4.3.1 General considerations

Codeine is one of the naturally occurring alkaloids found in opium. Depending on where the poppies were grown, samples of opium may contain from 0.7 to 2.5% codeine. Codeine was first isolated from opium by Robiquet in 1832, 27 years after Sertürner isolated morphine. Most of the codeine that is consumed in antitussive and analgesic mixtures is of semisynthetic origin, produced by the methylation of morphine. The DAWN report lists 501 codeine related deaths in 1990.

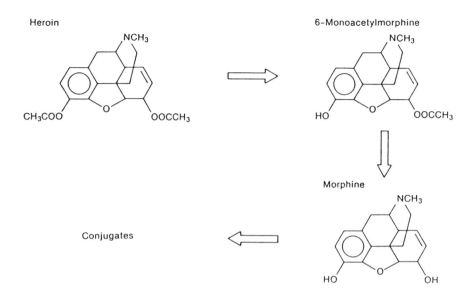

Figure 5.4.2 Heroin metabolism
Adapted from Baselt: Disposition of Toxic Drugs and Chemicals in Man, Vol. 1,
Canton, Conn, Biomedical Publications, 1978, p. 11.

Tons of this compound are consumed annually, but very important
questions about codeine metabolism and toxicity remain unanswered.
There is, for instance, some evidence that codeine's pain-relieving
properties, which are only about a fifth of morphine's, arise from the
fact that it is converted to morphine (Sanfilippo 1948). More important,
at least so far as investigations of toxicity are concerned, is the fact that
substantial variation exists in individuals' ability to metabolize codeine
(Yue, Hasselström et al. 1991) (Yue, Svensson et al. 1991) (Chen,
Somogy et al. 1991).

The major metabolic pathways for codeine are glucuronidation
and demethylation, but most of a given dose is converted to codeine-6-
-glucuronide, an inactive metabolite. Much smaller amounts may be converted to norcodeine, which is thought to be psychoactive (Fraser, Isbell
et al. 1960). It has only recently become apparent that, depending on the
individual's genetic makeup, significant amounts of codeine may be
shunted to pathways yielding pharmacologic active products. N-demethylation produces norcodeine that is converted to glucuronide or to
normorphine. The O-demethylation route is much more important,
because it leads to the production of morphine, and codeine that has
been converted to morphine is, in turn, converted to morphine-3-glucur-

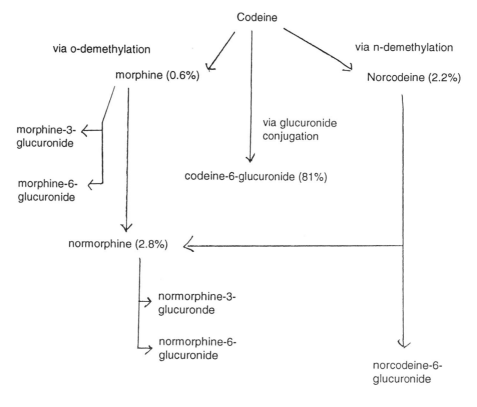

Figure 5.4.3.1 Human metabolism of codeine
Based on results observed after giving 30 mg of codeine phosphate to 8
volunteers. Percentages of metabolite formed are in brackets. Some individuals
lack cytochrome P450 IID6 and cannot dealkylate codeine to morphine. From
Vree, Corrien, Verwey-Van Wissen, 1992.

onide or morphine-6-glucuronide. All of these compounds are excreted
in the urine, where somewhat less than 90% of a single dose can be
recovered within 48 hours, mostly as codeine-6-glucuronide (Chen,
Somogy et al. 1991). The important consideration here is that codeine
metabolism yields three different compounds with known psychoactivity
(morphine, normorphine, and morphine-6-glucuronide).

5.4.3.2 Routes of administration

Pharmacokinetic studies of codeine's fate have been published,
but the radioimmune assays used very likely produced spuriously high
concentrations of codeine in the plasma and urine (Chen, Somogy et al.
1991). Similar considerations apply to many of the earlier studies on the
fate of morphine. Measurements in healthy volunteers given a 50-mg
oral dose of codeine show a plasma half-life of 2.4 to 3.2 hours (Yue,

Hasselström et al. 1991; Yue, Svensson et al. 1991) (Chen 1991). When measured with high-pressure liquid chromatography, peak blood levels after an oral dose of 50 mg in healthy, normal metabolizers averaged 140 ng/mL (Yue, Svensson et al. 1991). A second study, also using HPLC, yielded similar results (Chen 1991). Interestingly, the peak concentration of codeine in the saliva is nearly three times that measured in the blood, even though the half-life in both fluids is approximately 3.2 hours (Chen, Somogy et al. 1991). Resultant blood levels after alternate routes of administration have not been reported.

5.4.3.3 Role of genetic polymorphism

After oral dosing, plasma levels of codeine-glucuronide are 5–10 times higher than codeine levels. After chronic dosing the pharmacokinetics of both codeine and its principal metabolite, codeine-6-glucuronide, are unchanged. Even though chronic usage seems to have no effect, an individual's genetic makeup does, both in terms of analgesic properties and toxic effects.

TABLE 5.4.3.1

	Hydroxylators	Non-hydroxylators
Codeine	411 ± 219	239 ± 60
C6G	4090 ± 3380	3890 ± 949
NC	48 ± 26	48 ± 13
NCG	108 ± 44	146 ± 8
M3G	186 ± 121	9.1 ± 8.2
M6G	41 ± 23	non-detectable
NM	41 ± 33	non-detectable
M	27 ± 23	non-detectable

Values are in nmol/dL. All measurements were from healthy volunteers who had been previously screened for the ability to hydroxylate debrisoquine. *Data derived from Yue.*

Codeine metabolism is under monogenic control. The ability to form morphine-6-glucuronide, morphine and norcodeine from codeine can be predicted by an individual's ability to hydroxylase debrisoquine (debrisoquine phenotype). Approximately 10% of Caucasians, and a much larger percentage of Chinese, are poor hydroxylators. The majority of Caucasians, referred to as extensive hydroxylators, convert 6% of a given dose of codeine by demethylation and subsequent conjugation, eventually producing small amounts of morphine. Plasma levels of morphine-6-glucuronide, normorphine, and morphine peak at levels that are about one tenth the peak codeine level (see table below). In poor hydroxylators, much less than 0.5% is metabolized in this manner, and no morphine, morphine-6-glucuronide, or morphine is detectable in the plasma.

The forensic significance of these observations needs further elaboration, but it should be apparent that some individuals will have more psychoactive material in their bloodstreams than simple measurements of morphine or codeine levels would indicate. The obverse is also true. Individuals likely to be slow hydroxylators should have little or no morphine detectable in their blood if the only drug taken was codeine.

Interpreting the presence of small amounts of codeine and morphine in urine specimens is something of a problem (see above). It had been thought that small amounts of morphine were metabolically converted to codeine, but in fact that is not the case. The codeine detected in urine gets there because it is present in morphine in trace amounts, even in pharmaceutical grade morphine preparations. Thus the presence of codeine should not be presumed to be evidence for anything but the ingestion of codeine. The presence of trace amounts of morphine, on the other hand, can be accounted for by the metabolic conversion of codeine to morphine. Before accepting such an explanation, some attempt should be made to determine whether that individual is, in fact, capable of such a metabolic conversion. Fully 10% of the Caucasian population, and a much larger proportion of the Asian population may not be, and in those cases the presence of morphine may be evidence for the use of morphine or heroin.

5.4.3.4 Codeine tissue disposition

Data on codeine's tissue distribution is sparse, and difficult to interpret in light of what is now known about the role of active metabolites such as morphine and morphine-6-glucuronide. Nearly all the reports in the literature are from the 1970's, before the role of genetic variation was recognized and before the importance of metabolically active glucuronides was appreciated.

TABLE 5.4.3.4
TISSUE LEVELS IN REPORTED CASES OF CODEINE OVERDOSE DEATHS

	Blood	Bile	Liver	Kidney	Urine
Codeine	2.8	17.6	6.8	11.7	103.8
	(1–8.8)	(5–43)	(0.6–45)	(2.3–36)	(29–229)
Morphine	0.2	37.6	1.5	2	19.6
	(0–0.5)	(3–117)	(0–6.3)	(0.3–5.2)	(0–58)

Data adapted from Baselt

5.4.3.5 Excretion and detectability

The elimination half-life of both codeine and its main metabolite, codeine-6-glucuronide, is slightly over 3 hours. Both compounds should be detectable in the bloodstream for more than 12, but less than 24 hours. Urinary excretion of codeine may be longer than that of morphine.

5.4.4 METHADONE

Methadone belongs to a class of compounds referred to as diphenylpropylamine derivatives. Drugs in this class have the general formula which at first glance bears little relationship to the basic morphine molecule, but which in fact contains the same basic structures common to morphine analgesics. Until 1965, when it was introduced as a maintenance drug for heroin addicts, it enjoyed little popularity, probably because, in some individuals, its half-life can exceed 50 hours. Today it is the drug of choice for the treatment of heroin addiction, and it is frequently prescribed to cancer patients. Tolerance is quick to develop, but it does so in an unpredictable fashion. In one cluster of ten methadone related fatalities, the deaths appear to have been the result of excessively rapid dosage increases (Drummer, Opeskin, Syrjanen & Cordner, 1992). There were 421 methadone-related deaths in 1990 (National Institute on Drug Abuse 1990b). Methadone is supplied as a racemic mixture, but almost all of the opiate activity is due to the *l* form.

5.4.4.1 General considerations

Drawing conclusions about the toxicity of a given dose of methadone, or of a particular methadone blood level, without additional historical and clinical information, is impossible. In one study, heroin addicts treated with doses ranging from 180 mg to 260 mg/day experienced no adverse effects (Walton 1978). The results of other studies done to assess the central nervous system response to graded doses of methadone suggest that neurophysiologic responses do not correlate well with blood levels. In non-tolerant individuals, methadone doses that are only a fraction as high as those taken by individuals on replacement therapy, can induce fatal respiratory depression. Drummer described a group of ten patients who died shortly after being enrolled in a methadone maintenance program. Historical and autopsy findings were consistent with the diagnosis of respiratory arrest, but the average dose being taken by these individuals was only 57 mg per day, with mean blood levels of 600 ng/mL. In other series of methadone related deaths, average blood levels have been closer to 1,000 ng/mL (Robinson and Williams, 1971) (Norheim, 1973) (Segal and Catheman, 1974) (Manning, Bidanset, Cohen, Lukash 1976) (Drummer, Opeskin, Syrjanen & Cordner 1992).

Nonetheless, recent studies on methadone kinetics have shown that (1) there is fairly good correlation between the dose given and the resultant plasma level (Wolff and Hay 1991; Wolff, Hay et al. 1991), and that (2) addicts are likely to complain of withdrawal symptoms if their blood level drops much below 50 ng/mL (Wolff, Hay et al. 1992).

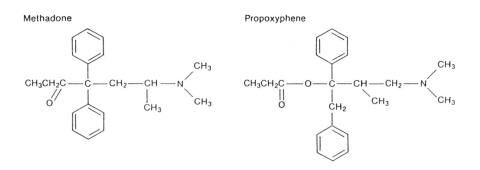

Figure 5.4.4 Methadone and propoxyphene
Even though it is not obvious, the methadone molecule contains the same basic
structures as all the other ¯morphine related analgesics. Propoxyphene is a
derivative of morphine.

The results of other studies suggest that the best results, both
in terms of preventing HIV seroconversion and in deterring heroin use,
are seen when a patient takes at least 90 mg/day (Loimer and Schmid,
1992). Both because methadone is a potent respiratory depressant, and
because methadone treatment is ineffective if doses are too low, many
argue that therapeutic drug monitoring should be an integral component
of all methadone treatment programs.

5.4.4.2 Routes of absorption

Oral absorption of methadone is excellent, and there is a very
good correlation between the dose administered and the plasma level
that results. Over the range of 3–100 mg plasma methadone concentrations increase by 263 ng/mL for every milligram of methadone per
kilogram of body weight administered (Wolff, Hay et al. 1991). This
same, nearly linear, concentration increase is also observed in saliva,
though the peak levels are somewhat higher and the half-life somewhat
longer (Wolff and Hay 1991).

The results of intravenous methadone injections have been
studied in cancer patients. In one case a 10-mg bolus produced a peak
plasma level slightly above 500 ng/mL immediately after injection, falling
to below 100 ng/mL at one hour (Inturrisi, Colburn et al. 1987). In a
group of addicts maintained on methadone, saliva levels were found to
be somewhat higher than simultaneously measured blood levels (Wolff
and Hay 1991). Levels after the less common routes of administration
have not been measured. Once in the body, methadone is transformed
via N-demethylation to a group of metabolites, all of which are inactive.

There is wide individual variation in its half life, with reported values ranging from 13 to 58 hours (Goldstein 1971) (Inturrisi 1972).

Methadone clearance is altered when it is taken with other drugs. In theory some of these interactions could lead to toxicity, but when alcohol and methadone are taken together, they enhance each other's metabolism, so that the most likely outcome of this combination is the onset of withdrawal symptoms (Kreek 1981).

5.4.4.3 Autopsy findings

Individuals in methadone maintenance programs are likely to have some cutaneous stigmata of past intravenous heroin abuse. Since all opiates are respiratory depressants, bronchopneumonia would not be a surprising finding. It has been suggested that chronic persistent hepatitis is a frequent finding in methadone related deaths, however that probably is not the case. Inflammatory infiltrates, without evidence of necrosis, are commonly seen in the portal triads of heroin abusers (see section 5.9.3.1).

5.4.4.4 Tissue levels

Tissue levels, using various techniques, have been measured in about 50 cases, most of them in the early 1970's (Robinson and Williams, 1971), (Norheim, 1973), (Segal and Catheman, 1974), (Manning, Bidanset, Cohen & Lukash, 1976), (Drummer, Opeskin, Syrjanen & Cordner, 1992). Methadone tends to concentrate in the liver, but often blood levels equal or exceed hepatic levels when measured at autopsy. In the most recent study, blood and liver concentrations were measured in individuals whose methadone dosage was known (Drummer, Opeskin, Syrjanen & Cordner, 1992).

Table 5.4.4.3
DOSAGE AND TISSUE LEVELS IN 10 METHADONE RELATED DEATHS

Dosage Range	Blood Level	Liver Level	Urine Concentration
45–70 mg/day	260–2,500 ng/mL	670–5,500 ng/mL	15,000–116,000 ng/mL

adapted from Drummer et al. 1992

The concentrations observed in fatal cases overlap the methadone concentrations that have been observed in patients participating in methadone maintenance programs (Garriott 1973) (Robinson 1971). Given the degree of overlap it is difficult, if not impossible, to distinguish between overdose and maintenance on the basis of toxicology testing alone (Baselt 1989). If tissue levels of methadone metabolites are high, than that suggests chronic use, but the breakdown rate of methadone metabolites postmortem has not been characterized.

5.4.5 PROPOXYPHENE

5.4.5.1 General considerations

Chemists have used manipulations of the methadone molecule to create a series of related analgesics, the most important of which is propoxyphene. Unlike methadone, which is a potent analgesic, propoxyphene has only mild analgesic properties. In spite of that it is widely prescribed, and overdose has been associated with large numbers of fatalities (Soumerai, Avorn et al. 1987). Propoxyphene is particularly toxic because, in addition to exerting the usual respiratory depressant effects common to all μ agonist narcotics, propoxyphene and its principal metabolites also act as local anesthetics, with potent membrane stabilizing effects.

Intravenous propoxyphene abuse has been all but eliminated by reformulating the drug. Essentially all cases of toxicity are now due to oral ingestion. It is absorbed rapidly out of the gastrointestinal tract (Flanagan, Ramsey et al. 1984) (Gibson, Giacomini et al. 1980) (Young 1983), with peak plasma concentrations occurring within 1 to 2 hours after a single oral dose. Peak concentrations of propoxyphene itself are usually not very high, because the drug undergoes extensive first-pass metabolism in the liver where it is oxidized to norpropoxyphene. Peak propoxyphene levels after a single 65-mg dose in healthy young volunteers ranged from 260 to 900 ng/mL with a mean of 590 ng/mL. In this same group the half-life ranged from 6.4 to 26.4 hours, with a mean of 13 hours. Simultaneous measurements of nordextroropoxyphene showed peak levels ranging from 510 to 2,140 ng/mL with a mean of 1,950 ng/mL. The half-life for the metabolites is much longer than that of the parent compound, with a mean value of 22.2 hours.

There are no detectable differences between the sexes, but age has definite effects on how propoxyphene is metabolized. The half-life for both parent compound and metabolite is more than twice as long in the elderly than in the young. The half-life of dextroporopoxyphene in the young is only 13 hours, but it rises to over 35 hours in the elderly. Similarly, the half-life for norpropoxyphene in the young is approximately 22 hours, but it rises to over 40 hours in the elderly (Flanagan, Ramsey et al. 1984). This pattern is not unique, and is often encountered with drugs that undergo hepatic oxidation and then renal elimination. The prolonged course of excretion in the elderly may have some bearing on reported cases of toxicity, since norpropoxyphene has the same membrane stabilizing properties as propoxyphene itself (Nickander, Emmerson et al. 1984).

Excretion is also prolonged in the elderly and individuals with liver impairment. In the latter group, first-pass oxidation can be reduced resulting in increased levels of propoxyphene in the circulation. Since both parent and metabolite have equal membrane stabilizing ability, there probably is no increase in cardiotoxicity, though the opiate effects of propoxyphene may be exaggerated (Giacomini, Giacomini et al. 1980). There is some evidence that, when used with ethanol, first-pass transformation is decreased and that higher blood levels of propoxyphene result (Orguma and Levy 1981), but this effect is modest, and when large numbers of propoxyphene-related deaths are analyzed, consistent correlations between propoxyphene and alcohol levels have not been demonstrated (Theilade 1989).

5.4.5.2 Tissue distribution

Propoxyphene is highly lipid soluble, and very large amounts can be sequestered in fat tissue. Fatalities were frequent during the mid 1970's, and levels at autopsy have been reported for hundreds of cases (Caplan, Thompson et al. 1977) (McBay 1976) (Finkle, Caplan et al. 1981) (Finkle, McCloskey et al. 1976) (Baselt, Wright et al. 1975) (Cravey, Shaw et al. 1974). In the past it was generally assumed that serious toxicity was associated with levels greater than 1 mg/L, and fatalities are associated with levels of over 2 mg/L. But, as with all opiates, there is tremendous overlap, and fatalities have occurred at much lower levels while, at the same time, higher values have been observed as incidental findings.

Even though blood and tissue levels have been measured and reported many times, the results of a recent study suggest that post-mortem measurements are unpredictable and that measured concentrations depend entirely on where in the body the blood samples are drawn (Yonemitsu & Pounder, 1992). Multiple blood and tissue samples from 4 different individuals who had died after overdosing with dextropropoxyphene and paracetamol were analyzed after taking samples from various sites within each cadaver. Then the sampling was repeated at 24 and 48 hours. In every case the lowest blood levels were observed in peripheral blood samples. When the levels in the peripheral blood measured 3.5 mg/L the concentration in the aorta was 1.9 grams/L, nearly 55 times higher! When blood was drawn from the pulmonary artery the propoxyphene concentration increased two-fold at 24 hours and three-fold at 48 hours. When repeat samples were drawn from the inferior vena cava, there were variable increases in measured blood levels. In one individual there was a seven-fold increase over 24 hours.

Given the wide variations in values that can be measured in the same individual, drawing any sorts of conclusions from quantitative propoxyphene levels would appear to be very risky. For forensic purposes it might be more useful to look at the individual's electrocardiogram. Truly toxic propoxyphene levels will produce some fairly distinctive EKG changes (Whitcomb 1989), and these might reveal more about the cause of death than quantitation of blood levels.

Thus in a group of 29 patients who committed suicide by taking propoxyphene orally, the median total level of propoxyphene was 9.4 mg/L versus a total of only 2.2 mg/L in accident victims (Kaa, Dalgaard, 1989). In another study propoxyphene and norpropoxyphene levels were measured in a group of opiate addicts who were being maintained on propoxyphene instead of methadone. They received, on average, 800 to 1,600 mg of propoxyphene napsylate daily for anywhere from 13 to 50 months. Serum propoxyphene levels ranged from 127 to 1,070 mg/L and norpropoxyphene levels measured from 814 to 2,638 ng/mL, while the ratio of the two compounds ranged from 0.1 to 0.4. Since these levels are well in excess of what were thought to be toxic levels, it is obvious that tolerance occurs, and at very significant levels (Hartman, Miyada, Pirkle et al. 1988).

At autopsy, observed concentrations are both site and time dependent. In one study of suicidal patients who had overdoses with a medication containing parecetamol and dextropropoxyphene, concentrations of the latter varied seven- to ten-fold. Propoxyphene concentrations in the pulmonary artery increased 2x over 24 hours and 3x over 48 hours. Samples from the interior vena cava varied in an unpredictable fashion, sometimes increasing as much as 7x. Propoxyphene levels in the aorta were 55 times as high as in the peripheral blood (Yonemitsu, Pounder 1992).

5.4.5.3 Excretion and detectability

Propoxyphene is not a "NIDA drug". Furthermore, none of the standard immunologic screening tests for opiates react with propoxyphene to any significant degree, so it wouldn't even be detected on a standard NIDA urine-screening test (Cone, Dickerson et al. 1992). Nonetheless, it remains present in the urine for very long periods of time, and given a half-life of 22 hours for norpropoxyphene, the drug or its metabolite should still be detectable in the blood stream for more than 4 days after the last dose was taken. The window of detectability in the urine might be even longer.

5.4.5.4 Mechanisms of toxicity

Propoxyphene-induced respiratory depression is treated effectively with opiate antagonists, but most of the patients reaching the hospital die of cardiotoxicity (Sorenson 1984), and cardiotoxicity is not reversed with naloxone. Evidence for propoxyphene-induced cardiotoxicity includes electrocardiographic changes such as QRS prolongation, bundle branch block, and, in extreme cases, asystole. Myocardial contractility decreases and, as a result, cardiac output and blood pressure both drop. Neither treatment with beta adrenergic agents, nor pacing, have proven very effective (Whitcomb 1989). All of these electrophysiologic changes can be accounted for by propoxyphene's ability to block the inward sodium current (I_{Na}). The orderly sequence of depolarization is disrupted, conduction is delayed across the myocardium, and insufficient calcium enters the myocytes, preventing them from contracting maximally. Very much the same thing happens in cases of cocaine toxicity, which is hardly surprising, since cocaine is also a local anesthetic agent that binds to receptors controlling the I_{Na} channel. The reason that this sort of toxicity is more evident in the case of propoxyphene is probably related to relative receptor affinity at the site of the sodium influx channel.

5.4.6 FENTANYL AND OTHER SYNTHETIC AGENTS

5.4.6.1 General considerations

Fentanyl is a μ agonist, a synthetic phenylpiperidine derivative closely related in structure to meperidine (Demerol). Fentanyl was first introduced into clinical practice in the early 1960's. On a weight for weight basis, it is 50 to 100 times more potent than morphine. The first two fentanyl-related deaths were reported in 1979. In both cases the deceased had died with their paraphernalia at their sides, and at autopsy both were noted to have needle tracks and pulmonary edema. Surprisingly, toxicologic tests on both bodies and on the injection paraphernalia were negative for opiates. Six additional deaths occurred before it was finally determined that the individuals had overdosed on alpha-methylfentanyl (Kram, 1981) (Allen, Cooper et al. 1981). During the last decade there have been over 100 additional deaths from fentanyl or one of its illicitly produced homologues (Henderson 1991). Recent cases have occurred as a cluster in New York City and Philadelphia. In February of 1991 heroin mixed with fentanyl, selling for $10 a bag, suddenly appeared on the streets in New York, resulting in the hospitalization of 200, and at least 22 deaths. Literally hundreds of different fentanyl analogues can be synthesized and detection is difficult. At least 12 different analogues are known to have been sold on the illicit drug market (World Health Organization 1990).

5.4.6.2 Routes of absorption

The fentanyls are mostly used intravenously. After an oral dose of 15 μg/kg, peak plasma concentrations in healthy volunteers were 3.0 ng/mL. Peak plasma levels after giving that same amount intravenously were nearly 10 times higher, however the terminal elimination half-life is approximately 7 hours in either case (Streisand 1991). Other studies have shown that loss of consciousness occurs at levels of 34 ± 7 ng/mL (Lunn 1979), but that respiratory depression may be detected at levels as low as 1–5 ng (Fung 1980) (Andrews 1983). The minimal effective plasma concentration to produce analgesia averages 0.63 ± 0.25 ng/mL, but there is considerable variation in sensitivity from individual to individual (Gourlay, Kowalski et al. 1988).

In the rhesus monkey, which appears to parallel human responses quite well, 4 μg/kg given intravenously results in a plasma fentanyl concentration of 2.7 $\pm$ 0.9 ng/mL. A dose of 64 μg/kg results in a blood level of 43.4 $\pm$ 26. 0 ng/mL. These animals become apneic at blood levels much over 40 ng/mL (Nussmeier et al. 1991). Fentanyl can also be smoked or snorted, and there are reports that clandestine labs sometimes manufacture two forms of the drug, one for "shooters" and one for "snorters" (World Health Organization 1990). In either case, small amounts of fentanyl are mixed with very large amounts of manitol, lactose, and occasionally, heroin. There are no published studies on absorption by non-traditional routes such as rectal, vaginal, or nasal application.

Because fentanyl is lipophilic and of low molecular weight, it is readily absorbed through the skin. Transdermal delivery systems are now marketed in the United States and Europe. The degree of absorption depends on where the patch is placed and varies from person to person. Measurements indicate that 46–66% of a given dose applied to the skin will be absorbed. After applying a patch, serum levels are undetectable for 2 hours, then rise gradually for 12–14 hours, reaching a steady state at 24 hours. Studies done in surgical patients show mean levels ranging from 0.3 ng/mL to 2.7 ng/mL at various times after patch application (Calis, Kohler et al. 1992). Patches have already been diverted to the illicit market and are now available on the streets.

5.4.6.3 Metabolism

After an initial rapid uptake by lung and fat, fentanyl is slowly released with a mean terminal half-life of 2 to 4 hours in healthy volunteers, and anywhere from 2.5 to 8 hours in surgical patients (Mather 1983). It is metabolized in the liver and transformed by N-dealkylation to norfentanyl (Goromaru, Matsura et al. 1981). Both fentanyl and its metabolite can undergo hydroxylation to inactive hydroxypropionyl derivatives. The conversion is rapid, and within 30 minutes of intravenous administration metabolite concentration is higher than fentanyl concentration (McClain and Hug 1980). Other metabolic routes are possible but their significance in man is still not clear. Approximately 50% of a given dose is eliminated in the urine within the first 8 hours, and 85% will be recovered in the urine within 72 hours (World Health Organization 1990). Less than 8% of a given dose is excreted unchanged in the urine (Schleimer, Benjamini et al. 1978).

5.4.6.4 Tissue levels

All of the fentanyls are highly lipid soluble and they distribute widely throughout the body (Hess, Hertz et al. 1972; Hess, Stiebler et al. 1972). Fentanyl's relatively short duration of action is, in fact, explained by rapid lipid uptake. In animal studies, high levels are achieved quickly in well perfused tissues such as lung, kidney, heart, and brain. Approximately 3–4% of an intravenous dose will be secreted into the gastric juice from where there is minimal reabsorption (Stoeckle, Hengstmann et al. 1979). Fentanyl tissue/blood partition coefficients have been measured in the rat model, and there is good evidence to suggest that tissue distribution in this model reflects the distribution pattern seen in humans. The values in Table 5.4.6.1 were measured after a 6-hour infusion. Levels in the liver and brain were 4 times higher than in the plasma. Levels measured in the stomach can be misleading because, as previously mentioned, fentanyl is actively secreted into the stomach (Stoeckel, 1979) (Björkman 1990).

In Henderson's series of 112 deaths from illicit fentanyl preparations, fentanyl concentrations in blood ranged from 0.2 ng/mL to > 50 ng/mL, and urine concentrations ranged from 0.2 to > 800 ng/mL. If the few individuals with extremely high levels are excluded, than the mean fentanyl level at autopsy was 3.0 ± 3.1 ng/mL in the blood and 3.9 ± 4.3 ng/mL in the urine. In the handful of deaths due to fentanyl citrate (the pharmaceutical grade product used as an intravenous anesthetic), blood concentrations have ranged from 3 to 27 ng/mL (Garriott 1973).

TABLE 5.4.6.1
STEADY STATE TISSUE/BLOOD PARTITION COEFFICIENTS FOR FENTANYL IN THE RAT

Organ/Tissue	Level
Plasma	1
Brain	4
Liver	4
Heart	5
Stomach	14
Kidneys	14
Lungs	15
Pancreas	24
Fat	30

Adapted from Björkman et al. 1990.

(Rodriguez et al. 1984) (Matejezyk 1988). McGee et. al. compared blood and tissue levels in 7 overdose deaths with fentanyl levels observed in anesthetized patients dying at surgery (McGee, Marker et al. 1992). In most cases the overdose deaths had levels that were 5 to 10 times higher than levels in anesthetized patients.

TABLE 5.4.6.2
**COMPARISON OF BLOOD LEVELS IN FENTANYL RELATED "OVERDOSE"
DEATHS AND LEVELS SEEN IN ANESTHETIZED PATIENTS DYING OF SURGICAL
COMPLICATIONS**

	Deaths from Fentanyl overdose	Deaths at surgery
Blood	11 – 233 ng/mL	5 – 45 ng/mL
Brain	20 – 194 ng/mL	18 – 85 ng/mL
Liver	28 – 1,000 ng/mg	41 – 158 ng/mg

Adapted from McGee et al. 1992.

The plasma level required to produce effective analgesia in surgical patients is 1–3 ng/mL, but there is wide interpatient variability. Values in this range can also be associated with severe respiratory depression, but the relationship between fentanyl and carbon dioxide levels is inconsistent (Lehmann, Freier et al. 1982). Respiratory depression is observed in human volunteers when levels are between 2 and 3 ng/mL (Cartwright, Prys-Ropberts et al. 1983). Effects of the illicit fentanyl homologues have never been assessed in humans.

As is true in all opiate-related deaths, other drugs are frequently detected. In nearly 40% of the fentanyl-related deaths, alcohol is also present, frequently at high levels. In 20% of cases, cocaine was also detected. At one time, most fentanyl-related deaths were reported from California. That is no longer true and, increasingly, cases are now being reported from the East Coast. Supplies of this drug remain quite limited. Of 3,000 blood samples submitted to Henderson's reference laboratory at U.C. Davis, only 112 were positive for fentanyl or one of its known illicit analogues (alpha-methylfentanyl, paraflurofentanyl, 3-methylfentanmyl and thienmylfentanyl) (Henderson 1991).

Most reported fentanyl-related deaths have been in males (78%) with a mean age of 32.5 years ± 6.7 years. This is in contrast to the typical heroin overdose victim who is usually in his mid 20's. Unlike heroin users, who are often found on the street, fentanyl overdoses usually occur at home, in the bedroom or bath. Like heroin-related deaths, 60% of the time the deceased is found with their paraphernalia at their side. Otherwise, autopsy findings are the same as in heroin overdose. Mean lung weights are 726 grams.

5.4.7 OTHER OPIATES
Other opiates are abused with some frequency, but the associated incidence of untoward events is quite low. These other agents cause fewer than 2% of the deaths, and less than 2% of the emergency-room visits reported to the DAWN survey (National Institute on Drug Abuse 1990b) (National Institute on Drug Abuse 1990a). These drugs are not

reliably detected by the immunologic screening tests used to detect morphine and codeine (Cone, Dickerson et al. 1992), and under NIDA rules, the presence of these drugs couldn't be reported anyway (Most Federally regulated drug programs only test for 5 drugs: cocaine, pcp, marijuana, methamphetamine, and morphine. Even if propoxyphene were detected, its presence could not be reported out. Different rules apply to the nuclear and transportation industries).

5.4.7.1 Hydromorphone (Dilaudid™)

This is a semisynthetic opiate, the hydrogenated ketone derivative of morphine. On a weight-per-weight basis it is 7–10 times more potent than morphine (Mahler and Fottdry 1975), but otherwise it shares most of morphine's properties. Hydromorphone has been available for many years, but it has recently become popular in the management of chronic pain syndromes. It is more potent than morphine, and it can be prepared in more concentrated aqueous solutions than morphine. In spite of its potency, and persistent strong underground demand for this drug, it is seldom associated with toxicity. Of the 2,800 deaths attributed to narcotic analgesics in the 1990 DAWN report only 9, or 0.3% of all cases, were due to hydromorphone.

Hydromorphone is well absorbed by all routes. After an intravenous injection, more than 90% is cleared from the plasma and redistributed into tissue stores within 10 minutes of injection. This is almost exactly the same thing that happens after giving intravenous morphine, and methadone (Hill, Coda et al. 1991). Elimination of the drug then depends on how fast it diffuses back into the blood stream. The average elimination half-life is 3 hours, but there is very substantial intersubject variation. In the most recently published study, a 40-μg/kg bolus given intravenously produced average blood levels of 7 ng/mL at 15 minutes, 5 ng/mL at 30 minutes, and 4 ng/mL at one hour. The kinetics are not dose dependent. Humans excrete mainly the 3-glucuronide (Cone, Phelps et al. 1977). Less than 6% of a given dose is excreted unchanged in the urine. The 6-hydroxy metabolite is probably not produced in man. Older measurements of blood and tissue levels are difficult to interpret, because the radioimmunoassays that were used cross-react with the glucuronide metabolites, resulting in final concentrations that were probably falsely high.

Hydromorphone is a μ agonist and produces all of the classic symptoms of opiate intoxication. The minimum plasma concentration necessary to relieve severe pain is 4 ng/mL (Ridenberg, Goodman et al. 1988). Studies in abusers have not been made. There is a paucity of autopsy data and no evidence to suggest that hydromorphone abuse causes any unique pathologic alterations. Since oral tablets are often crushed and injected, angiothrombotic lung disease could be a sequela of long-term use, but this has not been substantiated.

5.4.7.2 Hydrocodone (Hycodan™, Tussend™, Tussionex™)

This compound is structurally almost identical with codeine, the only difference being a =O group substitution for a hydroxyl group at position 6. Alone or in combination with other drugs, hydrocodone was responsible for 45 deaths in 1990. It is well absorbed from the gastrointestinal tract, and according to Baselt it has a half-life of 3.8 hours. Hydrocodone is cleared from the system by conversion to hydromorphone (Cone, Darwin et al. 1978). It is also a μ agonist capable of causing respiratory depression and death. As is true for hydromorphone, there is almost no autopsy information available, but there is no reason to suppose that this drug causes lesions any different from the other opiate agents.

5.4.7.3 Oxycodone (Tylox™, Percodan™)

This compound is a semi-synthetic derived from codeine. It is thought to be widely abused, but in all of 1990 only 25 deaths were recorded in the DAWN survey. Its potency and duration of action are comparable to that of morphine. Peak levels after oral administration are reached in one hour (Inturrisi 1982).

5.4.7.4 Oxymorphone (Numorphan™)

This is a semisynthetic opioid with pure μ agonist properties, and a potency that is seven to ten times as great as morphine. In 1990 it accounted for less than 0.2% of all narcotic related fatalities. More recently this agent has seen increasing use as an intravenous anesthetic agent. Since it is capable of producing profound respiratory depression for over 5 hours after administration, more fatalities may be anticipated (Patt 1988).

5.4.7.5 Meperidine (Demerol™, Pethidine™)

A synthetic phenylpiperidine derivative, this is the only member of this class known to cause toxicity or death with any regularity. In 1990 meperidine accounted for slightly more than 0.5% of narcotic-related deaths reported in the United States. On a weight-for-weight basis meperidine has only one-sixth the analgesic potency of morphine. Unlike the naturally occurring opiates, meperidine in large doses can be neurotoxic. This toxicity is manifested as muscle twitching or convulsions (Boros, Chaudry et al. 1984) (Morisy and Platt 1986) (Hershey 1983). Meperidine-induced neurotoxicity is not reversed by opiate antagonists, but meperidine-induced respiratory depression is. There are reports in the literature of prolonged narcosis, especially in elderly patients receiving high doses (Chan, Kendall et al. 1975).

Meperidine is well absorbed by all conventional routes of administration. Peak plasma levels occur 1 to 2 minutes after intra-

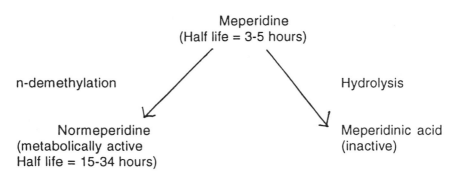

Figure 5.4.7 Meperidine metabolism
The metablite normeperidine has about half the analgesic potency of meperidine and is also neurotoxic. Normeperidine's half-life is much longer than meperidine's, and toxic levels may accumulate in individuals with renal impairment.

venous administration, and within 1 hour after it is given orally. After intravenous administration there is extensive first-pass uptake of meperidine (as is true for most, but not all, of the other opiates) by the lung. Measurements have shown that as much as 75% of a given dose of meperidine is taken up in the lung during the first pass. The drug is then released back into the circulation at a variable rate (Roerig, Kotrly et al. 1987). This first-pass phenomenon does not occur with morphine or heroin. After oral dosing, maximum plasma levels are seen from 0.5 to 1.5 hours later (Pond, Tong et al. 1981).

Meperidine is hydrolyzed in the liver to form meperidinic acid (Asatoor, London et al. 1963) (Pond, Tong et al. 1981). N-demethylation leading to the formation of normeperidine has also been documented. Normeperidine is metabolically active. It has about one half the analgesic potency of meperidine but is several times more neurotoxic (Miller and Anderson 1984). It also has a much longer half-life (Pond, Tong et al. 1981). Under normal circumstances the half-life of meperidine is 3 to 5 hours (Koska, Krasmer et al. 1981) (Mather, Tucker et al. 1975), but the clearance rate depends somewhat on the amount given. In individuals with extensive liver disease meperidine is metabolized more slowly. The half-life of meperidine in such cases can be as long as 11 hours (Pond, Tong et al. 1981).

When large doses of meperidine are administered, normeperidine accumulates in the plasma in large quantities (Koska, Krasmer et al. 1981). In normal individuals the terminal half-life of normeperidine is anywhere from 15 to 34 hours, but in individuals with renal impairment it may be three or four days. Thus toxicity, when it occurs, may be prolonged (Szeto, Inturrisi et al. 1977). In control studies, 5% of a given dose was excreted unchanged in the urine. One quarter of the dose will be excreted as meperidinic acid or normeperidinic acid.

Like all the opiates, meperidine and normeperidine distribute widely throughout the body. Meperidine blood levels measured at autopsy in the 6 cases reported by Siek ranged from 4,300 ng/mL to 12,000 ng/mL. Hepatic levels were twice the blood levels in patients who were intravenous users, but only one half the blood level if the individual had taken the meperidine orally. Clinical evidence of normeperidine toxicity is seen with levels ranging from 425 to 1,900 ng/mL, with normeperidine to meperidine ratios of 0.79 to 5.4 (Szeto 1977). Even higher ratios have been observed. In the autopsy case reported by Jiraki, an addict with end-stage renal failure was found to have a meperidine blood level of only 60 ng/mL, while at the same time his normeperidine level was 3,000 ng/mL (Jiraki 1992).

5.4.7.6 Pentazocine

Pentazocine differs from the other agents discussed in that is both a narcotic agonist and antagonist. It is active at kappa and delta receptor sites, but antagonizes effects at the μ receptor site. It has less than half the potency of morphine. While there is no question that pentazocine (Talwin™) can be abused, the practice is extremely uncommon. No pentazocine-related deaths were noted in the DAWN survey for 1990, and pentazocine accounted for fewer than 0.2% of all drug related emergency-room visits in that same year (National Institute on Drug Abuse 1991). The low incidence of reports may well have to do with the fact that the oral form of pentazocine has been reformulated by the manufacturer and now contains the opiate antagonist, naloxone.

Earlier discussions of pentazocine abuse emphasized the high incidence among medical professionals, and the fact that pentazocine was often used with other drugs, especially alcohol, and the antihistamine tripelennamine (Ellenhorn and Barceloux 1988). In some areas this latter combination was especially popular among pregnant women. One of the older pentazocine tablets crushed together with 2 tripelennamine tablets would be dissolved in water and injected (Carlson 1982). The combination was referred to as "T's and Blues"). That pattern of usage also seems to have changed, as evidenced by the fact that the most recent DAWN report contains no mentions of pentazocine use in conjunction with any other drug.

With the exception of a tendency to produce myositis and fibrosis (Oh 1975) (Schiff 1977), long-term parenteral abuse of the drug results in the same set of complications produced by the long-term parenteral abuse of any other opiate (King 1978). Unlike other opiates, pentazocine causes increased release of epinephrine from the adrenals (Fukumitsu 1991) and elevates circulating catecholamines. That may explain why high doses increase both heart rate and blood pressure, a rather dangerous combination for individuals with preexisting coronary artery disease (Alderman 1972). The results of these experimental studies raise the possibility that, in pentazocine-related deaths, there might be anatomic findings consistent with catecholamine toxicity, such as contraction band necrosis. Such alterations are yet to be reported, but it is not clear if they have ever been systematically sought.

Peak pentazocine blood levels occur 15 minutes to 1 hour after intramuscular administration, but after oral administration peak levels may not be reached for several hours. Oral administration can produce levels that are almost as high as those seen after intramuscular injection. The peak level after a 75-mg dose given orally averages 160 ng/mL (Berkowitz 1969). Peak levels after 45 mg intramuscularly was 140 ng/mL. Five to 10 minutes after a 30-mg intravenous dose, blood levels as high as 1,000 ng/mL may be seen (Agurell 1974). Baselt states that plasma levels in fatalities range from 1 to 5 mg/L (Baselt 1989), but patients have survived with blood levels as high as 9 mg/L (Stahl 1983). The same difficulties apply to the interpretation of pentazocine levels as apply to any opiate. Tolerance occurs, and without knowledge of the individual's past history, attributing a specific event or outcome to an isolated toxicologic finding is impossible.

Pentazocine's terminal half-life is between 2 and 4 hours (Berkowitz 1969), but there is considerable variation from individual to individual. Very high levels can also be measured in the brain, where the concentration may exceed that found in the blood. High levels are also seen in the liver, bile, and kidney (Pittman 1973). There is extensive first-pass metabolism in the liver, where both oxidation and glucuronidation occur. Less than 10% of a given dose is excreted unchanged (Pittman 1970).

References

Alderman, E., Barry, W., Graham, A. and D. Harrison (1972). Hemodynamic effects of morphine and pentazocine differ in cardiac patients. N Engl J Med, 287, 623–627.

Aherne, G. and P. Littleton (1985). Morphine-6-glucuronide, an important factor in interpreting morphine radioimmunoassays. Lancet. ii:210–211.

Allen, A., D. Cooper and T. Kram (1981). "China White":alpha-Methylfentanyl. Microgram. 14(3):26–32.

Andrews, C. and Prys-Roberts, C. (1983). Fentanyl-a review. Clin Anaesthesiol, 1: 97–122.

Anon (1861). A new theory of poisoning. Lancet. i:93.

Asatoor, A., D. London, M. Milne and M. Simenhoff (1963). The excretion of pethidine and its derivatives. Br J Pharmacol. 20:285–298.

Agurell, S. Boréus, L., E. Gordon et al. (1974). Plasma and cerebrospinal fluid concentrations of pentazocine in patients; assay by mass fragmentography. J Pharm Pharmacol, 26:1–8.

Ball, M., McQuay, H., M. Moore et al. (1985). Renal failure and the use of morphine in intensive care. Lancet. 1:784–786.

Baselt, R., J. Wright, J. Turner and R. Cravey (1975). Propoxyphene and norpropoxyphene tissue concentrations in fatalities associated with propoxyphene hydrochloride and propoxyphene napsylate. Arch Tox. (34):145–152.

Berkowitz, B., S. Ngai, J. Yang et al. (1975). The disposition of morphine in surgical patients. Clin Pharmacol Ther. 17:629–635.

Berkowitz, B., Asling, J., E. Way et al. (1969). Relationship of pentazocine plasma levels to pharmacological activity in man. Clin Pharmacol Ther, 10:320–328.

Björkman, S., Stanski, D., Verotta, D. and H. Harashima. (1990). Comparative tissue concentration profiles of fentanyl and alfentanil in humans predicted from tissue/blood partition data obtained in rats. Anesthesiology, 72:865–873.

Boerner, U., Abbott, S. and R. Roc (1975).The metabolism of morphine and heroin in man. Drug Metab Rev, 4:39–73.

Boros, M., I. Chaudhry, H. Nagashima et al. (1984). Myoneural effects of pethidine and droperidol. Br J Anesth. 56:195–202.

Brunk, F. and M. Delle (1974). Morphine metabolism in man. Clin Pharm Ther. 16: 51–57.

Calis, K., D. Kohler and D. Corso (1992). Transdermally administered fentanyl for pain management. Clin Pharm. 11:22–36.

Caplan, Y., B. Thompson and R. Fisher (1977). Propoxyphene fatalities: blood and tissue concentrations of propoxyphene and norpropoxyphene and a study of 115 medical examiner cases. J Analyt Toxicol. 1:27–35.

Carlson, C. (1982). The drug victim too often the same: The fetus. JAMA, 248: 409–410.

Cartwright, P., C. Prys-Roberts, K. Gill et al. (1983). Ventilatory depression related to plasma fentanyl concentrations during and after anesthesia in humans. Anesth Analg. 62:966–974.

Chan, K., M. Kendall, M. Mitchard and W. Well (1975). The effect of age on plasma pethidine concentrations. Br J Clin Pharmacol. 2:297–302.

Chan, S., E. Chan and H. Kaliciak (1986). Distribution of morphine in body fluids and tissues in fatal overdose. J Forensic Sci. 31(4):1487–1491.

Chen, Z., A. Somogyi, G. Reynolds and F. Bochner (1991). Disposition and metabolism of codeine after single and chronic doses in one poor and seven extensive metabolizers. B J Clin Pharm. 31:381–390.

Cone, E., B. Phelps and C. Gorodetzky (1977). Urinary excretion of hydromorphone and metabolites in humans, rats, dogs, guinea pigs, and rabbits. J Pharm Sci. 66:1709–1713.

Cone, E., W. Darwin, C. Gorodetzky et al. (1978). Comparative metabolism of hydrocodone in man, rat, guinea pig, rabbit, and dog. Drug Metab Dispos. 6: 488–493.

Cone, E., (1990). Testing human hair for drugs of abuse. I. Individual dose and time profiles of morphine and codeine in plasma, saliva, urine, and beard compared to drug-induced effects on pupils and behavior. J Analyt Toxicol. 14:1–7.

Cone, E., P. Welch, B. Paul and J. Mitchell (1991a). Forensic drug testing for opiates, III. Urinary excretion rates of morphine and codeine following codeine administration. J Analyt Toxicol. 15:161–166.

Cone, E., P. Welch, J. Mitchell and B. Paul (1991b). Forensic drug testing for opiates: I. Detection of 6-acetylmorphine in urine as an indicator of recent heroin exposure; drug assay and considerations and detection times. J Analyt Toxicol. 15:1-7.

Cone, E., S. Dickerson, B. Paul and J. Mitchell (1992). Forensic drug testing for opiates. IV. Analytical sensitivity, specificity, and accuracy of commercial urine opiate immunoassays. J Analyt Toxicol. 16:72-78.

Cravey, R., R. Shaw and G.Nakamura (1974). Incidence of propoxyphene poisoning. A report of fatal cases. J Forensic Sci. 19:72-80.

Dahlström, B. and Paalzow, L. (1978). Pharmacokinetic interpretation of the enterohepatic recirculation and first-pass elimination of morphine in the rat J Pharmacokinet Biopharm, 6:505-529.

De Schepper, A. and Degryse, H. (1990). Imaging findings in a patient with pentazocine-induced myopathy. Am. J. Roent, 154:343-344.

Drummer, O., Opeskin, K., Syrjanen, M. and Cordner, S. (1992). Methadone toxicity causing death in ten subjects starting on a methadone maintenance program. Am J Forensic Med Pathol, 13:346-350.

Ellenhorn, M. and D. Barceloux (1988). Medical Toxicology: the diagnosis and treatment of human poisoning. New York, Elsevier, 1st edition. p 734.

Ellison, N. and G. Lewis (1984). Plasma concentrations following single doses of morphine sulfate in oral and rectal suppository. Clin Pharm. 3:614-617.

Felby, S., H. Christensen and A. Lund (1974). Morphine concentrations in blood and organs in cases of fatal poisoning. Forensic Sci. 3:77-81.

Finkle, B., Y. Caplan, J. Garriott et al. (1981). Propoxyphene in postmortem toxicology 1976-1978. J Forensic Sci. 26:739-757.

Finkle, B., K. McCloskey, G. Kiplinger and I. Bennett (1976). A national assessment of propoxyphene in postmortem medicolegal investigation, 1972-1975. J Forensic Sci. 21:706-742.

Flanagan, R., J. Ramsey and I. Jane (1984). Measurement of dextropropoxyphene and nordextropropoxyphene in biological fluids. Hum Toxicol. 3:103S-114S.

Fraser, H., H. Isbell and G. Van Horn (1960). Human pharmacology and addiction liability of norcodeine. J Pharm Exp Ther. 129:172-177.

Fukumitsu, K., Sumikawa, K., Hayashi, Y. et al. (1991). Pentazocine-induced catecholamine efflux from the dog perfused adrenals. J Pharm Pharmacol, 43: 331-336.

Fung, D. and J. Eisele (1980). Narcotic concentration-respiratory effect curves in man. Anesthesiology, 53:S397.

Garriott, J., Sturner, W., and Mason, M. (1973). Toxicologic findings in six fatalities involving methadone. Clin Toxic 6:163-173.

Garriott, J., R. Rodriguez and V. DiMaio (1984). A death from fentanyl overdose. J Analyt Toxicol. 8:288-289.

Giacomini, K., J. Giacomini, T. Gibson and G. Levy. (1980). Propoxyphene and norpropoxyphene plasma concentrations after oral propoxyphene in cirrhotic patients with and without surgically constructed portacaval shunt. Clin Pharm Ther. 28:417-424.

Gibson, T., K. Giacomini, W. Briggs et al. (1980). Propoxyphene and norpropoxyphene plasma concentrations in anephric patients. Clin Pharm Ther. 27: 665-670.

Goldstein, A. (1991). Measuring compliance in methadone maintenance patients: use of a pharmacologic indicator to estimate methadone plasma levels. Clin Pharmacol Ther, 50:199–207.

Goromaru, T., T. Furuta, S. Baba et al. (1981). Metabolism of fentanyl in rats and man. Anesthesiology. 55:A173.

Gottschalk, L. and R. Cravey (1980). Toxicological and pathological studies in psychoactive drug-involved deaths. Davis, CA, Biomedical Publications.

Gourlay, G., D. Cherry and M. Cousins (1986). A comparative study of the efficacy and pharmacokinetics of oral methadone and morphine in the treatment of severe pain in patients with cancer. Pain. 25:297–312.

Gourlay, G., S. Kowalski, J. Plummer et al. (1988). Fentanyl blood concentration-analgesic response relationship in the treatment of postoperative pain. Anesth Analg. 67:329–337.

Gourlay, G. and R. Boas (1992). Fatal outcome with use of rectal morphine for postoperative pain control in an infant. Br Med J, 304:766–777.

Graham, K., G. Koren, J. Klein et al. (1989). Determination of gestational cocaine exposure by hair analysis. JAMA. 262(23):3328–3330.

Greene, M., Luke, J., DuPont, R. (1974). Opiate overdose deaths in the District of Columbia. Part II - methadone-related deaths fatalities. J Forensic Sci. 19:575–584.

Hanks, G., P. Hoskin, G. Aherne et al. (1988). Enterohepatic circulation of morphine. Lancet. I:469.

Harding-Pink, D. and O. Fryc (1988). Risk of death after release from prison: a duty to warn. Br Med J. 297:596.

Hartman B., Miyada D., Pirkle, H. et al. (1988). Serum propoxyphene concentrations in a cohort of opiate addicts on long-term propoxyphene maintenance therapy. Evidence for drug tolerance in humans. J Analyt Toxicol, 12:25–29.

Hartvig, P., B. Lindberg, A. Lilja et al. (1989). Positron emission tomography in studies on fetomaternal disposition of opioids. Dev Pharmacol Ther. 12:74–80.

Henderson, G. (1991). Fentanyl-related deaths: demographics, circumstances, and toxicology of 112 cases. J Forensic Sci. 2 36:422–433.

Hershey, L. (1983). Meperidine and central neurotoxicity. Ann Intern Med. 98:548–549.

Hess, R., A. Hertz and K. Friedel (1972). Pharmacokinetics of fentanyl in rabbits in view of the importance for limiting the effect. J Pharmacol Exp Ther. 179: 474–484.

Hess, R., G. Stiebler and A. Herz (1972). Pharmacokinetics of fentanyl in man and the rabbit. Euro J Clin Pharmacol 4:135–141.

Hill, H., B. Coda, A. Tanaka and R. Schaffer (1991). Multiple-dose evaluation of intravenous hydromorphone pharmacokinetics in normal human subjects. Anesth Analg. 72:330–336.

Hine, C., J. Wright, D. Allison et al. (1982). Analysis of fatalities from acute narcotism in a major urban area. J Forensic Sci. 27:372–384.

Hoskin, P., G. Hanks, G. Aherne et al. (1989). The bioavailability and pharmacokinetics of morphine after intravenous, oral, and buccal administration in healthy volunteers. Br J Clin Pharmacol. 27:499–505.

Inturrisi, C. and Verebely, K. (1972). The levels of methadone in the plasma in methadone maintenance. Clin Pharmacol Ther, 13:633–647.

Inturrisi, C. (1982). Narcotic drugs. Med Clin North AM. 66:1061–1071.

Inturrisi, C., W. Colburn, R. Kaiko et al. (1987). Pharmacokinetics and pharma-codynamics of methadone in patients with chronic pain. Clin Pharm Ther. 41: 392–401.

Iwamato, K. and C. Klaassen (1977). First-pass effect of morphine in rats. J Pharmacol Exp Ther. 200:236–244.

Jiraki, K. (1992). Lethal effects of normeperidine Am J Forensic Med & Pathol, 13: 42–43.

Kaa, E., Dalgaard, J. (1989). Fatal dextropropoxyphene poisonings in Jutland, Denmark. Zeitschrift für Rechtsmedizin, 102:107–115.

King, A., Betts, T. (1978). Abuse of pentazocine. Br Med J, 2:21.

Kintz, P., P. Mangin, A. Lugnier and A. Chaumont (1989). Toxicological data after heroin overdose. Hum Toxicol. 8:487–489.

Koren, G., Butt, W., Pape, K. and H. Chiryanga (1983). Morphine induced seizures in newborn infants. Vet Hum Toxicol, 27:519–520.

Koska, A., W. Kramer, A. Romagnoli et al. (1981). Pharmacokinetics of high dose meperidine in surgical patients. Anesth Analg. 60:8–11.

Kram, T., Cooper, D., and Allen, A. (1981). Behind the identification of China White. Analyt Chem, 53(12) 1379A–1386A.

Kreek, M. (1973). Plasma and urine levels of methadone: comparison following four medication forms used in chronic maintenance treatment. N Y State J Med, 73:2773–2777.

Kreek, M. (1988). Medical complications in methadone patients. Ann N.Y. Acad Sci, 311:110–134.

Laitinen, L., J. Kanto, M. Vapaavuori and M. Viljanen (1975). Morphine concen-trations in plasma after intramuscular injection. Br J Anaesth. 47:1265–1267.

Lehmann, K., J. Freier and D. Daub (1982). Fentanyl-Pharmacokinetics and postoperative respiratory depression. Anaesthesia. 31:111–118.

Lindahl, S., Olsson, A, and D. Thomson (1981). Rectal premedication in children. Anesthesia, 36:376–379.

Little, B., L. Snell, V. Klein and L. Gilstrap.,III (1989). Cocaine abuse during pregnancy: maternal and fetal implications. Obstet Gynecol. 73(2):157–160.

Lorimer, N. and Schmid, R. (1992). The use of plasma levels to optimize methadone maintenance treatment. Drug Alcohol Depend, 30:241–246.

Lun, J., Stanley, T., Eisele, J. et al. (1979). High dose fentanyl anesthesia for coronary artery surgery: plasma fentanyl concentrations and influence of nitrous oxide on cardiovascular responses. Anest Analg, 58:390–395.

Mahler, D. and W. Forrest Jr. (1975). Relative analgesic potencies of morphine and hydromorphone in postoperative pain. Anesthesiology. 42:602–607.

Manning, T., Bidanset, S. J, Cohen B S et al. (1976). Evaluation of Abuscreen for methadone. J For Sc, 21:112–120,

Matejczyk, R. (1988). Fentanyl related overdose. J Analyt Toxicol. 12:236–238.

Mather, L. (1983). Clinical pharmacokinetics of fentanyl and its newer deriva-tives. Clin Pharmacokinet. 8:422–426.

Mather, L., G. Tucker, A. Pflug et al. (1975). Meperidine kinetics in man. Clin Pharmacol Ther. 17:21–30.

Mazoit, J., P. Sandouk, J. Scherrmann and A. Roche (1990). Extrahepatic meta-bolism of morphine occurs in humans. Clin Pharmcol Ther. 48:613–618.

McBay, A. (1976). Propoxyphene and norpropoxyphene concentrations in blood and tissues in cases of fatal overdose. Clin Chem. 22:1319–1321.

McClain, D. and C. Hug (1980). Intravenous fentanyl kinetics. Clin Pharmacol Ther. 28:106–114.

McGee, M., E. Marker, M. Jovic and M. Stajic (1992). Fentanyl related deaths in New York City. Annual Meeting American Academy of Forensic Science. New Orleans, LA, February 1992.

Miller, J. and H. Anderson (1954). The effect of N-demethylation on certain pharmacologic actions of morphine, codeine and meperidine in the mouse. J Pharmacol Exp Ther. 112:191–196.

Mitchell, J., B. Paul, P. Welch and E. Cone (1991). Forensic drug testing for opiates. II. Metabolism and excretion rate of morphine in humans after morphine administration. J Analyt Toxicol. 15:49–53.

Mo, B. and Way, E. (1966). An assessment of inhalation as a mode of administration of heroin by addicts. J Pharm and Exp Ther, 154:142–151.

Morisy, L. and D. Platt (1986). Hazards of high dose meperidine. JAMA. 255:467–468.

Mulder, G. (1992). Pharmacological effects of drug conjugates: is morphine 6-glucuronide an exception? Trends Pharm Sci, 131:302–303.

Murphy, M. and C. Hug (1981). Pharmacokinetics of intravenous morphine in patients anesthetized with enflurane-nitrous oxide. Anesthesiology 54:187–192.

Nakamura, G. and J. Choi (1983). Morphine in lymph nodes of heroin users. J Forensic Sci. 28(1):249–250.

National Institute on Drug Abuse (1990a). Annual Emergency Room Data. Data from the Drug Abuse Warning Network. Statistical Series I, Number 10-A. Rockville, Maryland, U.S. Department of Health and Human Services.

National Institute on Drug Abuse (1990b). Annual Medical Examiner Data. Data from the Drug Abuse Warning Network. Statistical Series I, Number 10-B. Rockville, Maryland, U.S. Department of Health and Human Services.

Nickander, R., J. Emmerson, M. Hynes et al. (1984). Pharmacologic and toxic effects in animals of dextropropoxyphene and its major metabolite, norpropoxyphene: a review. Hum Toxicol. 3:13S–36S.

Nordberg, G. (1984). Pharmacokinetic aspects of spinal morphine analgesia. Acta Anaesth Scand. 28 (Suppl 79):7–38.

Norheim, G. (1973). Methadone in autopsy cases. Z. Rechtsmed, 73:219–224.

Nussmeier, N., Benthuysen, J., Steffey, E. et al. (1991). Cardiovascular, respiratory, and analgesic effects of fentanyl in unanesthetized Rhesus monkeys. Anesth Analg, 72:221–226.

Oh, S., Rollins, J., and I Lewis (1975). Pentazocine -induced fibrous myopathy. JAMA, 231:271–273.

Oneil, P. and J. Pitts (1992). Illicitly imported heroin products (1984 to 1989) - some physical and chemical features indicative of their origin. J Pharm Pharmacol. 44(1):1–6.

Oguma, T. and G. Levy (1981). Acute effect of ethanol on hepatic first-pass elimination of propoxyphene in rats. J Pharm Exp Ther. 219:7–13.

Osborne, R., S. Joel, D. Trew and M. Slevin (1988). Analgesic activity of morphine-6-glucuronide. Lancet. I:828.

Osborne, R., S. Joel, D. Trew and M. Slevin (1990). Morphine and metabolite behavior after different routes of morphine administration: demonstration of the importance of the active metabolite morphine-6-glucuronide. Clin Pharmacol Ther. 47:12–19.

Pacifici, G. and A. Rane (1982). Renal glucuronidation of morphine in the human foetus. Acta Pharmacol Toxicol. 50:155–160.

Patt, R. (1988). Delayed postoperative respiratory depression associated with oxymorphone. Anesth Analg. 67:403–404.

Pittman, K. (1970). Human metabolism of orally administered pentazocine. Biochem Pharmacol, 19:1833–1836.

Pittman, K. (1973). Pentazocine in rhesus monkey. Plasma and brain after parenteral and oral administration. Life Sci, 12:131–143.

Pond, S., T. Tong, N. Benowitz et al. (1981). Presystemic metabolism of meperidine to normeperidine in normal and cirrhotic subjects. Clin Pharmacol Ther. 30: 183–188.

Reed, D., V. Spiehler and R. Cravey (1977). Two cases of heroin-related suicide. Forensic Sci. 9(1):49–52.

Richards, R., D. Reed and R. Cravey (1976). Death from intravenously administered narcotics: A study of 114 cases. J Forensic Sci. 21:467–482.

Robinson, A. and Williams, F. (1971). The distribution of methadone in man. J. Pharm Pharmac 23:353–358.

Reidenberg, M., H. Goodman, H. Erle et al. (1988). Hydromorphone levels and pain control in patients with severe chronic pain. Clin Pharm Ther. 44:376–382.

Ritschel, W., Parab, P., D. Denson et al. (1987). Absolute bioavailability of hydromorphone after peroral and rectal administration in humans: saliva/plasma ratio and clinical effects. J Clin Pharmacol, 27:647–653.

Roerig, D., K. Kotrly, E. Vucins et al. (1987). First pass uptake of fentanyl, meperidine, and morphine in the human lung. Anesthesiology. 67:466–472.

Rurak, D., M. Wright and J. Axelson (1991). Drug disposition and effects in the fetus. J Dev Physiol. 15:33–44.

Sanfilippo, G. (1948). Contributo sperimenteale all'ipotesi della smetilazione della codeina nell'organismo. I. Influenza della dose sull'assuefazione alla codeina. II. Assuefazione alla codeina ottenuta con somministrazione prolungata di morfina. Boll Soc Ital Biol Sper. 24:723–726.

Säwe, J. (1986). High dose morphine and methadone in cancer patients. Clinical pharmacokinetic considerations of oral treatment. Clin Pharmacokinet. 11:87–106.

Säwe, J., B. Dahlstrom, L. Paalzow and A. Rane (1981). Morphine kinetics in cancer patients. Clin Pharm Ther. 30:629–635.

Säwe, J., L. Kager, J. Svensson, A. Rane (1985). Oral morphine in cancer patients: in vivo kinetics and in vitro hepatic glucuronidation. Br J Clin Pharmacol. 19: 495–501.

Sawyer, W., G. Waterhouse, D. Doedens and R. Forney (1988). Heroin, morphine, and hydromorphone determination in post-mortem material by high performance liquid chromatography. J Forensic Sci. 33:1146–1155.

Schiff, B., Kern, A. (1977). Unusual cutaneous manifestations of pentazocine addiction. JAMA, 238:1542–1543.

Schleimer, R., E. Benjamini, J. Eisle and G. Henderson (1978). Pharmacokinetics of fentanyl as determined by radioimmunoassay. Clin Pharmacol Ther. 23(2): 188–194.

Schramm, W., Smith, R., Craig, P. and Kidwell, D. (1992). Drugs of abuse in saliva: a review. J Analyt Toxicol, 16:1–9.

Segal, R., Catherman, R. (1974). Methadone - a cause of death? J Forensic Sci, 19:64–71.

Sharp, M., Wallace, S., Hindmarsh, K., and Peel, H. (1983). Monitoring saliva concentrations of methaqualone, codeine, secobarbital, diphenhydramine and diazepam after single oral doses. J Analyt Toxicol. 7:11-14

Siek, T. (1978). The analysis of meperidine and normeperidine in biological specimens. J Forensic Sci, 23:6–13.

Steentoft, A., Kaa, E., Worm, K. (1989). Fatal intoxications in the age group 15–34 years in Denmark in 1984 and 1985. A forensic study with special reference to drug addicts. Zeitschrift für Rechtsmedizin, 103:93–100.

Szeto, H., Inturrsi, C., Houde, R. et al. (1977). Accumulation of normeperidine, an active metabolite of meperidine in patients with renal failure or cancer. Ann Intern Med, 86:738–741.

Soumerai, S., J. Avorn, S. Gortmaker and S. Hawley (1987). Effect of government and commercial warnings on reducing prescription misuse: the case of propoxyphene. Am J Public Health. 77:1518–1523.

Spector, S. and E.Vesell (1971). Disposition of morphine in man. Science. 174:421–422.

Spiehler, V. (1989). Computer-assisted interpretation in forensic toxicology: morphine-involved deaths. J Forensic Sci. 34(5):1104–1115.

Spiehler, V. and R. Brown (1987). Unconjugated morphine in blood by radioimmunoassay and gas chromatography/mass spectrometry. J Forensic Sci. 32:906–916.

Stahl, S., Kasser, I. (1983). Pentazocine overdose. Ann Emerg Med, 12:28-31

Stanski, D., D. Greenblatt and E. Lowenstein (1978). Kinetics of intravenous and intramuscular morphine. Clin Pharm Ther. 24:52–59.

Steentoft, A., K. Worm and H. Christensen (1988). Morphine concentrations in autopsy material from fatal cases after intake of morphine and/or heroin. J Forensic Sci Soc. 28:87–94.

Streisand, J., Varvel, J., Stanski, D. et al. (1991). Absorption and bioavailability of oral transmucosal fentanyl citrate. Anesthesiology, 75:223–229.

Stoeckle, H., J. Hengstmann and J. Schüttler (1979). Pharmacokinetics of fentanyl as a possible explanation for recurrence of respiratory depression. Br J Anesth. 51:741–745.

Szeto, H., C. Inturrisi, R. Houde et al. (1977). Accumulation of norpemeridine, an active metabolite of meperidine, in patients with renal failure or cancer. Ann Intern Med. 86:738–741.

Svensson, J., Rane, A., Säwe, J. and Sjöqvist F. (1982). Determination of morphine, morphine-3-glucuronide, and (tentatively) morphine-6-glucuronide in plasma and urine using ion-pair high-performance liquid chromatography. J Chromatogr 230:427–432.

Theilade, M. (1989). Death due to dextropropoxyphene: Copenhagen experiences Forensic Sci Int. 40:143–151.

Walton, R., Thornton, T., Whal, G. (1978). Serum methadone as an aid in managing methadone maintenance patients. Int J Addict. 13:689–694.

Whitcomb, D., Gilliam, F. 3d, Starmer, C., Grant, A. (1989). Marked QRS complex abnormalities and sodium channel blockade by propoxyphene reversed with lidocaine. J. Clin Invest 84:1629–1636.

Westerling, D., S. Lindahl, K. Andersson et al. (1982). Absorption and bioavailability of rectally administered morphine in women. Eur J Clin Pharmacol. 23: 59–64.

Wolff, K. and A. Hay (1991). Methadone in saliva. Clin Chem. 37(7):1297–1298.

Wolff, K., A. Hay, D. Raistrick et al. (1991). Measuring compliance in methadone maintenance patients: use of a pharmacologic indicator to estimate methadone plasma levels. Clin Pharmacol Ther. 50:199–207.

Wolff, K., A. Hay, D. Raistrick (1992). Plasma methadone measurements and their role in methadone detoxification programs. Clin Chem 38:420–425.

World Health Organization (1990). Fentanyl analogues. Information manual on designer drugs. World Health Organization, Geneva.

Yonemitsu, K., Pounder, D. (1992). Postmortem toxico-kinetics of co-proximol. Int J Leg Med, 104:347–353.

Young, R. (1983). Dextropropoxyphene overdosage: pharmacological considerations and clinical management. Drugs. 26:70–79.

Yue, Q., J. Svensson, F., Alm, C. et al. (1989). Codeine O-demethylation co-segregates with polymorphic debrisoquine hydroxylation. B J Clin Pharm, 28; 639–645.

Yue, Q., J. Hasselström, J. Sevensson and J. Säwe (1991). Pharmacokinetics of codeine and its metabolites in Caucasian healthy volunteers: comparisons between extensive and poor hydroxylators of debrisoquine. Br J Clin Pharm. 31: 635–642.

Yue, Q., J. Svensson, F. Sjöqvist and J. Säwe (1991). A comparison of the pharmacokinetics of codeine and its metabolites in healthy Chinese and Caucasian extensive hydroxylators of debrisoquine. Br J Clin Pharm. 31:643–647.

5.5 INTERPRETING TISSUE AND BLOOD LEVELS

5.5.1 INTRODUCTION

Whenever there is an investigation of a drug-related death or injury, two important questions arise: How much drug was present, and was it responsible for the outcome? Toxicology testing can answer the first question, but not the second. Whether or not a specific blood level caused death, morbidity, or even significant impairment, depends not only on the findings at autopsy, but also on what is observed at the scene, and on the individual's past medical and drug history (Stafford 1983) (Harding-Pink 1991). In poisoning cases information may be available from many sources, including the emergency room, and the physicians who attended the patient in the past. Valuable historical information is almost always available, and in some cases, such historical sources can provide information not obtained at autopsy. This is especially true in cases of advanced decomposition, and where the individual is HIV seropositive (Harding, Pink 1991).

There are other situations where only the first question is at issue. Workplace drug testing is done only to determine whether or not a certain drug is present; whether impairment and disability are present is irrelevant. Answering the first question can be more complex than it appears, because chemical testing does not always yield unequivocal results.

5.5.2 TESTING URINE

The procedures followed for drug testing in the workplace are somewhat different from those followed by the medical examiner. If the testing is being done under Federal rules, then screening for opiates must be done with a test that can differentiate specimens that contain more than 300 ng/mL from those that do not. Because the body metabolizes codeine to morphine, both can appear in the urine at the same time, and then it becomes a question of determining whether the origin of the drug was licit or illicit. The most widely used screening tests (TDx™ Opiates, Abuscreen™ Radioimmunoassay for Morphine, and Emit™-d.a.u.) all cross-react with other opiates besides morphine, but the Coat-A-Count™ for Morphine in Urine is highly selective for free morphine (Cone, Dickerson et al. 1992).

The accurate interpretation of urine opiate testing results usually requires quantitation of the amount of codeine and morphine present. Thus a prescription for codeine could explain the presence of some, but not massive amounts, of morphine in the urine. After oral dosing with codeine, 5%–15% will be excreted in the urine as free or conjugated morphine (Moffat, Jackson et al. 1986) (Gjerde and Morland 1991). Morphine to codeine ratios that are much higher than that strongly suggest that the origin of the morphine was not codeine. Heroin use can explain the presence of both morphine and codeine in the urine, because heroin is rapidly converted to morphine and because heroin is often contaminated with small amounts of codeine (Yong and Lik 1977). In humans, morphine is not metabolized to codeine (Mitchell, Paul et al. 1991). The best way to prove heroin use is to detect 6-acetyl morphine, but the half-life of this compound is so short that this option is rarely available. Even without being able to detect 6-acetyl morphine, heroin use will result in substantial levels of morphine that, even allowing for a 300-ng/mL cut off, will be detectable for several days.

Codeine-containing cough syrups (one syrup sold in Japan and S.E. Asia is responsible for a large percentage of positive tests at the Army's testing lab in Hawaii), and poppyseed-containing pastries, both cause positive urine tests for opiates. Poppy seeds contain both morphine and codeine, and very high levels can be seen if substantial amounts (several teaspoons) are eaten (ElSohly, ElSohly et al. 1990;

Ketchum, Stabler et al. 1990; Selavka 1991). Things become a bit confusing if the tested individual has a prescription for codeine and also claims to have eaten poppy seeds. In that case his urine might well have more morphine than codeine in it, even if he were not abusing drugs!

The general characteristics of the commercial opiate assays are such that semisynthetic opiates are unlikely to be detected. The EMIT test for morphine, for instance, cross-reacts well with codeine, but hardly at all with oxymorphone or oxycodone. The Roche Abuscreen test cross-reacts with codeine, but not with 6-acetyl morphine, hydromorphine, hydrocodone, oxymorphone, or oxydocodone (Mitchell, Paul et al. 1991). Since none of these latter compounds are metabolized to codeine or morphine, they will not be detected on routine urine screens, and, even if they were, they could not be reported out under current National Institute on Drug Abuse testing guidelines (which only permit the reporting of morphine or codeine).

5.5.3 TESTING BLOOD

Opiate abusers become tolerant of the drug's respiratory depressant effects. The fact that tolerance occurs makes interpretation of blood levels difficult. In cases of acute overdose, where death is obviously due to respiratory depression or pulmonary edema, blood levels have ranged anywhere from 100 to 2,800 ng/mL (Felby, Christensen et al. 1974) (Richards, Reed et al. 1976) (Reed, Spiehler et al. 1977) (Moffat, Jackson et al. 1986) (Logan, Oliver et al. 1987) (Sawyer, Waterhouse et al. 1988) (Steentoft, Worm et al. 1988) (Kintz, Mangin et al. 1989). All of these reported values were measured before it was appreciated that morphine--6-glucuronide was as metabolically active as morphine itself. Thus the range of reported values in these cases is very broad, and probably not very accurate. The same value may be associated with death in one individual and minimal symptoms in another. Even though fatalities have often been associated with codeine levels of over 500 ng/mL, a recent case report describes a man arrested for erratic driving who was found to have a codeine level of 8,600 ng/mL! Final determinations as to the mode and manner of death cannot be made on the basis of toxicological data alone.

5.5.4 INTERPRETING TEST RESULTS

Even in cases where the results of testing appear to be straightforward, the results must not be considered in isolation. Examination of the death scene may reveal findings that can confirm or cast doubt on the toxicology results. Helperin was one of the first to point out that there was a sameness about heroin-related deaths. More often than not the heroin user is found on the street, or in an alley, injecting himself and dying in isolation (Halpern 1972). His paraphernalia is likely to be at his side and, in some instances, the needle may still be in his arm.

More than three quarters of the victims are males, mostly in their mid-twenties (Louria 1967) (Cherubin 1967) (Froede and Stahl 1971) (Wetli, Davis et al. 1972). Under such circumstances, if the blood morphine level were found to be quite low, then an examiner would be justified in wondering if heroin overdose were really the cause of death. Conversely, if a well-dressed middle-aged woman was found dead in a doorway, with no injection apparatus, but with high levels of morphine, then the examiner would, again, be justified in wondering if opiate overdose was all that was going on.

The situation is quite different in fentanyl-related deaths where the victim is usually found at home, in his bedroom (Henderson 1991). The individual is still most likely to be a man, but the average age at death is 32.5 years, older than in heroin users who tend to be in their mid-twenties and tend not to die in their own home, or the home of a friend or relative. Heroin-related deaths are much more likely to occur on the streets. Nearly a third of fentanyl deaths occur in employed individuals, many of them professionals, while heroin-related deaths are more frequent in the unskilled and the unemployed. The probability of finding drug paraphernalia is about the same (>60%) in both fentanyl and heroin-related deaths. In both cases, if there are other individuals present at the time of death, it is likely they will make every effort to remove any evidence of illicit drug use.

Historical information is also important because deaths in opiate abusers are more likely to occur when they have been abstinent for some time. It is important to establish whether the individual has just been released from jail or a detoxification program (Harding-Pink and Fryc 1988). Another important historical finding is whether or not the individual used alcohol. This combination is notoriously lethal, but the mechanism is unexplained. In Ruttenber's large series of 505 heroin-related deaths, those who had not been drinking had higher morphine levels in their blood and bile (500 ng/mL and 7,500 ng/mL) than those individuals who had been drinking (levels of 300 ng/mL and 3,000 ng/mL). These findings suggest that opiate abusers who also use alcohol are occasional users, with lower levels of tolerance, which place them at greater risk for overdose (Ruttenber 1990).

The findings at autopsy may or may not be helpful in opiate-related deaths. If the lungs are frothy, weigh 2,000 grams, and the morphine blood level is 1,000 ng/mL, then the diagnosis is obvious. But pulmonary edema is not present in every case of heroin overdose, blood levels much lower than 1,000 ng/mL can cause respiratory depression, and there may be no cutaneous stigmata (Kintz, Mangin et al. 1989). Indeed, death from narcotism has been diagnosed in cases where the blood morphine level was zero (Richards, Reed et al. 1976). Furthermore, even if there were some known, dependable, relationship between a given morphine blood level and a specific effect, levels measured at autopsy probably do not correspond to levels measured in life. Morphine levels may even vary depending on the location in the body from which the blood sample is obtained. That certainly is the case in cocaine-related deaths (Hearn, Keran et al. 1991), and there is evidence from animal studies that significant increases in blood morphine can be detected within minutes of death and continue for days afterwards (Sawyer and Forney 1988).

The results of toxicological testing can't be considered in isolation. Other than the fact that the drug was taken, not much else can be inferred from a single blood level. The notion that the likelihood of death can be determined by consulting a reference table, if it was ever valid, certainly is no longer so. Quantitative measurement of drugs at autopsy is only of value when the results are combined with evidence obtained by thoroughly examining the death scene, reviewing the deceased's history, and examining the body. The final diagnosis depends on appropriately weighing all these factors. In 1972 Helpern wrote that "a diagnosis of an acute death from narcotic addiction is more reliably arrived at from the investigation of the circumstances under which the body is found and the findings of the complete postmortem examination than from the toxicologic analysis, which has proved revealing in less than half the cases." The passage of twenty years has produced no evidence to contradict Helpern's original impression.

References

Cherubin, C. (1967). The medical sequelae of narcotic addiction. Ann Intern Med. 67:23–33.

Cone, E., S. Dickerson, B. Paul and J. Mitchell (1992). Forensic drug testing for opiates. IV. Analytical sensitivity, specificity, and accuracy of commercial urine opiate immunoassays. J Analyt Toxicol. 16:72–78.

ElSohly, H., M. ElSohly and D. Stanford (1990). Poppy seed ingestion and opiates urinalysis: a closer look. J Analyt Toxicol. 14 (September/October):308–310.

Felby, S., H. Christensen and A. Lund (1974). Morphine concentrations in blood and organs in cases of fatal poisoning. Forensic Sci. 3:77–81.

Froede, R. and C. Stahl (1971). Fatal narcotism in military personnel. J Forensic Sci. 16(2):199–218.

Gjerde, H. and J. Morland (1991). A case of high opiate tolerance: implications for drug analyses and interpretations. Int J Leg Med. 104(4):239–240.

Helpern M. (1972). Fatalities from narcotic addiction in New York City. Incidence, circumstances, and pathologic findings. Hum Pathol. 3(1):13–21.

Harding-Pink, D. and O. Fryc (1988). Risk of death after release from prison: a duty to warn. Br Med J. 297:596.

Harding-Pink, D. and O. Fryc (1991).Assessing death by poisoning: does the medical history help? Med Sci Law, 31:69–75.

Hearn, W., E. Keran, H. Wei and G. Hime (1991). Site-dependent postmortem changes in blood cocaine concentrations. J Forensic Sci. 36(3):673–684.

Henderson, G. (1991). Fentanyl-related deaths: demographics, circumstances, and toxicology of 112 cases. J Forensic Sci. 2:422–433.

Ketchum, C., T. Stabler, K. Upton and C. Robinson (1990). Positivity rate of urine opiate tests following ingestion of poppy seeds. Clin Chem. 36(6):1026.

Kintz, P., P. Mangin, A. Lugnier and A. Chaumont (1989). Toxicological data after heroin overdose. Hum Toxicol. 8:487–489.

Logan, B., J. Oliver and H. Smith (1987). The measurement and interpretation of morphine in blood. Forensic Sci Int. 35:189–195.

Louria, D., Hensle, T., and J. Rose (1967). The major medical complications of heroin addiction. Ann Int Med. 67:1–22.

Mitchell, J., B. Paul, P. Welch and E. Cone (1991). Forensic drug testing for opiates. II. Metabolism and excretion rate of morphine in humans after morphine administration. J Analyt Toxicol. 15:49–53.

Moffat, A., J. Jackson, M. Moss and B. Widdop (1986). Clarke's isolation and identification of drugs in pharmaceuticals, body fluids, and postmortem material London, The Pharmaceutical Press.

Reed, D., V. Spiehler and R. Cravey (1977). Two cases of heroin-related suicide. Forensic Sci. 9(1):49–52.

Richards, R., D. Reed and R. Cravey (1976). Death from intravenously administered narcotics: A study of 114 cases. J Forensic Sci. 21:467–482.

Ruttenber, A., Kalter, H. and P. Santinga (1990). The role of ethanol abuse in the etiology of heroin-related death. J Forensic Sci, 35:891–900.

Sawyer, W. and R. Forney (1988). Postmortem disposition of morphine in rats. Forensic Sci Int. 38:259–273.

Sawyer, W., G. Waterhouse, D. Doedens and R. Forney (1988). Heroin, morphine, and hydromorphone determination in postmortem by high performance liquid chromatography. J Forensic Sci. 33:1146–1155.

Selavka, C. (1991). Poppy seed ingestion as a contributing factor to opiate-positive urinalysis results: the Pacific perspective. J Forensic Sci. 36(3):685–696.

Stafford, D., Prouty, R., and W. Anderson (1983). Current conundrums facing forensic pathologists and toxicologists. Am J Forensic Med Pathol, 4:103–104

Steentoft, A., K. Worm and H. Christensen (1988). Morphine concentrations in autopsy material from fatal cases after intake of morphine and/or heroin. J Forensic Sci. 28:87–94.

Wetli, C., J. Davis and B. Blackbourne (1972). Narcotic addiction in Dade County , Florida - an analysis of 100 consecutive autopsies. Arch Pathol. 93:330–343.

Yong, L. and N. Lik (1977). The human urinary excretion pattern of morphine and codeine following the consumption of morphine, opium, codeine and heroin. Bull Narc. 29:45–74.

5.6 DERMATOLOGIC SEQUELAE OF OPIATE ABUSE

There are dermatologic sequelae associated with all sorts of intravenous drug abuse, but skin lesions are more common in opiate, than in stimulant abusers. This is somewhat surprising, because stimulant abusers inject much more frequently than do opiate abusers.

Some of the difference has to do with the properties of the drugs themselves. Stimulants, for instance, do not cause histamine release and so are seldom associated with pruritus or excoriations. For the most part, the higher incidence of cutaneous complications seen in intravenous opiate abusers can be explained by the adulterants and expients injected along with the opiates.

5.6.1 FRESH PUNCTURE SITES

Recent injection sites are usually present, though in sophisticated users these marks may be hard to find. While not quite as dramatic as finding a needle still in the user's arm, the presence of dried blood on the surface of the skin surrounding a puncture is considered almost equally strong evidence that sudden death occurred following an injection (Hirsch 1972). The antecubital fossa is the most common location, but punctures may be detected at the wrist, under a watch band, or between the toes. The presence of injection tracks may be confirmed by making a skin incision immediately adjacent to the suspected site. This will reveal the presence of small subcutaneous hemorrhages that occur after venipuncture (Helpern 1972). Alternatively, a single longitudinal incision can be made on the flexor surface of the arm from midbiceps to distal forearm, and the subcutaneous tissues exposed by either blunt or sharp dissection (Hirsch 1972). Subcutaneous hemorrhage will not be evident in every case, but chemical analysis of tissue around the needle track often yields evidence of the drug injected. As the practice of "snorting" becomes more popular (it appears that fear of AIDS has sparked increased interest in this route), the situation may well arise where there are no track marks to be seen. If there is even the remotest suspicion that a narcotic was used, the nasal cavity should be examined and then swabbed with saline for toxicology testing.

5.6.2 ATROPHIC SCARRING

Novice abusers, and the occasional experienced abusers who can't find a vein, will inject subcutaneously, usually on the flexor aspect of the arm. Absorption of heroin is fairly good by this route, but the deposition of expients in the subcutaneous tissue eventually leads to the development of oval or irregularly shaped lesions that may measure 1–3 cm. These lesions are slightly depressed and often hyperpigmented. Most of these lesions are located at the site of healed abscesses, but they may be produced without proceeding abscess formation. These lesions have been recognized for more than a half century, but the dermatopathology remains poorly characterized and the etiology unclear. Early workers suggested that they were a direct result of heroin's effect on the skin (Light, Torrance et al. 1929), but adulterants or infectious agents are just as likely to be the cause. It may be the pH of the solution, rather than the drug itself, that determines whether tissue injury occurs

(Pollard 1973). Microscopic examination of healed atrophic lesions usually reveals subcutaneous fibrosis. Foreign body granulomas may or may not be present, but birefringent material, such as talc or starch crystals, is likely to be seen (Hirsch 1972).

5.6.3 ABSCESS AND ULCERATIONS

Abscesses are common and result from infection at the injection site (Orangio, Pitalick et al. 1984; Webb and Thadepalli 1979) (Minkin and Cohen 1967). Lesions are found mostly on the extensor surfaces and lateral aspects of the arms and hands, but they may also be seen almost anywhere else on the body. Injection into the subclavian area and the femoral triangle can lead to life-threatening infections (Pace, Doscher et al. 1984). Similar complications occur after injection into the intercostal vessels (Gyrtrup 1989). Active ulcers have a punched out configuration and indurated borders surrounding a floor of granulation tissue. There is nothing to distinguish the appearance of injection site abscesses from any other sort of soft tissue abscess. In the past, the organisms most commonly encountered were various species of *staphylococci* and *streptococci* (Sapira, 1968), but many different gram-negative organisms have also been cultured and polymicrobial infections are not uncommon (Webb and Thadepalli 1979). In the most recent study, which is nearly 10 years out of date, *Staphylococcus aureus* and beta-hemolytic streptococci were found to be the most common cause of soft tissue infections in parenteral drug abusers, but enteric gram negative aerobes and oral flora were also common (Orangio, Pitalick et al. 1984).

Most of the material injected is adulterant. Depending on the part of the country, an assortment of different chemicals may be used to "cut" the heroin. Commonly encountered agents include lactose, manitol, procaine, and quinine. These compounds predominate, but substances such as methaqualone, caffeine, and phenobarbitone (Oneil and Pitts 1992) (see tables 5.3.2.1 and 5.3.3.1) can also be encountered. Most of the compounds added to adulterate heroin are not very soluble in water. When these insoluble materials extravasate out into the area surrounding an injection site, foreign-body reactions occur. Even if the material doesn't extravasate, repeated injections can lead to the formation of needle "tracks" (see below).

5.6.4 "TRACK" MARKS

This lesion was first described in 1929. It was observed in a heroin addict who had contracted malaria from his intravenous injections (Biggam 1929). The author who first described them thought that the lesions resembled railroad tracks. Lesions are linear, indurated and hyperpigmented. What the tracks will look like, and how rapidly they will form, depends on what is being injected. The expients found in illicit cocaine and methamphetamine are usually water soluble, so "track" marks are an uncommon finding in this group of abusers (Wetli 1991). Paregoric, on the other hand, causes an intense sclerotic reaction, and when paregoric injecting was popular in the 1960's, addicts ran out of peripheral veins so quickly they resorted to injecting themselves in the neck and groin (Lerner and Oerther 1966). Heroin, even in its adulterated form, is less sclerotoxic than paregoric, but prolonged use will eventually cause thickening and sclerosis of the subcutaneous veins.

The skin overlying the affected veins becomes hyperpigmented, probably as a result of the underlying chronic inflammatory process (Vollum 1970). The degree of hyperpigmentation depends largely on the individual's coloration, and not necessarily on how long the addict has been injecting himself. Discoloration of the area can also be the result of inadvertent tattooing. Addicts may try to sterilize their needles with a match flame. This causes small amounts of soot to be deposited on the outside of the needle, and this soot is carried into the skin at the time of injection. Addicts have traditionally tried to conceal these marks by tattooing, or even by burning themselves in the hopes of scarring the whole area.

The histologic appearance of sclerotic veins varies (Schoster and Lewis 1968). There may be only fibrous thickening of the vein wall, consistent with a low-grade, chronic inflammatory process. In other instances thrombophlebitis, sterile or septic, may occur. The results are hard to predict, and Helpern even commented that on occasion the veins repeatedly used by addicts "show less evidence of closure by thrombosis than the veins of patients subjected to repeated punctures by physicians for medical purposes" (Helpern 1972).

5.6.5 TATTOOS

Tattoos are sometimes used to conceal the scars and track marks associated with intravenous drug abuse, though that hardly explains the frequency of this finding in addict subpopulations. The practice derives its name from the Tahitian word "tatau" which means "the results of tapping", describing the fashion in which tattoos were applied. The practice dates back to antiquity. Tattoos have been found on Egyptian mummies from the Eleventh Dynasty, making the practice at least 4,000 years old (Sperry 1991). Tattoos are applied in jail using the "melted--toothbrush" technique. Any pointed object, such as a bedspring or matchbook staple, can be used as a needle. The end of a plastic toothbrush is then melted in a flame and the smoky residue collected. The residue is mixed with soap and water to form an ink (Martinez and Wetli, 1989).

Chronic abusers sometimes apply tattoos in order to obscure old track marks, but most of the time tattoos are applied for other reasons, usually while the individual is in jail. In the past, much significance was attributed to the design and location of tattoos. Symbols on the thumb webbing were popularly said to indicate criminal specialties. The results of more recent studies suggest that hand-web tattoos probably have significance only in the prison where they are applied (Martinez and Wetli 1989). In some specific subpopulations, such as the Marielitos, tattoos may represent religious symbols or themes, but these interpretations are not generalizable to other subgroups.

5.6.6 "PUFFY" HANDS

Lymphedema is sometimes seen in chronic users. The condition was first described in the 1960's. Both hands become smooth and slightly edematous with obliteration of the normal anatomic landmarks. Pitting edema is absent. In contrast to the changes seen in the hands of myxedematous patients, the skin in addicts with "puffy" hands is thin and smooth. The skin on the volar aspect of the forearm will be normal, even though evidence of repeated injections can be seen in both antecubital fossa (Abeles 1965) (Ritland and Butterfield 1973).

5.6.7 NECROTIZING FASCITIS

This lethal infection was first described over 120 years ago. As commonly used, the term refers to a severe infection of the superficial fascia and subcutaneous tissue. At least initially, the infection does not involve the overlying skin (Wojno and Spitz 1989). There have been no controlled studies, but it has been suggested that this disorder may be more prevalent in cocaine users (Webb and Thadepalli 1979) (Wetli 1987). In the absence of drug abuse, necrotizing fascitis is usually seen in diabetics, or patients with severe atherosclerosis, but the infectious process can be initiated by surgery, or even minor trauma. Individuals taking non-steroidal anti-inflammatory drugs are said to be at increased risk (Rimailho 1987).

Once infection becomes established, necrosis rapidly spreads through the of the fascia and subcutaneous tissues. The overlying skin looks normal until very late in the course of the disease, and the underlying muscle is usually not involved either (Tehrani and Ledingham 1977). Hematogenous seeding may occur, involving organs through the body. Even purulent myocarditis has been reported as a complication. The fact that the overlying skin looks normal may delay the diagnosis and lead to a fatal outcome (Wojno and Spitz 1989). At first it was thought that gram positive aerobes were the causative agent, but in more recently reported cases the etiology was polymicrobial. In the two heroin users described by Webb the causative organisms were *Enterobacter* and *Proteus*.

5.6.8 Histamine related urticaria

Skin excoriations are common, but it is not clear if the skin excoriations are the result of narcotic-induced pruritus or psychologic disorder (Young and Rosenberg 1971). Histamine release in narcotic abusers is not a true, IgE mediated, allergic response (Hermens, Ebertz et al. 1985) (Paton 1957). Opiates act, in some undetermined fashion, directly on mast cells to produce histamine release. The amount of histamine released depends on the dose of opiate administered. In some instances the amount of histamine liberated can be large enough to cause hypotension in addition to erythema and tachycardia. Not all narcotics are associated with histamine release. Substantial elevations in plasma histamine can be seen after dosing with intravenous morphine and meperidine, but not after treatment with fentanyl or sulfentanil (Flacke, Flacke et al. 1987).

5.6.9 Fungal lesions

Candida infections of the mouth, esophagus, upper airway, and lungs are recognized as "indicator" diseases for AIDS. The prevalence of oral thrush in AIDS patients is 40 to 90%. The prevalence of eso-phageal involvement is much lower, only 4 to 14% (Redfield, Wright et al. 1986) (Tavitian, Raufman et al. 1986). As a rule, in AIDS patients *C. albicans* infections are limited to the mucosa. Disseminated disease does not occur in AIDS patients unless they are also heroin addicts or have some other similar risk factor (steroid therapy, indwelling catheters, severe granulocytopenia) (Drouhet and Dupont 1991).

Candida related febrile septicemia with cutaneous involvement is a disorder that is confined to heroin addicts. Beginning 2 to 24 hours after the last heroin injection, there is onset of chills, fever, headache and profuse diaphoresis. Within 1 to 3 days, patients develop dissemi-nated folliculitis and scalp nodules. Any hair-bearing area may be invol-ved, but the scalp is the most common site (Dupont and Drouhet 1985). Painful cutaneous nodules, usually measuring less than 1 cm, erupt quite suddenly. As many as 100 of these nodules may be present, and it is said that the scalps of these individuals feel like "a sack of marbles." Smaller pustules may be seen adjacent to the nodules. The pustules look like they are the result of a staphylococcal or streptococcal infection, but microscopic examination will disclose yeast and filaments of *C. albicans*. Biopsy of the follicular nodules can be diagnostic for the syndrome: bi-furcated filaments of *C. albicans* will be seen admixed with an intense, mixed inflammatory infiltrate (Drouhet and Dupont 1991). C. albicans is the only species of candida that causes the syndrome (Dupont and Drouhet 1985).

5.6.10 MISCELLANEOUS CUTANEOUS ABNORMALITIES

Other skin disorders are occasionally seen, but none with sufficient frequency to be of any diagnostic value. Sapira described a rosette of cigarette burns around the neck. After injecting himself with opiate, the abuser may fall asleep with a cigarette in his mouth, burning his anterior chest when his head falls forward (Sapira 1968). Other sorts of lesions reflect usage patterns that were unique to a specific time and place and are as much historical curiosities as anything else. In the late 1800's, when opium smoking was still popular, the presence of cauliflower ears (swelling of the auricles), was considered almost pathognomonic for opium use. They were the result of lying for long periods on opium beds with hard wooden pillows (Owens and Humphries 1988).

References

Abeles, H. (1965). The puffy-hand sign of drug addiction. N Engl J Med. 273:1167.

Biggam, A. (1929). Malignant malaria associated with administration of heroin intravenously. Trans Royal Soc Trop Med and Hyg. 23 (2):147–153.

Drouhet, E. and B. Dupont (1991). Candidosis in heroin addicts and AIDS - new immunologic data on chronic mucocutaneous candidosis. Candida and Candidamycosis. 50:61–72.

Dupont, B. and E. Drouhet (1985). Cutaneous, ocular, and osteoarticular candidasis in heroin addicts:new clinical and therapeutic aspects in 38 patients. J Infect Dis. 152:577–591.

Flacke, J., W. Flacke, B. Bloor et al. (1987). Histamine release by four narcotics: a double blind study in humans. Anesth Analg. 66:723–730.

Frank, R. (1987). Drugs of abuse: data collection systems of DEA and recent trends. J Analyt Toxicol. 11:237–241.

Gyrtrup, H. (1989). Fixing into intercostal vessels: a new method among drug addicts. Br J Addict. 84:945–946.

Helpern, M. (1972). Fatalities from narcotic addiction in New York City. Incidence, Circumstances, and Pathologic findings. Hum Pathol. 3(1):13–20.

Hermens, J., J. Ebertz, J. Hanifin and C. Hirshman (1985). Comparison of histamine release in human skin mast cells induced by morphine, fentanyl, and oxymorphone. Anesthesiology. 62:124–129.

Hirsch, C. (1972). Dermatopathology of narcotic addiction. Hum Pathol. 3(1):37–53.

Lerner, A. and F. Oerther (1966). Characteristics and sequelae of paregoric abuse. Ann Intern Med. 65:1019–1030.

Light, A. and E. Torrance. (1929). Opium addiction - physical characteristics and physical fitness of addicts during administration of morphine. Arch Intern Med. 43:326–334.

Martinez, R. and W. CV. (1989). Tattoos of the Marielitos. Am J Forensic Med & Pathol. 10(4):315–325.

Minkin, W. and H. Cohen (1967). Dermatologic complications of heroin addiction. Report of a new complication. N Engl J Med. 277:473–475.

Oneil, P. and J. Pitts (1992). Illicitly imported heroin products (1984 to 1989) - some physical and chemical features indicative of their origin. J Pharm Pharmacol. 44(1):1-6.

Orangio, G., S. Pitlick, P. Latta et al. (1984). Soft tissue infections in parenteral drug abusers. Ann Surg. 199:97-100.

Owens, D. and M. Humphries (1988). Cauliflower ears, opium, and Errol Flynn. Br Med J. 297:643-644.

Pace, B., W. Doscher and I. Margolis (1984). The femoral triangle - a potential death trap for the drug abuser. N.Y. State J Med. 84:596-598.

Paton, W. (1957). Histamine release by compounds of simple chemical structure. Pharmacol Rev. 9:269-328.

Pollard, R. (1973). Surgical implications of some types of drug dependence. Br Med J. 1:784-787.

Rimailho, A. (1987). Fulminant necrotizing fascitis and nonsteroidal anti-inflammatory drugs J Infect Dis. 155:143-146.

Redfield, R., D. Wright and E. Tramont (1986). Walter Reed staging classification for HTLV-III/LAV infection. N Engl J Med. 314:131-132.

Ritland, D. and W. Butterfield (1973). Extremity complications of drug abuse. Am J Surg. 126:639-648.

Sapira, J. (1968). The narcotic addict as a medical patient. Am J Med. 45:555-588.

Shuster, M. and M. Lewis (1968). Needle tracks in narcotic addicts. N Y State J Med. 68:3129-3134.

Sperry, K. and McFeely, P. (1987). Medicolegal aspects of necrotizing fascitis of the neck. J Forensic Sci. 32:273-281.

Sperry, K. (1991). Tattoos and Tattooing. Am J Forensic Med and Pathol. 12 (4):313-319.

Tavitian, A., J. Raufman and L. Rosenthal (1986). Oral candidiasis as a marker for esophageal candidiasis in the acquired immunodeficiency syndrome. Ann Intern Med. 104:54-55.

Tehrani, M. and I. Ledingham (1977). Necrotizing fascitis. Postgrad Med J. 53:237-242.

Vollum, D. (1970). Skin lesions in drug addicts. Br Med J. 2:647-650.

Webb, D. and H. Thadepalli (1979). Skin and soft tissue polymicrobial infections from intravenous abuse of drugs. West J Med. 130:200-204.

Wetli, C. (1987). Fatal reactions to cocaine. Cocaine: a clinician's handbook. Washington, AM,Gold, MS, eds. New York, London, Guilford Press.

Wojno, K. and W. Spitz (1989). Necrotizing fascitis: a fatal outcome following minor trauma. Am J Forensic Med and Pathol. 10(3):239-241.

Young, A. and F. Rosenberg (1971). Cutaneous stigmas of heroin addiction. Arch Derm. 104:80-86.

5.7 CARDIOVASCULAR DISORDERS

5.7.1 INTRODUCTION

The frequency of heart disease in opiate abusers is not really known. Except for endocarditis, and the various complications associated with HIV infection, it is not even clear that heart disease is any more frequent among opiate abusers then it is in controls (Kringsholm and Christoffersen 1987). In Siegel and Helpern's classic paper on the "Diagnosis of death from intravenous narcotism", heart disease isn't even mentioned (Siegel, Helpern et al. 1966), nor were any significant cardiac abnormalities noted in Wetli's study of 100 consecutively autopsied narcotic abusers (Wetli, Davis et al. 1972). When Louria analyzed the discharge diagnosis of addicts admitted to Bellevue's general medicine service, the incidence of endocarditis was under 10% and no other cardiac disorders were noted (Louria 1967). At the other extreme is the comprehensive study by Dressler and Roberts. They analyzed 168 drug-related deaths and found that the incidence of cardiac abnormalities approached 100% (Dressler and Roberts 1989b)!

TABLE 5.7.1
TYPES OF CARDIAC LESIONS FOUND IN OPIATE ABUSERS COMING TO AUTOPSY

Disorder	Percentage
Cardiomegaly	68
Endocarditis (active or healed)	48
Coronary artery disease	21
Congenital	11
Acquired valvular disease	10
Myocardial disease	8

These figures are based on the report by Dressler and Roberts, published before HIV infection was widespread.

Interpreting the older studies, and even some of the newer ones, is difficult. The phrase "narcotic addict" has never been used consistently. Often it has been applied to any sort of intravenous drug abuse, even though the effects of sympathomimetics are manifestly different from those of opiates. In early studies, chemical confirmation of the diagnosis was lacking. The diagnosis of opiate abuse was based solely on clinical findings. Even after toxicologic screening first became available, the limits of detection were far higher than they are today. Another confounding factor is that almost all of the studies, both old and new, were uncontrolled. The very high frequency of cardiac lesions reported by Dressler and Roberts can't be generalized. Their study was uncontrolled, and many of the 168 cases they examined had been referred to the National Heart, Lung and Blood Institute, presumably because the original prosecutors suspected that cardiopulmonary abnormalities were present. Only one controlled study has compared the cardiopulmonary pathology in opiate-related deaths with the findings in a group of age-matched controls. Many changes could be identified in the opiate users' lungs, but the hearts of the addicts differed in no significant way from those of the controls (Kringsholm and Christoffersen 1987).

The observed frequency of a particular cardiac lesion depends on the pattern of drug abuse within the population being studied. When Rajs reviewed the cardiac pathology in a group of 25 intravenous drug users he found contraction band necrosis, fibrosis and inflammatory infiltrates (Rajs and Falconer 1979), but amphetamine abuse was common in the population he studied, and the changes that he observed are consistent with that fact. In some areas, especially Europe, the injection of pills meant for oral use is still a fairly common practice. In those localities, granulomatous lung disease and pulmonary hypertension are common. The spectrum of cardiac lesions seen at autopsy is likely to reflect that fact. An increasing number of drug-related deaths are due to violence, and not to any direct opiate-mediated effect or medical complication of opiate abuse. The frequency of incidental cardiac lesions in addicts dying of trauma has never been tabulated.

The lesions most likely to be seen in opiate abusers' hearts are listed in decreasing frequency in Table 5.7.1. No data has been compiled since HIV infection became widespread, and there is no doubt that a very significant percentage of HIV-positive opiate abusers will have lesions and opportunistic infections as a consequence of their disease. Similarly, in areas where mixed opiate-stimulant abuse is prevalent, changes associated with catechol toxicity, such as contraction band necrosis and myocardial fibrosis, are likely to be superimposed on any of the changes secondary to opiate abuse (Rajs and Falconer 1979).

5.7.2 PATHOLOGY ASSOCIATED WITH HIV INFECTION

In some areas of the United States more than one half of all intravenous drug abusers carry the HIV virus. The true percentage of intravenous heroin abusers who die from AIDS, rather than some complication of their drug abuse, is not known. Whatever the number, it is not inconsiderable. Given that fact, and the fact that endocarditis is the only cardiac disorder unequivocally associated with intravenous opiate abuse, it is highly probable that any myocardial lesion encountered in the heart of an intravenous heroin user is due to HIV infection, or an opportunistic infection related to HIV infection.

Pericardial effusion is the cardiac lesion most commonly seen in AIDS patients. One third of patients dying of AIDS have effusions, with or without pericarditis (Lewis 1989), and the probability is that the effusion will not have been symptomatic during life. The second most common AIDS related abnormality is right ventricular hypertrophy. Right ventricular hypertrophy is not particularly surprising in drug abusers who are likely to have both angiothrombotic lung disease from their drug abuse, and AIDS related fibrotic interstitial lung disease, at the same time. In Lewis's autopsy series of AIDS patients, mononuclear infiltrates were present in the myocardium of 10% of the patients, but none had evidence of healed or active myocarditis. Clinical experience suggests that the incidence of opportunistic infection, especially disseminated cryptococcosis and CMV infections is also high, and usually unsuspected during life. Kaposi's sarcoma involving the myocardium, and even the epicardial coronary arteries, has been observed in a small percentage of cases.

TABLE 5.7.2
**CARDIAC FINDINGS IN AIDS PATIENTS AT AUTOPSY,
IN ORDER OF FREQUENCY**
1. Pericardial effusion
2. Right ventricular hypertrophy
3. Infiltrates
4. Opportunistic infection
5. Kaposi's sarcoma
6. Nonbacterial thrombotic endocarditis

5.7.3 ENDOCARDITIS

After HIV infection, endocarditis is the only other cardiac disorder with a clearly higher incidence among intravenous drug abusers than in the population at large. There has been surprisingly little research with any bearing on what, exactly, makes the intravenous drug user more susceptible to valvular infection. Autopsy evidence suggests that most (>80%) vegetations occur on previously normal valves (Dressler and Roberts 1989a). However, recently published echocardiographic studies, comparing the valves of intravenous heroin users having no clinical evidence of endocarditis with the valves of healthy controls, have demonstrated tiny areas of thickening on both the mitral and tricuspid valves (Pons-Lladó, Carreras et al. 1992). This finding is consistent with the notion that some sort of endothelial trauma must occur to allow the deposition of the microscopic thrombi that appear to constitute the first stage of infection.

It has always been emphasized that addicts are prone to right-sided infection. While there is no question that the tricuspid and pulmonic valves are involved more often in addicts than in the general population, it is also true that in some series addicts actually have left-sided involvement more often than right (Dressler and Roberts 1989a) (Hubbell, Cheitlin et al. 1981). The origin of the infectious agent has also been a matter of some dispute. Addicts do not use sterile technique. Needles may be contaminated and the injected material unsterile. The injection site, especially if it is in the groin, may be colonized with pathogenic organisms. Thus there are a number of possible sources for infection. With the exception of Candida infection (Drouhet and Dupont 1991), studies have failed to link the heroin itself, or the paraphernalia used, with the infectious organism (Tuazon, Hill et al. 1974). More often than not, the infectious organism is derived from either the addict's normal surface flora (Tuazon, 1974), or from a preexisting infection such as cellulitis or suppurative thrombophlebitis.

Platelet deposition, for whatever cause, damages valvular epithelium, exposing the matrix of subendothelial connective tissue below, and allowing the further deposition of fibrin and platelet thrombi. The resulting vegetations are friable, white or tan, and most likely to be found along the line of valve closure. Bacterial vegetations tend to arise on the atrial aspect of the atrioventricular valves and on the ventricular surfaces of the aortic and pulmonary valves. With time they may proliferate and involve the opposite side of the valve, or spread to the chordae tendinae or onto the parietal pericardium. The lesions ulcerate, and the ulcerations seen in acute endocarditis tend to be larger and deeper than those associated with subacute disease (Silber 1987).

The size of vegetations is variable. Their size, color and appearance depend on the sort of infectious agent. Fungal lesions tend to be larger and bulkier than bacterial vegetations and are more likely to cause valvular insufficiency and embolization. *Streptococcal* vegetations grow more slowly than *Staphylococcal* vegetations, but they may get to be much larger. Much smaller sterile vegetations may be seen in up to 2% of patients coming to autopsy. Such small, sterile lesions are classified as nonbacterial thrombotic endocarditis (marantic endocarditis or NBTE), and there is a particularly strong association with carcinoma and general cathexia (Angrist and Oka 1963). On microscopic examination, NBTE lesions are seen to be composed of amorphous material that is free of bacteria. On rare occasions one of the larger sterile vegetations can dislodge, enter the circulation and cause infarction. Marantic endocarditis is seen in AIDS patients and so is to be anticipated in intravenous drug abusers.

Depending on how much fibrin has been deposited, the color of the vegetations can range from white to tan or gray. On microscopic examination there is no confusing the lesions of marantic endocarditis with those of infectious endocarditis. Masses of fibrin, platelets and polymorphonuclear leukocytes can be seen surrounding colonies of bacteria located directly on the valve's surface. Necrotic areas of valve are surrounded with a mixed cellular infiltrate that often includes giant cells. In older lesions capillary proliferation occurs, along with the formation of granulation tissue (Saphir 1960). Fibrous tissue eventually proliferates over the vegetations, the necrotic material becomes organized, and eventually endothelialized. Healed lesions are often calcified.

The pattern of valvular involvement is different in drug abusers than in the population at large, and so are the symptoms. In Dressler and Robert's series of 80 autopsied addicts with infectious endocarditis, the tricuspid valve was involved nearly half the time. Within the general population, tricuspid valve involvement is seen less than 5% of the time in subacute cases, and less than 15% of the time in acute endocarditis (Lerner and Weinstein 1966) (Johnson, Rosenthal et al. 1975) (El-Khatib, Wilson et al. 1976) (Reisberg 1979) (Pelletier and Petersdorf 1977) (Pankey 1962). Table 5.7.3.1 compares the frequency of involvement in addicts with the frequency seen in the general population. There is some evidence that the likelihood of infection depends upon the pressure to which the valve is subjected (Lepeschkin 1952), so the high incidence of low-pressure valve disease in addicts is puzzling and unexplained. Equally difficult to explain is the fact that a significant incidence of right-sided involvement has been reported in some non-drug using populations (Grover, Anand et al. 1991).

TABLE 5.7.3.1

FREQUENCY OF VALVE INVOLVEMENT IN ADDICTS VS. GENERAL POPULATION

SITE	Addicts	General (Recent)
Left-sided	41%	85%
Aortic	23%	15 – 25%
Mitral	19%	30 – 45%
Right–sided	30%	5 – 20%
Tricuspid	29%	1 – 15%
Pulmonic	1%	<1%
Right & Left	16%	5 – 10%

Data for addict population derived from Dressler and Roberts. Data for general population derived from published clinical studies

There is no satisfactory explanation for why the spectrum of organisms attacking the right heart should be so different, and so much more virulent, than the group of agents that infect the mitral and aortic valves. *Staphylococcus aureus* is the predominant organism infecting right-sided valves, while the causative organism on the left is a *Streptococcus Viridians sps* 60–80% of the time (Weinberger, Rotenberg et al. 1990). The predominant organisms in addicts and the general population are compared in Table 5.7.3.2.

Infection with multiple organisms is uncommon on the left, but polymicrobial involvement of the tricuspid valve is becoming more prevalent, especially among intravenous drug abusers. Until recently, polymicrobial infection was a distinctly rare entity. In one retrospective study of nearly 1,000 patients seen from 1951 to 1966 there was only one case (Weinstein and Rubin 1973). In more recent reports the incidence has been closer to 8% (Levine, Crane et al. 1986). As many as 7 different organisms may be involved at one time, and since many of these organisms are quite fastidious, all may not be diagnosed by routine laboratory methods (Adler, Blumberg et al. 1991).

Right-sided involvement produces symptoms that are more pulmonary than cardiac. Dislodged vegetations frequently embolize to the lung, producing multiple segmental infiltrates, especially in the lower lobes (Chan, Ogilby et al. 1989). Tricuspid vegetations can, on occasion, grow quite large and may even interfere with valve function. Papillary rupture, on the other hand, produces relatively few symptoms on the right because of the low intracavitary pressure (Conway 1969). Aneurysm of the sinus of Valsalva may result when infection dissects into the valve ring. This process is most often seen in cases of *staphylococcal* infection. *Staphylococcal* infections may also extend outward from the ring, and in addition to ring abscess, infection may also involve the interventricular septum (Conde, Meller et al. 1975) (Rawls, Shuford et al. 1968). Lethal arrhythmia can result. Extension of the infection outward may result in purulent pericarditis or even cardiac rupture.

TABLE 5.7.3.2
**PATHOGENS REPORTED IN ADDICTS WITH INFECTIOUS ENDOCARDITIS,
COMPARED WITH PATHOGENS OBSERVED IN NON-ADDICTED POPULATION**

Pathogen	% Addicts	% Non-addicts
Streptococci	15%	65%
Viridians (α-hemolytic)	<5%	35%
Group D	<5%	25%
Staphylococcus aureus	50 – 80%	25%
Pseudomonas aeruginosa	10 – 40%	<5%
Polymicrobial	10 – 20%	<1%

Purulent pericarditis is seen in nearly 20% of cases, and need not be the result a large abscess rupturing (Silber 1987). Smaller abscesses may be scattered throughout the myocardium, and even though abscess formation is more common in cases of acute endocarditis, it may be seen in subacute cases as well. Abscesses may be subendocardial or subpericardial, but are most likely to be found in the left ventricle (Arnett and Roberts 1976). A spectrum of other myocardial alterations, short of frank abscess formation, can also be seen. In acute cases there may be cloudy swelling of the myocytes, hemorrhage, or even tiny areas of infarction. Small infarcts occur in subacute cases where small emboli obstruct distal branches of the coronary arteries (Saphir, Katz et al. 1950).

The peripheral sequelae of valve infection have changed little since Osler described them in the Gulstonian Lectures in 1885 (Osler 1885). The peripheral complications associated with endocarditis in addicts differ in no significant way from the same complications when they occur in the general population. Many of the extracardiac manifestations are the result of arterial embolization of the friable vegetations. Mycotic aneurysm is the result of septic emboli, most of which occur at the bifurcation of medium-size arteries (Katz, Goldberg et al. 1974). This process is especially common in the brain, but can also occur elsewhere. In the kidneys, septic emboli can cause infarction, especially when *Staphylococcus* is the etiology. Glomerulonephritis seen in more than half the patients, and is the result of immune complex deposition (Bell 1932) (Gutman, Striker et al. 1972). In addition to the classic focal embolic changes seen in the kidneys of patients with endocarditis, diffuse proliferative glomerulonephritis may also be seen. In these latter cases there is strong evidence for an immune-related etiology. It may well be that other peripheral lesions, such as Roth sports and even Osler's nodes have an immune etiology (Bayer and Theofilopoulos 1990).

At autopsy, if there is any suspicion that the patient was suffering from infectious endocarditis, then aseptic technique should be used to ensure the collection of uncontaminated material. The major vessels should be clamped before removing the heart from the body. Then an area on the surface of the heart adjacent to the affected valve (e.g., entrance through the posterior right atrial wall would give access to the tricuspid valve) should be seared and the center of the area incised with a sterile scalpel, allowing direct access to the valve which can be sampled and cultured. If such an approach is not followed, the samples obtained may well be contaminated, though even then cultures are probably worth the effort. Hearts should not be placed in formalin prior to sectioning, because then it becomes impossible to rule out the presence of infected vegetations. Smears should be made of the vegetations. In addition to routine gram stains, slides should also be stained for fungi (Gomori stain) and acid-fast organisms. Even if no organisms are apparent on the stains, some material should still be cultured, since in partially treated cases the organism may lose the ability to take stain (Atkinson & Virmani, 1991)

5.7.4 MISCELLANEOUS DISORDERS

Intravenous heroin abusers have abnormal, atherogenic lipid profiles (Maccari, Bassi et al. 1991). Whether the incidence of coronary artery disease in heroin addicts is any different from that in age-matched controls is not known. Dressler and Roberts found significant coronary artery disease (>75% narrowing) in 8% of their referral cases (Dressler and Roberts 1989b), but this observation has not been confirmed. In fact, no mention of coronary artery disease is made in any published autopsy series (Helpern and Rho 1966) (Siegel, Helpern et al. 1966) (Louria 1967) (Froede and Stahl 1971) (Wetli, Davis et al. 1972).

Myocardial fibrosis is also a frequent finding in drug abusers' hearts, and certain patterns of fibrosis play a role in the generation of malignant rhythm disorders and sudden cardiac death (Strain, Grose et al. 1983) (Karch and Billingham 1986) (Lecomte, Fornes et al. 1992). Microfocal fibrosis is most typically seen in stimulant abusers (Rajs and Falconer 1979) (Tazelaar, Karch et al. 1987), where it is the result of healing contraction band necrosis. Myocardial fibrosis in opiate abusers, especially if it is perivascular, is more likely to represent a healed bout of endocarditis. Healed myocarditis as a cause of fibrosis cannot be ruled out, but there is no evidence to suggest that this disease is any more frequent in addicts than it is in the rest of the population. Larger zones of fibrosis are likely to represent healed areas of ischemia infarction. This process may also be related to healed endocarditis, as emboli may cause infarction in some of the smaller coronary artery branches (Silber 1987).

References

Adler, A., E. Blumberg, D. Schwartz et al. (1991). Seven-pathogen tricuspid endocarditis in an intravenous drug abuser. Chest. 99:490–491.

Angrist, A. and M. Oka (1963). Pathogenesis of bacterial endocarditis. JAMA. 183: 249–252.

Arnett, E. and W. Roberts (1976). Prosthetic valve endocarditis. Clinicopathologic analysis of 22 necropsy patients with comparison of observations in 74 necropsy patients with active infective endocarditis involving natural left-sided cardiac valves. Am J Cardiol. 38:281–292.

Atkinson, J. and Virmani, R. (1991) Infective endocarditis:changing trends and general approach for examination. in Virmani, R, Atkinson, J, and Fenoglio, J (eds). Cardiovascular Pathology, W.B. Saunders Company, Philadelphia.

Bayer, A. and A. Theofilopoulos (1990). Immunopathogenetic aspects of infective endocarditis. Chest. 97:204–212.

Bell, E. (1932). Glomerular lesions associated with endocarditis. Am J Pathol. 8: 639–663.

Chan, P., J. Ogilby and B. Segal (1989). Tricuspid valve endocarditis. Am Heart J. 117(5):1140–1145.

Conde, C., J. Meller, E. Donoso et.al. (1975). Bacterial endocarditis with ruptured sinus of Valsava and aorticocardiac fistula. Am J Cardiol. 35:912–917.

Conway, N. (1969). Endocarditis in heroin addicts. Br Heart J. 31:543–545.

Dressler, F. and W. Roberts (1989a). Infective endocarditis in opiate addicts: analysis of 80 cases studied at necropsy. Am J Cardiol. 63:1240–1257.

Dressler, F. and W. Roberts (1989b). Modes of death and types of cardiac diseases in opiate addicts: analysis of 168 necropsy cases. Am J Cardiol. 64:909–920.

Drouhet, E. and B. Dupont (1991). Candidosis in heroin addicts and AIDS - new immunologic data on chronic mucocutaneous candidosis. Candida and Candidamycosis. 50:61–72.

El-Khatib, R., F. Wilson and A. Lerner (1976). Characteristics of bacterial endocarditis in heroin addicts in Detroit. Am J Med Sci. 271:197–201.

Froede, R. and C. Stahl (1971). Fatal narcotism in military personnel. J Forensic Sci. 16(2):199–218.

Grover, A., I. Anand, J. Varma et al. (1991). Profile of right-sided endocarditis: an Indian experience. Int J Cardiol. 33:83–88.

Gutman, R., G. Striker, B. Gilliland and R. Cutler (1972). The immune complex glomerulonephritis of bacterial endocarditis. Medicine. 51:1–25.

Helpern, M. and Y. Rho (1966). Deaths from narcotism in New York City. N.Y. State Med J. 66:2391–2408.

Hubbell, G.,M. Cheitlin and E. Rappaport (1981). Presentation, management, and follow-up evaluation of infective endocarditis in drug addicts. Am Heart J. 102: 85–94.

Johnson, D., A. Rosenthal and A. Nadas (1975). A forty- year review of bacterial endocarditis in infancy and childhood. Circulation. 51:581–588.

Karch, S. and Billingham M. (1986). Myocardial contraction bands revisited. Hum Pathol. 17:9–13.

Katz, R., H. Goldberg and M. Selzer (1974). Mycotic aneurysm. Arch Intern Med. 134: 939–942.

Kringsholm, B. and P. Christoffersen (1987). Lung and heart pathology in fatal drug addiction. A consecutive autopsy study. Forensic Sci Int. 34:39–51.

Lecomte, D., P. Fornes and G. Nicolas (1992). Isolated myocardial fibrosis as a cause of sudden cardiac death and its possible relation to myocarditis. Presented at Annual Meeting of the American Academy of Forensic Sciences. New Orleans, La. February 20, 1992.

Lepeschkin, E. (1952). On the relation between the site of valvular involvement in endocarditis and the blood pressure resting on the valve. Am J Med Sci. 224: 318–319.

Lerner, P. and L. Weinstein (1966). Infective endocarditis in the antibiotic era (pts 1 through 4). N Engl J Med. 274:199–206.

Levine, D., L. Crane and M. Zervos (1986). Bacteremia in narcotic addicts at the Detroit Medical Center: II. infectious endocarditis: a prospective comparative study. Rev Infect Dis. 8:374–396.

Lewis, W. (1989). AIDS: cardiac findings from 115 autopsies. Prog Cardiovasc Dis. 32: 207–215.

Louria, D., T. Hensle, and J. Rose (1967). The major medical complications of heroin addiction. Ann Int Med. 67:1–22.

Maccari, S., C. Bassi, P. Zanoni and A. C. Plancher (1991). Plasma cholesterol and triglycerides in heroin addicts. Drug Alcohol Depend. 29(2):183–187.

Osler, W. (1885). Gulstonian lectures on malignant endocarditis. Lancet. 1:415–418, 459–464, 505–508.

Pankey, G. (1962). Acute bacterial endocarditis at the University of Minnesota Hospitals, 1939-1959. Am Heart J. 64:583–591.

Pelletier, L. and R. Petersdorf (1977). Infective endocarditis: a review of 125 cases from the University of Washington Hospitals. Medicine. 56:287–313.

Pons-Lladó, G., F. Carreras, X. Borras, J. et al.. (1992). Findings on doppler echocardiography in asymptomatic intravenous heroin users. Am J Cardiol. 69(3): 238–241.

Rajs, J. and B. Falconer (1979). Cardiac lesions in intravenous drug addicts. Forensic Sci Int. 13:193–209.

Rawls, W., W. Shuford, W. Logan et al. (1968). Right ventricular outflow tract obstruction produced by a myocardial abscess in a patient with tuberculosis. Am J Cardiol. 21:738–745.

Reisberg, B. (1979). Infective endocarditis in the narcotic addict. Prog Cardiovasc Dis. 22:193–204.

Saphir, O. (1960). Endocarditis. Pathology of the heart. Springfield, Ill, Charles C. Thomas.

Saphir, O., L. Katz and I. Gore (1950). The myocardium in subacute bacterial endocarditis. Circulation. 1:1155–1167.

Siegel, H., M. Helpern and T. Ehrenreich (1966). The diagnosis of death from intravenous narcotism, with emphasis on the pathologic aspects. J Forensic Sci 11(1):1–16.

Silber, E. (1987). Infective endocarditis, in Heart Disease. 2nd edition New York, Macmillan, 1192–1219.

Strain, J., R. Grose, S. Factor and J. Fisher (1983). Results of endomyocardial biopsy in patients with spontaneous ventricular tachycardia but without apparent structural heart disease. Circulation. 68(6):1171–1181.

Tazelaar, H., S. Karch , M. Billingham and B. Stephens (1987). Cocaine and the heart. Hum Pathol. 18 :195–199.

Tuazon, C., R. Hill and J. Sheagren (1974). Microbologic study of street heroin and injection paraphernalia. J Infect Dis. 129(3):327–329.

Weinberger, I., Z. Rotenberg, D. Zacharovitch et al. (1990). Native valve infective endocarditis in the 1970s versus the 1980s: underlying cardiac lesions and infecting organisms. Clin Cardiol. 13:94–98.

Weinstein, L. and R. Rubin (1973). Infective endocarditis - 1973. Prog Cardiovasc Dis. 16:239–274.

Wetli, C., J. Davis and B. Blackbourne (1972). Narcotic addiction, Dade County, Florida - an analysis of 100 consecutive autopsies. Arch Pathol. 93:330–343.

5.8 PULMONARY DISORDERS

5.8.1 NONINFECTIOUS COMPLICATIONS

5.8.1.1 Respiratory failure and pulmonary edema

Narcotic-related pulmonary edema was first described in the 1850's. A Dr. Lee, from New York City, described both cerebral edema and pulmonary congestion in a man dying from a laudanum overdose (Woodman and Tidy 1877). There is a general presumption that pulmonary edema in heroin abusers is in some way related to the respiratory depression, and respiratory failure, but the pathophysiology of this condition is far from clear. All opiates exert direct effects on brain stem respiratory centers, resulting in decreased responsiveness of the respiratory centers to increased levels of PCO_2. When enough drug is given, the respiratory drive disappears.

There is no way an addict can know the potency of the drug he is using. If the sample should be less adulterated than usual (Purity on the street is variable, but at anything less than 3% purity, withdrawal symptoms are likely) fatal respiratory depression may supervene. Addicts who have been abstinent for some time are particularly at risk, since they will have lost their tolerance. This situation is not uncommon in addicts who have been incarcerated and then returned to the streets (Harding-Pink and Fry 1988). Autopsy findings in typical cases reveal pulmonary congestion of varying degrees, but there need not always be florid pulmonary edema. Some addicts die with needles still in their arms (Siegel, Helpern et al. 1966). Such deaths are thought to be due to acute respiratory depression, even though the maximal effects of intravenous narcotics on the brain stem aren't seen for several minutes (Sanford, Gilman, Gilman 1990).

The edema fluid in these cases is rich in protein, and agonal respiratory efforts will cause the fluid to froth up, much like beaten egg whites. In extreme cases, congealed froth is seen in the mouth and nares. In one series, the average weight of the right and left lungs was 830 grams and 790 grams respectively (Levine and Grimes 1973). Siegel reported an average total weight of 1,400 grams for both lungs. The changes are lobular in distribution, with areas of congestion and edema alternating with other areas of air trapping and acute emphysematous change. The posterior lower lobes are most severely affected, especially if gastric aspiration has also occurred. Depending on the severity of the process, histologic examination may reveal a spectrum of changes. In less severe cases, the only abnormality found will be widening of the interstitial spaces, especially around the bronchi and extraalveolar vessels (Pietra 1991). In more extreme cases, the alveolar spaces are flooded with protein-rich fluid (Gottlieb and Boylen 1974).

If there is enough time for hypoxic heart failure to occur, blood vessels in the nose and pharynx rupture, giving a pink tinge to the edema fluid. After 24 hours, hyaline membranes will be visible in the alveoli. They are composed of necrotic alveolar cell debris, mixed with the protein-rich edema fluid deposited on the alveolar walls. This phase is followed by a recovery phase. During this final phase, the cut surface of the lung will be firm and brownish, suggesting the diagnosis of pneumonia. Type II alveolar cells and fibroblasts proliferate and the fibrinous exudate in the alveoli is replaced by granulation tissue.

The results of repeated long-term opiate use are readily apparent when the lungs of intravenous narcotic abusers are compared to age and sex matched controls (Rajs, Härm et al. 1984). Alveolar septa are thickened, fibrotic and hypercelullar. Hemosiderin-laden macrophages can often be seen in the alveolar walls and even in the lamina of the alveoli and respiratory passages. If any one morphologic finding in the lung is typical of narcotic drug abuse, it is the presence of iron-containing macrophages in the lung.

Why some individuals should develop florid pulmonary edema and others not is unexplained. It has been argued that heroin has direct toxic effects on pulmonary capillaries, or even the heart, leading to hypoxic-induced heart failure (Menon 1965) (Silver 1959). A role for altered capillary permeability is suggested by the fact that the protein content of the edema fluid is nearly twice that of serum (Katz, Aberman et al. 1972). Other theories that have been proposed include acute allergic reactions to heroin, the presence of contaminants in the heroin, histamine release, or some centrally mediated effect (Silber 1959). Current thinking favors a mechanism similar to that in high-altitude sickness: respiratory depression leads to hypoxia which in turn causes increased capillary permeability and fluid extravasation into the alveoli (Duberstein and Kaufman 1971).

5.8.1.2 Emphysema

Emphysematous changes are occasionally seen in the subset of intravenous abusers who inject medications meant for oral use. The process may involve both the upper (Goldstein, Karpel et al. 1986) (Paré, Fraser et al. 1980; Paré et al. 1989), and lower lobes (Smeenk, Serlie et al. 1990). In extreme cases involvement may be panacinar (Groth, Mackay et al. 1972). Usually the upper lobes show the most damage. Intravenous drug abusers with emphysema are in their late 30's, which distinguishes them from those whose emphysema is due to smoking or alpha-1-antitrypsin deficiency, who tend to be much older.

Emphysematous changes are more common in stimulant abusers than in individuals taking opiates (Schmidt, Glenny et al. 1991) (Guenter, Coalson et al. 1981). There is an experimental model where symptomatic bullae result from the coalescence of smaller bullae (Strawbridge 1960) (Guenter, Coalson et al. 1981). The smaller bullae could be a manifestation of septic emboli damaging the capillary beds, or possibly even a result of granuloma formation (Thomasahow, Summer et al. 1977), but proof is lacking. A more recent explanation for emphysematous changes is Pneumocystisis infection. The healing process in such infections may lead to pneumatoceles that are discovered only at a later date.

5.8.1.3 Needle and mercury emboli

Attempts at central vein injection may sometimes result in needle fragments embolizing to the lung. These events are usually not fatal, but the x-ray appearance can be quite frightening (Shapiro 1941) (Lewis and Henry 1984) (Angeolos, Sheets et al. 1986). In the late 1980's several reports were published that described the picture seen when mercury was injected intravenously (Murch 1989). According to street

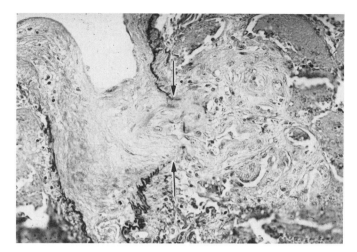

Figure 5.8.1.4 Thromboembolic arteriopathy
Repeated injection of particulate material can lead to pulmonary hypertension. Organizing and recanalizing thrombi in drug abusers can look very much like the plexiform lesions of primary pulmonary hypertension. The plexiform lesions of primary pulmonary hypertension, such as the above, are typically seen only at the branch points of stenotic small arteries. Lesions are composed of a complex network of small blood vessels and proliferating myofibroblasts. Courtesy of Giuseppe Pietra, Director, Division of Anatomic Pathology, Hospital of the University of Pennsylvania.

lore, such injection increased athletic ability and sexual prowess. There have been no recent reports and no autopsy studies. Chest x-rays of these individuals show striking metallic opacities outlining the pulmonary vascular bed and the apex of the right ventricle!

5.8.1.4 Foreign Body Granulomas

Foreign particle embolization is frequent in intravenous drug abusers, but clinical symptoms related to the practice are uncommon, and granuloma formation is an inconsistent finding at autopsy (Helpern and Rho 1966) (Sapira 1968) (Gottlieb and Boylen 1974) (Glassroth, Adams et al. 1987). Granulomas form when intravenous abusers repeatedly inject themselves with aqueous suspensions of pharmaceutical preparations designed to be taken orally. Heroin has been available since the turn of the century, and morphine for nearly 200 years, but pulmonary granulomatosis in drug users was first described only in 1950 (Spain 1950). The time lapse suggests that the injection of oral medications is a relatively recent innovation.

In some cases, cotton fibers are the culprit. Some addicts load their syringes by drawing up the liquid through a cotton ball; small fibers of cotton are drawn up at the same time. Most granulomas are due to magnesium trisilicate (talc), because talc is widely used in the pharmaceutical industry as a filler. The amount of active ingredient in most pills is often quite small, so talc is added so to create a pill of manageable size. When injected, talc particles become trapped in the pulmonary arterioles and capillaries, producing acute focal inflammation and thrombosis. The reported incidence of talc-containing granulomas ranges from 15% (Hopkins 1972) to as high as 90% in some series. The tissue reaction to cotton is about the same as the response to talc. The sort of lesions seen is determined by the general pattern of abuse within the population being studied. If the injection of crushed pills is common, then so will be the incidence of foreign-body granulomas (Tomashefski and Hirsch 1980) (Kringsholm and Christofferson 1987). Fungal spores can also cause granulomatous disease. The soil sapro-phyte *Scopulariopsis brumptii* was found to be the cause of hypersensitivi-ty pneumonitis in at least one addict (Grieble, Rippon et al. 1975), and analysis of confiscated heroin samples has shown the presence of many different fungal varieties.

TABLE 5.8.1.4.1
CHARACTERISTICS OF BIREFRINGENT MATERIALS FOUND IN THE LUNGS OF INTRAVENOUS DRUG USERS

Substance	Shape	Size	PAS staining
Talc	needle shaped	5 – 15 μm	negative
Potato starch	Maltese cross, eccentric center	20 – 200 μm	positive
Maize starch	Maltese cross, concentric	10 – 30 μm	positive
Microcrystalline cellulose	elongated rod	25 – 200 μm	positive
Cotton fibers	irregular	variable	negative

Talc and cellulose are frequently seen in conjunction with granulomatous reactions, but other agents are not. *Adapted from Kringsholm and Christoffersen, 1987.*

Whether the offending agent is talc, cotton, corn starch, or cellulose, the clinical course and pathologic findings are much the same. Trapped particles cause microthrombosis, and granulomas form. Some of the trapped material may migrate into the perivascular space where the process is repeated, and more granulomas form. If the process is ongoing, a reduction in the size of the pulmonary bed occurs, and pul-monary hypertension can result. Associated anatomic changes include medial hypertrophy, and eccentric/concentric intimal fibrosis. The tissue diagnosis can be confusing, because organizing and recanalizing thrombi seen in intravenous drug users can appear very much like the plexiform lesions of primary pulmonary hypertension. The two conditions can be distinguished by the fact that plexiform lesions are typically seen only at the branching points of stenosed small arteries (Pietra, Edwards et al. 1989).

Microcrystalline cellulose, a depolymerized form of cellulose, is also used as a filler and binder in the manufacture of oral medications. Cellulose crystals measure anywhere from 20 to 90 μm and are a good deal larger than talc or cornstarch crystals. The larger size of these crystals explains granuloma formation in the larger elastic pulmonary arteries, and even the right ventricle. Corn starch granulomas are particularly associated with the injection of oral pentazocine and secobarbitol preparations (Johnson, 1971) (Newell, Reginato et al. 1988). They can be identified by their distinctive Maltese-cross pattern visible with the polarizing microscope, and by the fact that they stain as carbohydrates (Tomashefski and Hirsch 1980). The presence of birefringent material in the interstitium is consistent with a long standing process, while material confined to the media of vessels is consistent with more recent use.

5.8.1.5 Injuries of the great vessels

Adulterants and expients mixed with illicit heroin can provoke an inflammatory reaction. As a result, peripheral veins become sclerotic, and abusers must use central veins for access. The two most popular sites are the vessels of the groin (Pace, Doscher et al. 1984) and neck (Lewis, Groux et al. 1980) (the "groin hit" and the "pocket shot"). The neck vessels are especially hard for the abuser to inject himself, and for a fee, other addicts will do the injecting. The results are predictable. Pneumothorax is a frequent occurrence, as is hemothorax from laceration to one of the great vessels (Lewis, Groux et al. 1980) (Douglas and Levison 1986). Pyohemothorax (Zorc, O'Donnell et al. 1988) and pseudoaneurysm (Navarro, Dickinson et al. 1984) (Johnson, Lucas et al. 1984) (McCarroll and Roszler 1991) are also seen. In Europe, the use of intercostal vessels seems to be a popular alternative to neck injections. Reported complications include both pneumothorax and infection (Gyrtrup 1989).

5.8.2 INFECTIOUS COMPLICATIONS

5.8.2.1 Aspiration pneumonia

The combination of depressed cough reflex and decreased level of consciousness, in conjunction with a general tendency to retain secretions, favors aspiration (Cherubin 1967). If the aspirated stomach contents are of very low pH, then acute chemical pneumonitis will result. If there is much particulate matter present, then acute airway obstruction is possible. Pneumonitis in such cases is usually a result of infection with gram-negative and anaerobic organisms. Aspiration pneumonia in narcotics abusers is in no way different from aspiration pneumonia in alcoholics or in people debilitated with chronic disease.

5.8.2.2 Community acquired pneumonia

Even before the HIV epidemic, intravenous drug abusers were at increased risk for pneumonia, and for infections in general (Cherubin 1971) (Harris and Garret 1972) (Hussey and Katz 1950) (Moustoukas, Nichols et al. 1983) (Scheidegger and Zimmerli 1989). If opiate users had normal immune function, which they do not (Novick, Ochshorn et al. 1989), the injection of unsterilized material through contaminated syringes would still cause a transient septicemia. The number of HIV-infected individuals in some areas is already over 50% (Quinn, Zacarias et al. 1989), and HIV-positive intravenous drug users are much more prone to develop community acquired pneumonia and tuberculosis than are their HIV-negative counterparts (Selwyn, Feingold et al. 1988). When HIV-positive individuals get community acquired pneumonia, their clinical course is said to be more severe (Hind 1990).

Among HIV-infected patients, even those without AIDS, the increased rate of infection can be quite striking. In one study the annual attack rate for *Streptococcus pneumoniae* was only 0.7–2.6/1,000 in the general population, compared to 21/1,000 in asymptomatic HIV infected intravenous abusers (Selwyn, Feingold et al. 1988). There is nothing to distinguish community acquired pneumonia among intravenous heroin abusers from their non-infected counterparts, but there is evidence that infections may be more severe and the mortality higher (Chaisson 1989). Opportunistic lung infections in HIV + intravenous drug abusers are similar in frequency and type to those seen in other HIV+ subgroups (Neidt and Schinella 1985) (Ambros, Lee et al. 1987).

5.8.2.3 Fungal pneumonia

Pulmonary fungal infections occur even in HIV-negative intravenous drug users (Rosenbaum, Barber et al. 1974) (Mellinger, DeBeauchamp et al. 1983) (Collignon and Sorrel 1983) (Orangio, 1984). Street heroin is often contaminated with a fungal species, and percipitins to *Aspergillus, Micropolyspora faeni, and Thermoactinomyces vulgaris* are frequently found in intravenous abusers (Smith, Wells et al. 1975). The preponderance of evidence suggests that most of the fungi found in illicit drug samples are there largely because of airborne contamination introduced when the users prepare their fix. The presence of specific fungi cannot be used to identify the origin of a sample, though some types of heroin seem to contain more contaminants than others (Domínguez-Vilches, Durán-González et al. 1991). Analysis of several outbreaks of fungal pneumonia among addicts suggests that the cause of infection was contaminated paraphernalia, including preserved lemon juice which is used to prepare the heroin injection (Clemons, Shankland et al. 1991). Some types of heroin (Mexican Brown) are poorly soluble in water and can only be dissolved after they have been acidified. The two most popular agents for acidifying are lemon juice and vinegar. Candida species are present as contaminants of the lemon rind. Infected patients most often present with lobar pneumonia. In a high percentage of cases peripheral nodules, with or without cavitation, may be seen. Lung abscess and empyema may also develop (Mellinger, DeBeauchamp et al. 1983). Hilar and mediastinal adenopathy can be a prominent finding that resolves over the course of weeks or months. Pleural effusions are seen in about 20% of cases, and pleural thickening may result (Lazzarin, Uberti-Foppa et al. 1985).

Disseminated candida infections have a rapid onset a few hours after injecting. The infection may be manifest as a self-limiting lobar pneumonia or as a generalized infection, with endocarditis, chorioretinitis, and hepatitis, with and without soft tissue abscesses. Occasionally the septicemia is manifested only as an isolated endopthalmitis (Shankland, Richardson et al. 1986). Repeat showers of emboli cause mycotic aneurysms of the pulmonary arteries, but these are usually asymptomatic and are only incidentally found at autopsy. Histologic diagnosis can sometimes be made by examination of scalp biopsy specimens which will show infiltration of the hair follicles with chronic inflammatory cells and Candida albicans.

5.8.2.4 Tuberculosis and meliodosis

There is an increased incidence of tuberculosis in both HIV positive and negative opiate abusers. Even without HIV infection, chronic heroin abuse is associated with a depressed immune response (Helpern and Rho 1966) (Brown 1974) (Reichman, Felton et al. 1979) (Novick, Ochshorn et al. 1989) (Hendrickse, 1989). The clinical course and pathologic findings are the same as in any other patients with tuberculosis. Pulmonary melioidosis (due to Pseudomonas pseudomallei), which can resemble tuberculosis on x-ray, also occurs in narcotics addicts (Cooper 1967). The diagnosis can be made by sputum culture.

5.8.2.5 Septic pulmonary emboli

This is a not infrequent finding in intravenous abusers. Recurrent emboli of infected material may be due to infected bone or soft tissue at the injection site, septic thrombophlebitis, or even endocarditis. The most probable source is vegetations on the tricuspid valve (Wendt, Puro et al. 1964) and in fact, recurrent septic pulmonary emboli must raise the possibility of tricuspid vegetations.

5.8.2.6 Anterior mediastinitis

Mediastinitis secondary to soft-tissue infection in the chest wall has recently been described in HIV-positive heroin users. In one case, the initial infection was sternoclavicular, and in another infection was sternochondrial. In both cases the infectious agent was *S. aureus*, and in both cases the infection of the anterior mediastinum caused sepsis and vascular compromise (Dreyfuss, Djedaini, et. al. 1992). Soft-tissue infections of the chest wall are relatively common among intravenous drug abusers, but spread to the mediastinum is not. Invasion of the mediastinum in these cases likely was a consequence of HIV infection.

References

Ambros, R., E. Lee, L. Sharer et al. (1987). The acquired immunodeficiency syndrome in intravenous drug abusers and patients with a sexual risk: clinical and postmortem comparisons. Hum Pathol. 18:1109–1114.

Angelos, M., C. Sheets and P. Zych. (1986). Needle emboli to lung following intravenous drug abuse. J Emerg Med. 4:391–396.

Brown, S., Stimmel, B.,Taub, R. et al. (1974). Immunologic dysfunction in heroin addicts. Arch Intern Med.134:1001–1006.

Chaisson, R. (1989). Bacterial pneumonia in patients with human immunodeficiency virus infection. Semin Respir Infect. 4:133–138.

Cherubin, C. (1967). The medical sequelae of narcotic addiction. Ann Intern Med. 67: 23–33.

Cherubin, C. (1971). Infectious disease problems of narcotic addicts. Arch Intern Med. 128:309–313.

Clemons, K., G. Shankland, M. Richardson and D. Stevens. (1991). Epidemiologic study by DNA typing of a *Candida albicans* outbreak in heroin addicts. J Clin Microbiology. 29(1):205–207.

Collignon, P. and T. Sorrel (1983). Disseminated candidiasis: evidence of a distinctive syndrome in heroin abusers. Br Med J. 287:861–862.

Cooper, E. (1967). Melioidosis. JAMA. 200:337–339.

Domínguez Vilches, E., R. Durán-González, F. Infante and A. Luna-Maldonado. (1991). Myocontamination of illicit samples of heroin and cocaine as an indicator of adulteration. J Forensic Sci. 36(3):844–856.

Douglass, R. and M. Levison (1986). Pneumothorax in drug users. An urban epidemic? Amer Surg. 52:377–380.

Duberstein, J. and D. Kaufman (1971). A clinical study of an epidemic of heroin intoxication and heroin-induced pulmonary edema. Am J Med. 51:704–714.

Glassroth, J., G. Adams and S. Schnoll (1987). The impact of substance abuse on the respiratory system. Chest. 91:596–602.

Goldstein, D., J. Karpel, D. Appel et al. (1986). Bullous pulmonary damage in users of intravenous drugs. Chest. 89:266–269.

Gottlieb, L. and T. Boylen (1974). Pulmonary complications of drug abuse. West J Med. 120:8–16.

Grieble, H., J. Rippon, N. Maliwan and V. Daun (1975). Scopulariopsosis and hypersensitivity pneumonitis in an addict. Ann Intern Med. 83:326–329.

Groth, D., G. Mackay, J. Crable and T. Cochran (1972). Intravenous injection of talc in a narcotics addict. Arch Pathol. 94:171–178.

Guenter, C., J. Coalson and J. Jacques (1981). Emphysema associated with intravascular leukocytesequestration. Comparison with papain-induced emphysema. Am Rev Respir Dis. 123:79–84.

Gyrtrup, H. (1989). Fixing into intercostal vessels: a new method among drug addicts. Br J Addict. 84:945–946.

Harding-Pink, D. and O. Fryc (1988). Risk of death after release from prison: a duty to warn. Br. Med J. 297(6648):596.

Harris, P. and R. Garret (1972). Susceptibility of addicts to infection and neoplasia. N Engl J Med. 287:310.

Helpern, M. and Y. Rho (1966). Deaths from narcotics in New York City. N.Y. State Med J. 66:2391–2408.

Hendrickse, R., Maxwell, S., Young, R. (1989). Aflatoxins and heroin. Br Med J. 299: 492–493.

Hind, C. (1990). Pulmonary complications of intravenous drug misuse .1. epidemiology and non-infective complications. Thorax 45(11):891–898.

Hopkins, G. (1972). Pulmonary angiothrombotic granulomatosis in drug offenders. JAMA. 221:909–911.

Hussey, H. and S. Katz (1950). Infections resulting from narcotic addiction. Am J Med. 9:186–193.

Johnson, J., C. Lucas, A. Ledgerwood and L. Jacobs (1984). Infected venous pseudoaneurysm: a complication of drug addiction. Arch Surg. 119: 1097–1098.

Katz, S., A. Aberman, U. Frand et al. (1972). Heroin pulmonary edema. Evidence for increased pulmonary capillary permeability. Am Rev Resp Dis. 106:472–474.

Kringsholm, B. and P. Christoffersen (1987). The nature and the occurrence of birefringent material in different organs in fatal drug addiction. Forensic Sci Int. 34:53–62.

Lazzarin, A., C. Uberti-Foppa, M. Gaslli et al. (1985). Pulmonary candidiasis in a heroin addict: some remarks on its aetiology and pathogenesis. Br J Addict 80:103–104.

Levine, S. and E. Grimes (1973). Pulmonary edema and heroin overdose in Vietnam. Arch Pathol. 95(5):330–332.

Lewis, J., N. Groux, J. Elliott et al. (1980). Complications of attempted central venous injections performed by drug abusers. Chest 74:613–617.

Lewis, T. and D. Henry (1985). Needle embolus: a unique complication of intravenous drug abuse. Ann Emerg Med. 14:906–908.

McCarroll, K. and M. Roszler (1991). Lung disorders due to drug abuse. J Thorac Imaging. 6(1):30–35.

Mellinger, M., O. DeBeauchamp, G. Gallien et al. (1982). Epidemiological and clinical approach to the study of candidiasis caused by *Candida albicans* in heroin addicts in the Paris region: analysis of 35 observations. Bull Narc. 34:61–68.

Menon, N. (1965). High-altitude pulmonary edema: a clinical study. N Engl Med J 273: 66–73.

Moustoukas, N., R. Nichols, J. Smith et al. (1983). Contaminated street heroin - relationship to clinical infections. Arch Surg. 118:746–749.

Murch, C. (1989). Quicksilver heart. Br Med J. 299:1056.

Navarro, C., P. Dickinson, P. Kondlapoodi and J. Hagstrom (1984). Mycotic aneurysms of the pulmonary arteries in intravenous drug addicts. Am J Med. 76: 1124–1131.

Neidt, G. and R. Schinella (1985). Acquired immunodeficiency syndrome: clinicopathologic study of 56 autopsies. Arch Pathol Lab Med. 109:727–734.

Newell, G., A. Reginato, D. Auerbach et al. (1988). Pulmonary granulomatosis secondary to pentazocine abuse mimicking connective tissue diseases. Am J Med. 85:890–892.

Novick, D., M. Ochshorn, V. Ghali et al. (1989). Natural killer cell activity and lymphocyte subsets in parenteral heroin abusers and long-term methadone maintenance patients. J Pharm and Exp Ther. 250(2): 606–610.

Orangio, G., Pitlick S., Latta, P. et al. (1984) Soft tissue infections in parenteral drug abusers. Ann Surg 199:97–100.

Pace, B., W. Doscher and I. Margolis (1984). The femoral triangle - a potential death trap for the drug abuser. N.Y. State J Med. 84:596–598.

Paré, J., R. Fraser, J. Hogg et al. (1979). Pulmonary mainline granulomatosis: talcosis of intravenous methadone abuse. Medicine 58:229–239.

Paré, J., and R. Fraser (1989). Long-term follow-up of drug abusers with intravenous talcosis. Am Rev Respir Dis. 139:233–241.

Pietra, G. (1991). Pathologic mechanisms of drug-induced lung disorders. J Thorac Imaging. 6(1):1–7.

Pietra, G., W. Edwards, J. Kay et al. (1989). Histopathology of primary pulmonary hypertension. A qualitative and quantitative study of pulmonary blood vessels from 58 patients in the National Heart, Lung, and Blood Institute Primary Pulmonary Hypertension Registry. Circulation. 80:1198–1206.

Quinn, T., F. Zacarias, P. St. John and R. St. John (1989). HIV and HTLV-1 infections in the Americas: a regional perspective. Medicine. 68:189–209.

Rajs, J., T. Härm and K. Ormstad (1984). Postmortem findings of pulmonary lesions of older datum in intravenous drug addicts. Virchows Arch. 402:405–414.

Reichman, L., C. Felton and J. Edsall (1979). Drug dependence, a possible new risk factor for tuberculosis disease. Arch Intern Med. 139:337–339.

Rosenbaum, R., J. Barber and D. Stevens (1974). *Candida albicans* pneumonia: diagnosis by pulmonary aspiration, recovery without treatment. Am Rev Respir Dis. 109:373–378.

Sanford, L. and Gilman, A.G. (1990). Goodman and Gilman's the pharmacologic basis of therapeutics. Eighth edition. New York. Pergamon Press.

Sapira, J. (1968). The narcotic addict as a medical patient. Am J Med. 45:555–588.

Scheidegger, C. and W. Zimmerli (1989). Infectious complications in drug addicts: seven-year review of 269 hospitalized narcotics abusers in Switzerland. Rev of Inf Dis. 11(3):486–493.

Schmidt, R., R. Glenny, J. Godwin et al. (1991). Panlobular emphysema in young intravenous Ritalin™ abusers. Am Rev Respir Dis. 143:649–656.

Selwyn, P., A. Feingold, D. Hartel et al. (1988). Increased risk of bacterial pneumonia in HIV-infected intravenous drug users without AIDS. AIDS. 1:267–272.

Shankland, G., M. Richardson and G. Dutton (1986). Source of infection in Candida endopthalmitis in drug addicts. Br Med J. 292:1106–1107.

Shapiro, S. (1941). Passage of a hollow needle into the venous blood stream to the heart, through the cardiac wall, and into the thorax. Am Heart J. 22:835–838.

Siegel, H., M. Helpern and T. Ehrenreich (1966). The diagnosis of death from intravenous narcotism, with emphasis on the pathologic aspects. J Forensic Sci 11(1):1–16.

Silber, R., Clerkin, E. (1959). Pulmonary edema in acute heroin poisoning: report of four cases. Am J Med 27, 187–192.

Smeenk, F., J. Serlie, E. Vanderjagt and P. Postmus (1990). Bullous degeneration of the left lower lobe in a heroin addict. Eur Resp J. 3(10):1224–1226.

Smith, W., I. Wells, F. Glauser and H. Novey (1975). High incidence of precipitins in sera of heroin addicts. JAMA. 232:1337–1338.

Spain, D. (1950). Patterns of pulmonary fibrosis as related to pulmonary function. Ann Intern Med. 33:1150–1163.

Strawbridge, H. (1960). Chronic pulmonary emphysema (an experimental study). III. Experimental pulmonary emphysema. Am J Pathol. 37:391–407.

Thomashow, D., W. Summer, J. Soin et al. (1977). Lung disease in reformed drug addicts: diagnostic and physiologic correlations. Johns Hopkins Med J. 141: 1–8.

Tomashefski, J. and C. Hirsch (1980). The pulmonary vascular lesions of intravenous drug abuse. Human Pathol. 11:133–145.

Wendt, V., H. Puro, J. Shapiro et al. (1964). Angiothrombotic pulmonary hypertension in addicts. JAMA. 188:755–757.

Woodman, W. and Tidy, C. (1877). Forensic medicine and toxicology. Lindsay & Blakiston, Philadelphia, pg 337–342.

Zorc, T., A. O'Donnell, R. Holt et al. (1988). Bilateral pyopneumothorax secondary to intravenous drug misuse. Chest, 93:645–647.

5.9 GASTROINTESTINAL DISORDERS

5.9.1 INTRODUCTION

Although there is some evidence to suggest that heroin may be directly hepatotoxic (de Araujo, Gerard, Chossergros, et al. 1990), most of the changes seen in the livers of opiate abusers are secondary in nature. These changes can be divided into several groups, depending on the underlying mechanism. The most commonly encountered pattern is that of hepatic and generalized visceral congestion. Portal fibrosis is also fairly common, its presence signifying previous viral infection. Foreign body granulomas are uncommon, but when they occur they are due to the intravenous injection of pills meant for oral use. None of these alterations are unique to opiate abusers, although the presence of enlarged nodes in the porta hepatitis is almost diagnostic for chronic narcotism.

5.9.2 BOWEL DISEASE

Narcotics decrease gut motility, resulting in severe constipation or obstipation. At autopsy, much of the colon may be distended with hard feces. The other bowel disease associated with narcotics is the "body packer" syndrome. This disorder was first noted in a cocaine courier by Suarez in 1977 (Suarez, Arango et al. 1977). Since that time, this mode of smuggling has been widely adapted (Pinsky, Ducas et al. 1978) (Sinner 1981) (Wetli and Mittleman 1981) (Gheradi, Baud et al. 1988) (Roberts, Price et al. 1986). Smugglers, known as "mules", ingest anywhere from 20–100 rubberized packets that contain multiple gram quantities of drug. At first the packets were made from condoms or balloons, or the fingers of surgical gloves. Now more care is devoted to the packaging, not only because the packets occasionally rupture and kill the courier, but also because the earlier packets were to easy to see on x-ray. Detection can be avoided by minimizing the contrast difference between the packets and the surrounding feces. To this end, more sophisticated smugglers may drink mineral oil to further reduce the contrast between the packets and the bowel contents. Even if they are hard to see with plain films, packets can be easily demonstrated using CT scanning (Vanarthros, Aizpuru et al. 1990). Urine testing is often positive, even if none of the packets rupture, because the rubber wrapping acts as a semipermeable membrane through which small amounts of the packet's contents gradually diffuse and enter the blood stream (Gheradi, Baud et al. 1988).

5.9.3 LIVER DISORDERS

When death is due to acute narcotic overdose, the liver is, more often than not, enlarged and congested. In typical cases the liver may weigh over 2,000 grams. Cut sections will be hyperemic. The other abdominal organs are also likely to be congested. Since these changes often occur in conjunction with pulmonary edema, it seems likely that the congestion is due to acute cardiac decompensation, though the issue has never been investigated satisfactorily, and it is far from proven that heroin-induced pulmonary edema is a consequence of heart failure.

5.9.3.1 Porta hepatis adenopathy

Enlargement of lymph nodes that are located in direct proximity of the liver is common, and nearly diagnostic for chronic intravenous heroin abuse. The exact incidence of these changes has never been tabulated, but some have placed it at over 75% (Edland 1972). The porta hepatis, subpyloric and peripancreatic lymph nodes, along with the cystic node at the neck of the gallbladder, and other nodes located along the common duct, may all be involved. Not infrequently the gastroduodenal and pancreatoduodenal nodes will also be enlarged. These nodes are gray, firm, sharply demarcated, and the degree of enlargement may be striking. Nodes measuring as much as 2 cm across are not uncommon. Microscopic examination of these nodes shows only a nonspecific pattern of reticuloendothelial hyperplasia. A puzzling aspect of this abnormality is why, even though systematic autopsies have been done on opiate abusers for nearly 150 years, this common abnormality was not recognized until Siegel and Helpern published their paper in 1966 (Siegel, Helpern et al. 1966), and their findings were reconfirmed by Wetli in 1972 (Wetli, Davis et al. 1972).

There are at least three possible explanations for this type of adenopathy, but they all are unproven. Node enlargement could be a reaction to the injection of particulate material. In one series, birefringent material was found in 39% of nodes from confirmed addicts (Kringsholm and Christoffersen 1987). Another possible explanation is recurrent infection. Changes consistent with nonspecific reactive hepatitis are found more than half the time in known drug users (Paties, Pezeri et al. 1987). Finally, there is the possibility that morphine, itself, exerts some direct effect on the nodes to cause enlargement. Morphine is easily detectable in nodes draining the portal areas, and in most cases the concentration of morphine is greater in the nodes than it is in the blood. Lymph node morphine concentrations measuring anywhere from 300 ng/mL to over 8,000 ng/mL have been recorded (Nakamura and Choi 1983). Whether lymph node enlargement is the result of some direct opiate effect has been a matter of conjecture for more than 50 years. The first paper suggesting the direct hepatotoxicity of heroin was published in 1935 (Baltaceano and Visilu 1935).

5.9.3.2 Non-specific alterations

Inflammation of the portal tracts is nearly a constant finding in long-term intravenous drug abusers. In one series the incidence was over 92% (Paties, Pezeri et al. 1987). The pattern of inflammation seen in addicts is commonly referred to as "triadiatis". There is a predominantly lymphocytic infiltrate, with fairly frequent plasma cells. On occasion, neutrophils may also be seen, but these infiltrates are usually devoid of eosinophils (Kaplan 1963) (Siegel, Helpern et al. 1966) (Edland 1972). Periportal fibrosis can be identified more than half the time in chronic intravenous heroin users (Paties, Pezeri et al. 1987).

Lobular inflammation is almost as common as "triaditis" (85%), but necrosis is less common (46%) and tends to be widely scattered. The changes in addicts are easily distinguishable from those seen in alcoholics, since there are no centrolobular lesions, no Mallory's hyaline, and only rare neutrophils. True bridging necrosis is also uncommon in these individuals. Infiltrates in areas of necrosis are composed mainly of monocytes. Steatosis, which earlier workers thought was uncommon, can be found over 70% of the time. The fatty accumulations may be microvesicular, macrovesicular, or mixed.

Hepatic foreign body granulomas are uncommon, since most injected contaminants are trapped in the pulmonary vascular bed and never enter the systemic circulation. Whether or not birefringent material will be found in the liver or hepatic nodes depends, in large part, on the population being studied. If the population of addicts is injecting pills meant for oral consumption, then the probability of finding birefringent material is greater. Of course, foreign bodies can be widely disseminated if there is a septal defect and a shunt, and there are occasionally reports of users with wide spread, systemic, granulomas (Riddick 1987).

TABLE 5.9.3.2
FREQUENCY OF HEPATIC LESIONS IN 150 RANDOMLY SELECTED DRUG ADDICTS

Lesion	Percentage
Steatosis	70%
Portal Fibrosis	47%
Portal Flogosis	93%
Piecemeal Necrosis	46%
Lymphoid Follicles	40%
Plasma Cells	34%
Acidophil Bodies	23%
Viral Antigens	16%
Bile Duct Proliferation	6%
Bridging Necrosis	5%
Granulomas	2%
Birefringent Material	<1%
Mallory's Hyaline	abs

Patients had mean age of 23.3 years and were predominantly male (86%). *Adapted from Paties.*

5.9.3.3 Hepatitis

In Paties' series of 150 addicts, changes consistent with chronic active hepatitis were found in 24%, and acute hepatitis was diagnosed in 12%. Most of these individuals had one or more viral antigens demonstrable with immunohistochemical techniques. In acute cases, scattered foci of parenchymal cell loss with acidophilic necrosis and swelling will be seen throughout the parenchymal, along with proliferating reticuloendothelial cells and mononuclear infiltrates.

In non-drug abusing populations, hepatitis B is, as a rule, a mild disease with a fatality rate of less than 2%, even among those requiring hospitalization. In addicts, fulminant hepatitis is much more frequent (Sheinbaum, Damus et al. 1974), probably a consequence of concurrent delta virus-hepatitis B confection. In the United States, at least, delta virus infection is mainly associated with parenteral drug abuse, but small numbers of cases are seen in the same groups that are at increased risk for hepatitis B (Lettau, McCarthy et al. 1987).

5.9.3.4 HIV infection and AIDS

For a variety of reasons, nearly two thirds of AIDS patients have hepatomegaly and abnormal liver function tests. The abnormalities may be a consequence of alcoholism, or of previously existing viral hepatitis, or even a manifestation of opportunistic infections or opportunistic tumors. Liver disease can also be a complication of sepsis, malnutrition, or drug therapy (Schneiderman 1988). The longer an individual has had AIDS, the higher the probability that histologic changes will be seen in the liver and that opportunistic infection will be present. High levels of alkaline phosphase should raise the suspicion of *M.avium-intracellulare* infection, with multiple granulomas obstructing the terminal branches of the biliary tree (Glasgow, Anders et al. 1985). In these cases diagnosis is often made more easily and rapidly by demonstrating mycobacteria on biopsy than by culture (Cappell, Schwartz et al. 1990). Besides tuberculosis, other opportunistic infections that have been reported include cytomegalovirus, *Cryptococcus neoformans,* and type 2 herpes simplex virus, to name but a few (Schneiderman 1988) (Devars du Mayne, Marche et al. 1985).

Elevation in total bilirubin in addition to elevation of alkaline phosphase suggests the presence of intrahepatic lymphoma (Schneiderman 1988). Kaposi's sarcoma, non-Hodgkin's lymphoma, and malignant fibrosarcoma all occur in AIDS patients (Reichert, O'Leary et al. 1983). Interestingly, HIV infected patients, like anabolic steroid abusers, may develop peliosis. This is a condition of unknown origin, characterized by the presence of many small, cystic, blood-filled areas, usually in the liver, but occasionally in the lungs or other organs. These blood-filled lesions are found randomly scattered throughout the liver, often in association with foci of hepatocellular necrosis. The condition was first recognized in conjunction with tuberculosis, but the connection with anabolic steroid abuse has been recognized for some time (Taxy 1978) (Bagheri and Boyer 1974). The mechanism by which theses lesions are formed is unknown. One theory is that these lesions may represent a transitional step preceding the more recognizable endothelial changes seen in Kaposi's sarcoma (Devars du Mayne, Marche et al. 1985). Others have speculated that in AIDS patients, Kaposi's sarcoma and peliosis are both manifestations of a system-wide vascular stimulation initiated by unknown causes (Devars du Mayne, Marche et al. 1985). The results of the most recent study raise the possibility that peliosis may be the result of an infectious process, related to, or possibly the same as, bacillary angiomatosis, a lesion usually found only in individuals with HIV infection (Leong, Cazen, Yu et al. 1992). The bacilli responsible for bacillary angiomatosis have staining and histologic similarities with the bacilli known to cause cat scratch disease, but whether infection with this agent is responsible for all cases of peliosis remains to be seen. Whatever the explanation, there is nothing to distinguish the changes seen in steroid abusers from the changes seen in AIDS patients, and in both groups the presence of these lesions can be symptomatic.

References

Bagheri, S. and J. Boyer (1974). Peliosis hepatis associated with androgenic-anabolic steroid therapy. Ann Intern Med. 81:610–618.

Baltaceano, G. and C. Visiliu (1935). Intoxication of hepatic cells by diacetylmorphine and its effects on bile. Can Royal Soc Biol. 120:229–244.

Cappell, M., M. Schwartz and L. Biempica (1990). Clinical utility of liver biopsy in patients with serum antibodies to the Human Immunodeficiency Virus. Am J Med. 88:123–130.

de Araujo, M., Gerard, F., Chossegros, P. et al. (1990). Vascular hepatotoxicity related to heroin addiction. Virchows Archiv. a. Path Anat Histol, 417:497–503.

Devars du Mayne, J., C. Marche et al. (1985). Hepatic involvement in acquired immune deficiency syndrome: a study of 20 cases. Presse Med. 14:1177–1180.

Edland, J. (1972). Liver disease in heroin addicts. Hum Pathol. 3(1):75–84.

Gheradi, R., F. Baud, P. Leporc and B. Marc (1988). Detection of drugs in the urine of body-packers. Lancet. 1(May 14):1076–1077.

Glasgow, B., K. Anders, L. Layfield et al. (1985). Clinical and pathologic findings of the liver in the acquired immune deficiency syndrome (AIDS). Am J Clin Pathol. 83:582–588.

Kaplan, K. (1963). Chronic liver disease in narcotics addicts. Am J Dig Dis. 8:402–410.

Kringsholm, B. and P. Christoffersen (1987). Lymph-node and thymus pathology in fatal drug addiction. Forensic Sci. Int. 34:245–254.

Leong, S., Cazen, R., Yu, G., et al. (1992). Abdominal visceral peliosis associated with bacillary angiomatosis. Ultrastructural evidence for endothelial destruction by bacilli. Arch Pathol Lab Med, 116:866–871.

Lettau, L., J. McCarthy, M. Smith et al. (1987). Outbreak of severe hepatitis due to Delta and Hepatitis B viruses in parenteral drug abusers and their contacts. New Engl J Med. 317:1256–1261.

Nakamura, G. and J. Choi (1983). Morphine in lymph nodes of heroin users. J Forensic Sci. 28(1):249–250.

Paties, C., V. Peveri and G.Falzi (1987). Liver histopathology in autopsied drug addicts. Forensic Sci.Int. 35:11–26.

Pinsky, M., J. Ducas and M. Ruggere (1978). Narcotic smuggling: the double condom sign. J Can Assoc Radiol. 29:78–81.

Reichert, C., T. O'Leary, D. Levens et al. (1983). Autopsy pathology in the acquired immune deficiency syndrome. Am J Pathol. 112:357–382.

Riddick, L. (1987). Disseminated granulomatosis through a patent foramen ovale in an intravenous drug user with pulmonary hypertension. Am J Forensic Med and Pathol. 8(4):326–333.

Roberts, J., D. Price, L. Goldfrank and L. Hartnett (1986). The bodystuffer syndrome: a clandestine form of drug overdose. Am J Emerg Med. 4:24–27.

Schneiderman, D. (1988). Hepatobiliary abnormalities of AIDS. Gastroenterol Clin North Am. 17:615–630.

Sheinbaum, A., K. Damus, T. Michael and G. Gitnick (1974). Acute fulminant hepatitis: a clustering of cases. Arch Intern Med. 134:1093–1094.

Siegel, H., M. Helpern and T. Ehrenreich (1966). The diagnosis of death from intravenous narcotism, with emphasis on the pathologic aspects. J Forensic Sci 11(1): 1–16.

Sinner, W. (1981). The gastrointestinal tract as a vehicle for drug smuggling. Gastrointest Radiol. 198(6):319–323.

Suarez, C., A. Arango and J. Lester (1977). Cocaine-condom ingestion. JAMA. 238: 1391–1392.

Taxy, J. (1978). Peliosis: a morphologic curiosity becomes an iatrogenic problem. Hum Pathol. 9:331–340.

Vanarthos W.,R. Aizpuru and H. Lerner (1990). CT demonstration of ingested cocaine packets. Am J Radiol. 155:419–420.

Wetli, C., J. Davis and B. Blackbourne (1972). Narcotic addiction in Dade County , Florida - an analysis of 100 consecutive autopsies. Arch Pathol 93:330–343.

Wetli, C. and R. Mittleman (1981). The body packer syndrome; toxicity following ingestion of illicit drugs packaged for transportation. J Forensic Sci. 26:492–500.

5.10 RENAL DISORDERS

5.10.1 INTRODUCTION

Chronic intravenous narcotic use can cause renal disease, though the factors determining individual susceptibility remain poorly understood. Symptomatic individuals are almost always middle-aged hypertensives with variable degrees of proteinuria, hematuria and pyuria. These abnormalities merely represent a final common pathway for a very diverse group of disorders. In the past, focal segmental glomerulosclerosis was the most frequent cause of nephrotic syndrome in addicts. It appears that morphine may have a direct role on mesangial cell growth and expansion. Opiate receptors have been found on mesangial cells and, at least in tissue culture, their proliferation appears to be stimulated by exposure to morphine (Singhal, Gibbons, Abramovici 1992). Today, in some populations at least, renal amyloidosis is the predominant histopathologic lesion. Table 5.10.1 lists the more common renal disorders that have been identified in narcotic abusers.

TABLE 5.10.1
RENAL DISORDERS ASSOCIATED WITH OPIATE ABUSE
    Focal glomerulosclerosis
    Membranoproliferative glomerulonephritis
    Renal amyloidosis
    Necrotizing angiitis with renal involvement
    Interstitial nephritis
    Acute tubular necrosis due to rhabdomyolysis

5.10.2 ACUTE RENAL FAILURE DUE TO NONTRAUMATIC RHABDOMYOLYSIS

This syndrome was first described in narcotic users just over 20 years ago (Richter, Challenor et al. 1971), but cases have been reported regularly since then (Schreiber, Liebowitz et al. 1971) (Penn, Rowland et al. 1972) (Dolich, 1973) (Koffler, Freidler et al. 1976) (Rao, Nicastri et al. 1978) (Akmal and Massry 1983) (Blain, Lane et al. 1985) (DeGans, Stam et al. 1985) (Curry 1989) (Otero, Esteban, Martine et al. 1992). Rhabdomyolysis accounts for much of the renal disease seen in addicts. Most cases of rhabdomyolysis are caused by a combination of factors including hypotension, fluid imbalance, and pressure necrosis. The result is muscle destruction and the liberation of myoglobin into the blood stream. However, as Richter observed, the syndrome can occur in patients who are neither comatose, nor subject to muscle compression, and in those cases it seems likely that mycotoxic adulterants play a role (Yuen-Fu, Wong et al. 1990). Whatever the etiology, rapid onset of oliguria is followed by azotemia, acidosis, hypophosphatemia, hyperuricemia, and all the other electrolyte and chemical disorders associated with renal failure. Since the condition is rarely fatal, these patients don't come to autopsy, or even biopsy. There is no reason to suppose that the histologic changes are in any way different from those encountered in cases due to traumatic rhabdomyolysis.

5.10.3 SECONDARY AMYLOIDOSIS

The first reports of amyloidosis in heroin abusers were published in 1978 (Jacob, Charytan et al. 1978). Since then it has become apparent that the incidence of renal amyloid in heroin addicts is significantly higher than the incidence of amyloid found at autopsy in the general population (Dubrow, Mittman et al. 1985). Furthermore, the incidence seems to be increasing. Amyloid is more common in older, long-term abusers. Those affected suffer from massive proteinuria, with or without azotemia. Over 90% of addicts with renal amyloid will have had clinical evidence of repeated skin infections with suppurative cutaneous lesions

(Neugarten, Gallo et al. 1986) (Menchel, Cohen et al. 1983) (Meador, Sharon et al. 1979) (Jacob, Charytan et al. 1978). Most of the reported cases have been from New York City, raising the possibility that some local practice has a role. It has been suggested that subcutaneous injecting, and the inevitable chronic skin infections that result, are the cause (Dietrick and Russi 1958) (Campistol, Montoliu et al. 1988). Renal amyloid is hardly unique to heroin users and a proven mechanism in these patients is still wanting (Maury and Teppo 1982). Routine light microscopy with H&E or PAS staining shows large amounts of eosinophilic material within the glomerulus. Confirmation that the material is, in fact, amyloid, can be obtained by Congo red staining, or by using polarizing microscopy. Amyloid has a typical apple-green birefringence. Electron microscopy shows amyloid fibrils.

5.10.4 HEROIN ASSOCIATED NEPHROPATHY (HAN)
AND OTHER GLOMERULAR DISORDERS

The possibility that opiate abuse might cause renal damage was recognized even before the advent of intravenous heroin (Light and Torrance 1929), and it has been known for many years that long-term heroin users can develop a relentlessly progressive variety of nephrotic syndrome, unresponsive to therapy, terminating in renal failure within a few months to a few years (Rao, Nicastri et al. 1978) (Cunningham, Zielezny et al. 1983) (Dubrow, Mittman et al. 1985). Consistent with the general pattern that has been observed in other types of drug toxicity (Sanders and Marshall 1989a), the predominant histologic alteration in intravenous heroin users is focal segmental glomerulosclerosis (Grishman, Churag et al. 1976) (Sanders and Marshall 1989b) (Stachura 1985).

IgM and C3 complement protein can both be identified in abnormal segments of the glomerulus, and electron microscopic studies show fusion of the foot processes (Treser, Chenibis et al. 1974). The mechanism for these changes is not clear, and appropriate animal models are lacking. Rats given high doses of heroin develop interstitial disease (Stachura 1985), but that pattern of injury does not reflect what is seen in human heroin users. Glomerulosclerosis has not been reproduced in an animal model. Because the human lung filters out foreign bodies before they ever reach the kidneys, granulomatous interstitial nephritis isn't seen in addicts either. Suggested mechanisms for the changes that have been observed in humans include increased glomerular capillary permeability (May and get 1986), and chronic immune complex deposition (Sanders and Marshall 1989a). Whatever the cause, progression of the lesions ultimately leads to glomerular destruction and symptomatic renal disease. Lesions consist primarily of intracapillary deposits of eosinophilic, PAS positive material involving isolated or multiple segments of the glomerulus.

HIV infection, even in the absence of opiate abuse, can cause a picture very similar to that seen in HAN. Without actually demonstrating the presence of virus, distinguishing HAN from HIV may be nearly impossible. However, there are some features that can be used to distinguish the two groups. Tissue from the heroin abusers usually shows marked interstitial fibrosis and interstitial infiltrates of lymphocytes and plasma cells. Bowmans capsule may be markedly thickened, and mesangial hypercellularity may also be a feature. Focal segmental glomerulosclerosis in AIDS patients, on the other hand, is usually devoid of cellular infiltrates, even when there is supervening opportunistic infection. There is mesangial hypocellularity, and interstitial fibrosis is absent. Nonetheless, specialized electron microscopic studies or even gene probes may be required to confirm the diagnosis (Chander, Soni et al. 1987) .

TABLE 5.10.4.1
DIFFERENTIATING HAN FROM HIV

Heroin Associated Nephropathy	HIV
mesangial hypercellularity	mesangial hypocellularity
interstitial infiltrates present	interstitial infiltrates absent
interstitial fibrosis prominent	interstitial fibrosis absent

Other disease processes can also involve the glomerulus. A high proportion of addicts with endocarditis have focal or diffuse glomerulonephritis as a result of circulating antigen-antibody complex deposition (Rao, Nicastri et al. 1978). The deposition of immune complexes causes diffuse proliferative changes and even classic crescent formation. Most reported cases are in the older literature, and occurred in individuals with *Staphylococcal* endocarditis (Gutman, Striker et al. 1972) (Louria 1967). The true incidence of glomerulonephritis in addicts has never been established, but reports are uncommon. In Sapira's autopsy study, the incidence of chronic glomerulonephritis in known addicts was 8% (Sapira, Ball et al. 1970). More recent experience suggests that the incidence of acute disease may be much lower. In most cases of endocarditis, renal embolization with infarction is probably much more common than immune complex deposition, but these lesions rarely cause significant disease.

5.10.5 NECROTIZING ANGIITIS

A polyarteritis-like syndrome in intravenous drug abusers was first reported by Citron in 1970 (Citron, Halpern et al. 1970). As originally described, medium-sized and small arteries in most organs, as well as the arterioles in the brain, were involved. The elastic arteries, capillaries, and veins were all spared. Acutely there was fibrinoid necrosis of the media and intima, with prominent infiltrates of eosinophils and lymphocytes. Occlusive thrombi were also described. The subacute process was marked by intimal proliferation and luminal narrowing, with saccular aneurysms, especially at vessel bifurcations. There is very little evidence that such a disorder ever occurs in opiate abusers. Most of the patients described by Citron were intravenous amphetamine abusers, or polydrug abusers taking combinations of amphetamine with other drugs. Of the patients Citron studied, none that used only heroin developed the syndrome, and there have been no reports in heroin users since.

References

Akmal, M. and S. Massry (1983). Peripheral nerve damage in patients with nontraumatic rhabdomyolysis. Arch Intern Med. 143:835–836.

Blain, P., R. Lane, D. Bateman and M. Rawlins (1985). Opiate-induced rhabdomyolysis. Hum Toxicol. 4:71–74.

Campistol, J., J. Montoliu, J. Soler-Amigo et al. (1988). Renal amyloidosis with nephrotic syndrome in a Spanish subcutaneous heroin abuser. Nephrol Dial Transplant. 3:471–473.

Chan, Y., P. Wong and T. Chow (1990). Acute myoglobinuria as a fatal complication of heroin addiction. Am J Forensic Med & Pathol. 11(2):160–164.

Chander, P., A. Soni, A. Suri et al. (1987). Renal ultrastructural markers in AIDS-associated nephropathy. Am J Pathol. 126:513–526.

Citron, B., M. Halpern, M. McCarron et al. (1970). Necrotizing angiitis associated with drug abuse. N Engl J Med. 283(19):1003–1011.

Cunningham, E., M. Zielezny and R. Venuto (1983). Heroin-associated nephropathy, a nationwide problem. JAMA. 250:2935–2936.

Curry, S., Chang, D and D. Connor (1989). Drug and toxin-induced rhabdomyolysis. Ann Emerg Med. 18:1068–1084.

DeGans, J., J. Stam and G. Van Wijngaarden (1985). Rhabdomyolysis and concomitant neurological lesions after intravenous heroin abuse. J Neurol Neurosurg Psychiatr. 48:1957–1059.

Dietrick, R. and S. Russi (1958). Tabulation and review of autopsy findings in fifty-five paraplegics. JAMA. 166:41–44.

Dubrow, A., N. Mittman, V. Ghali et al. (1985). The changing spectrum of heroin-associated nephropathy. Am J Kidney Dis. 5:36–41.

Grishman, E., J. Churg and J. Porush (1976). Glomerular morphology in nephrotic heroin addicts. Lab Invest. 35:415–424.

Gutman, R., G. Striker, B.Gilliland and R. Cutler (1972). The immune complex glomerulonephritis of bacterial endocarditis. Medicine. 51:1–25.

Jacob, H., C. Charytan, J. Rascoff et al. (1978). Amyloidosis secondary to drug abuse and chronic skin suppuration. Arch Intern Med. 138:1150–1151.

Koffler, A., R. Friedler and S. Massry (1976). Acute renal failure due to nontraumatic rhabdomyolysis. Ann Intern Med. 85:23–28.

Light, A. and E. Torrance (1929). Opium addiction - physical characteristics and physical fitness of addicts during administration of morphine. Arch Intern Med. 43:326–334.

Louria, D., T. Hensle, and J. Rose (1967). The major medical complications of heroin addiction. Ann Int Med. 67:1–22.

Maury, C. and A. Teppo (1982). Mechanism of reduced amyloid-A-degrading activity in serum of patients with secondary amyloidosis. Lancet. 2:234–237.

May, D., J. Helderman, E. Eigenbrodt, and F. Silva (1986). Chronic sclerosing glomerulopathy (heroin-associated nephropathy) in intravenous T's and blues abusers. Am J Kid Dis. 8:404–409.

Meador, K., Z. Sharon and E. Lewis (1979). Renal amyloidosis and subcutaneous drug abuse. Ann Intern Med. 91:565–567.

Menchel, S., D. Cohen, E. Gross et al. (1983). AA protein related renal amyloidosis in drug addicts. Am J Pathol. 112:195–199.

Neugarten, J., G. Gallo, J. Buxbaum et al. (1986). Amyloidosis in subcutaneous heroin abusers ('Skin Poppers' Amyloidosis'). Am J Med. 81:635–640.

Otero, A., Esteban, J., Martine, J., Cejudo, C. (1992). Rhabdomyolysis and acute renal failure as a consequence of heroin inhalation. Nephron, 62:245.

Penn, A., L. Rowland and D. Fraser (1972). Drugs, coma, and myoglobinuria. Arch Neurol. 26:336–343.

Richter, R., Y. Challenor, J. Pearson et al. (1971). Acute myoglobinuria associated with heroin addiction. JAMA. 216:1172–1176.

Sanders, M. and A. Marshall (1989a). Acute and chronic toxic nephropathies. Ann Clin Lab Sci. 19(3):216–220.

Sapira, J., J. Ball and H. Penn (1970). Causes of death among institutionalized narcotic addicts. J Chron Dis. 22:733–742.

Schreiber, S., M. Liebowitz, L. Bernstein et al. (1971). Limb compression and renal impairment (crush syndrome) complicating narcotic overdose. N Engl J Med. 284:368–369.

Singhal, P., Gibbons, N, Abramovici, M. (1992). Kidney international, 41:1560–1570.

Sreepeda Rao, T., Nicastri, A. and E. Friedman (1977). Renal consequences of narcotic abuse. Adv Nephrol 7:261–290.

Stachura, I. (1985). Renal lesions in drug addicts. Pathology Annual., 20 (2), 83–99 New York, Appleton-Century-Crofts.

Treser, G., C. Cherubin, E. Lonegran et al. (1974). Renal lesions in narcotic addicts. Am J Med. 57:687–694.

5.11 NEUROPATHOLOGY

5.11.1 INTRODUCTION

When the first reports of heroin toxicity were published at the turn of the century, opiates were thought to be neurotoxic. Creutzfeldt, Nissl, and other pioneers argued that they could see unique pathologic changes in the brains and spinal cords of narcotics abusers (Nissl 1897) (Creutzfeldt 1926). Fatty degeneration, particularly of neurons in the deeper layers of the frontal cortex and Ammon's horn, was thought to be diagnostic for morphinism. Subsequent studies have shown that the changes observed were either nonspecific or artifactual. In the 1970's it was argued that heroin abusers were uniquely prone to infarction of the basal ganglia (Jervis and Joyce 1948) (Strassmann, Sturner et al. 1969) (Pearson, Challenor et al. 1972). The nonspecific nature of this finding is also now appreciated. With the exception of perivascular pigment deposition within macrophages, which probably is the result of repeated intravenous injection of foreign material (Gray et al. 1992), no one lesion is diagnostic for narcotic abuse. Nonetheless, drug abusers do subject their nervous systems to a variety of insults, and some of these insults do produce lesions. The better-known neuropathologic complications of narcotic abuse are listed in Table 5.11.1.

5.11.2 HYPOXIC ENCEPHALOPATHY

Deaths from acute opiate toxicity are usually associated with cerebral edema, meningeal congestion, and flattening of the gyri. (Pearson and Richter 1975) (Adelman and Aronson 1969) (Levine and Grimes 1973). As a rule these deaths occur so rapidly that morphologic evidence of cellular injury is not apparent. With longer periods of survival, characteristic patterns of tissue necrosis emerge. The injuries seen are not so much a result of hypoxia, but rather a result of the arterial hypotension that ensues because of the hypoxia (Brierley 1972).

TABLE 5.11.1
NEUROPATHOLOGIC COMPLICATIONS OF NARCOTIC ABUSE
   1. Hypercapnic hypoxia
         a. Cerebral edema
         b. Venous congestion
         c. Focal hemorrhage
   2. Infectious
         a. Complications of endocarditis
         b. Complications of HIV infection
               i. Encephalopathy
               ii. Opportunistic infections
               iii. Opportunistic tumors
         c. Phycomycosis
   3. Spongiform encephalopathy
   4. Transverse myelopathy
   5. Peripheral neuropathy
   6. Rhabdomyolysis
   7. Stroke
   8. Necrotizing angiitis
   9. Parkinsonism

In almost all cases there will be terminal changes such as nerve cell ischemia and vascular congestion (Slater 1862) (Gray 1992), but, under certain circumstances, the pattern of injury may reveal a great deal about the clinical events that preceded death. A major abrupt decrease in systemic blood pressure typically produces necrosis in the arterial boundary zones between the major arteries. The area most frequently involved is the parieto-occipital region. If the drop in blood pressure is more gradual and of longer duration, then laminar necrosis may be seen. This lesion is most prominent in the deeper layers of the cortex and cerebellum. A pattern of continuous necrosis, often accentuated in arterial border zones, may also be observed. The Purkinje cells of the cerebellum are particularly vulnerable to injury, as are the cells of Sommer's sector, located in the hippocampus (Adams, Brierley et al. 1966) (Brierley 1972). Some time must elapse before these patterns become apparent. If death occurs within 3 to 6 hours, the probability of detecting anything but chronic changes is small. With the passage of more time, typical eosinophilic degenerative changes become apparent in scattered neurons. The cells of the caudate and putamen may or may not be involved. If changes are to be detected in those nuclei, then sampling from multiple sites will be required.

Chronic hypoxic episodes from repeated overdoses result in necrosis and scarring of the hippocampus, though the finding is hardly unique to narcotic abuse. And, of course, acute lesions may be superimposed on preexisting chronic or subacute changes. Thus parietal--occipital lesions may be seen along with areas of laminar necrosis, suggesting an initial acute hypotensive episode followed by prolonged hypotension and decreased cerebral flow, a sequence not uncommon in heroin addicts.

5.11.3 INFECTIOUS DISEASE

5.11.3.1 Complications of endocarditis

Narcotics abusers get infectious diseases because of their unhealthy life styles, because their sterile injection technique is not good, and because chronic opiate use causes immunosuppression. This combination of factors occasionally leads to some very bizarre infections, such as mucormycosis. Such infections are uncommon, and are not major causes of morbidity. On the other hand, septicemia and endocarditis are fairly common, and both disorders have neurologic sequelae. In fact, the incidence of neurologic complications from subacute endocarditis has changed hardly at all since the introduction of antibiotics (Ziment 1969).

Vegetations on the aortic and tricuspid valves can shed, producing disseminated microabscesses throughout the central nervous system. Small lesions center around septic emboli that lodge in terminal vessels, producing cerebral infarction (Grindal et al. 1978). In more severe cases, foci of metastatic suppuration may be seen throughout the leptomeninges, but intracranial hemorrhage secondary to the rupture of a mycotic aneurysm is a relatively uncommon event (Jones et al. 1969). The main sites of infection are the capillaries and small venules. They are usually surrounded by perivascular collections of polymorphonuclear leukocytes. Microabscesses do not produce severe or focal symptoms, and their presence may often be masked by other, more obvious disease processes (Adams, Corsellis et al. 1984).

5.11.3.2 Complications of HIV infection

Many intravenous drug abusers are HIV-infected, and most HIV-infected patients have central nervous system abnormalities detectable at autopsy. The AIDS associated disorders can be divided into three groups: (1) AIDS encephalopathy, due to the direct effects of the virus itself, (2) Opportunistic viral, fungal, parasitic and bacterial infections and (3) Opportunistic neoplastic processes, particularly primary brain lymphoma.

The most frequently seen abnormality in the brains of AIDS patients is atrophy with diffuse or focal lesions in the white matter. There is pallor of the myelin, and necrosis is prominent in the centrum semiovale. There may also be diffuse or focal neuronal loss in the caudate and putamen (Navia, Cho et al. 1986) (Petito, Cho et al. 1986). In cases where there is diffuse white matter damage, multifocal microgranulomatous lesions and multinucleated giant cells can be seen. Immunohistochemical techniques will almost invariably demonstrate the presence of the virus itself (Budka 1991).

Cytomegalovirus infection is also common. Evidence of infection is apparent in one quarter of all autopsied AIDS cases (Petito, Cho et al. 1986), but these patients often have minimal symptoms during life. Infection is evidenced by the presence of microglial nodules. Viral inclusions may or may not be obvious, but the presence of the virus can be detected with immunohistochemical techniques (Magello, Cho et al. 1987).

Toxoplasmosis infection is much less common than CMV infection, but it is more likely to produce symptomatic disease (Navia, Petito et al. 1986). In life, the diagnosis is made with CT scanning. It typically shows hypodense lesions with ring contrast enhancement. Serologic testing confirms the diagnosis. The findings at autopsy will depend on how long the disorder has been present, and whether it has been under treatment. Early on, there will be poorly demarcated foci of necrosis with surrounding edema and mixed inflammatory infiltrates. There may or may not be evidence of arteritis. The diagnosis of toxoplasmosis is confirmed by the demonstration of extracellular tachyzoites and bradyzoite containing cysts. In longer-standing cases, organization of the necrotic material occurs and well-demarcated areas of coagulation necrosis can be seen. In long-standing cases, cysts and tachyzoites may be very hard to find.

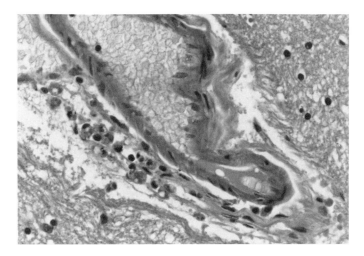

Figure 5.11.1 Hemosiderin laden macrophages
This micrograph is from the brain of an HIV negative heroin addict. Similar cells are often seen in the lungs. In both locations they appear to be the result of repeated intravenous injections of particulate material. Courtesy of Professor Françoise Gray, Départment de Pathologie, Hôpital Henri Mondor, Creteil, France.

The principal opportunistic neoplasm seen in AIDS patients is high-grade B cell lymphoma. The diagnosis is often difficult to make, especially in individuals who are already suffering from opportunistic infections (So, Beckstead et al. 1986) (Gill, Levine et al. 1985). Diffusely infiltrating masses may be seen that are indistinguishable from any other sort of glioma. Alternatively, lesions may consist of small necrotic foci that can be confused with microabscesses. A variegated picture is seen microscopically, and malignant cells are likely to be mixed in with benign inflammatory infiltrates.

5.11.3.3 Primary phycomycosis

This fungal infection is usually associated with poorly controlled diabetes, or the presence of some disorder, such as leukemia or severe burns, that depresses immunity. A handful of reports have linked phyco-mycosis to intravenous drug abuse, usually in heroin users (Chmel and Grieco 1973; Hameroff, Eckholdt et al. 1970; Kasantikul, Shuangshoti et al. 1987; Masucci, Fabara et al. 1982) (Adelman and Aronson 1969) (Micozzi and Wetli 1985) (Pierce, Solomon et al. 1982) (Wetli, Weiss et al. 1984). Infection begins in the nasal cavities and then, by invasion of the turbinates and the veins that drain them, infection extends into the paranasal sinuses, eventually reaching the orbital area. In other instances the infection reaches the brain by a hematogenous route. It may be that the brain supplies a particularly conducive environment in which the fungus can grow. Whatever the route of infection, the result is edema, proptosis, and ultimately destruction of the trigeminal and facial nerves. At least in drug addicts, the disease follows a fulminant course. Most patients die within two weeks of onset. Diagnosis in life may require brain biopsy, because fungi are not detected in the cerebro-spinal fluid. CT scanning may be suggestive, but it is not diagnostic. Lesions are usually multiple, symmetric, and involve the basal ganglia. Material removed at surgery or autopsy is composed of aggregates of macrophages, lymphocytes and multinucleated giants cells. Even routine H&E staining will show the broad, branching, nonseparate fungal mycelia (Schwartz 1982).

5.11.4 SPONGIFORM LEUKOENCEPHALOPATHY

The classification of this disorder is somewhat obscure. It has never been established whether its etiology is toxic or infectious. In 1982 an epidemic outbreak of spongiform leukoencephalopathy occurred in the Netherlands. Nearly 50 patients were involved, and the only factor common to all those affected was that they were addicts who smoked heroin. In most cases the disorder ran a two to three month course. In the initial stages, motor restlessness and apathy with obvious cerebellar signs rapidly gave way to hypertonic hemiplegia or even quadriplegia. In some cases patients developed myoclonic jerks or choreoathetoid movements. Onset of hemiplegia seemed to mark a turning point in the progression of the disease. Half the patients stabilized or improved, while the other half progressed to a final, fatal stage with central pyrexia, spastic paresis, and akinetic mutism. These individuals died of respiratory failure (Wolters, Wijngaarden et al. 1982). Since then other cases have occurred in England, Germany and Spain (Sempere, Posada et al. 1991) (Haan, Muller et al. 1983) (Wolters, Wijngaarden et al. 1982) (Hugentobler and Waespe, 1990) (Roulet Perez, Maeder, Rivier and Deonna, 1992) (Shiffer, Brignolio, Giordana et al. 1985), though not in the United States.

All patients had obvious edema with flattening of the convolutions and brain weights of 1,380–2,560 grams. In all cases, microscopic examination showed damaged white matter filled with vacuoles. In some areas the vacuoles had coalesced to form larger cavities. Around the cavities could be seen a fine network of attenuated myelin. The number of oligodendroglia was reduced, but no myelin breakdown products were evident. Inflammatory cells were also absent. Electron microscopy done in several cases showed multivacuolar degeneration of the oligodendroglia, with swollen mitochondria and distended endoplasmic reticulum. Light microscopic examination did not disclose it, but the electron micrographs showed abnormalities of the myelin lamellae and axoplasm, which also contained swollen, abnormal mitochondria.

The changes in these individuals are easily distinguishable from those seen in AIDS-associated leukoencephalopathy, where there is obvious evidence of demyelination, often with aggregates of microglial nodules. In addition, AIDS leukoencephalopathy is associated with changes in the microvasculature, including mural thickening, pleomorphism of the endothelial cells, and prominent perivascular collections of HIV-positive monocytes and multinucleated cells. AIDS can also be associated with very severe vacuolar changes, but these changes are confined to the posterior columns of the spinal cord (Petito, Navia et al. 1985). Toxicologic evaluation of all patients has been unremarkable, and chemical analysis of samples of local heroin used by the addicts showed only the usual adulterants: caffeine, lidocaine, procaine, phenobarbital and methaqualone. None of these agents have ever been shown to be neurotoxic.

5.11.5 TRANSVERSE MYELITIS

This rare entity was first described in 1926. Its etiology also remains undetermined, but its occurrence has been noted in conjunction with a heterogeneous group of disorders, including viral infections, AIDS, systemic lupus erythematosus, smallpox vaccination, trauma, extreme physical exertion, and heroin abuse. The association with heroin abuse was first noted in 1968 (Richter and Rosenberg 1968). Since the index report, transverse myelitis has been observed on a number of occasions (Schein, Yessayan et al. 1971) (Rodriguez, Smokvina et al. 1972) (Thompson and Waldman 1970) (Pearson, Challenor et al. 1972) (Hall and Karp 1973). Judging from the number of recent reports, the incidence of this disorder seems to be decreasing.

The patients first described by Richter had not been taking heroin for a number of months, and they developed neurologic symptoms only after they began injecting heroin again. In all of the cases, onset of symptoms was quite rapid, ranging anywhere from a few hours to a few days. Victims developed flaccid paralysis and complete sensory loss ascending from the lower extremities to thoracic or even cervical levels. In the addict subpopulation, at least, fairly rapid improvement seems to be the norm, though there were usually residual deficits. Myelography in acute cases is unremarkable (Arlazoroff, Klein et al. 1989) and the disorder is sufficiently uncommon so that patients have yet to be evaluated with NMR or CT scanning. Cerebrospinal fluid analysis has also been unremarkable. Autopsy studies are rare, but when they have been done, the only findings have been extensive, but non-specific necrosis.

At first, transverse myelitis was thought to be the result of anterior spinal artery occlusion, but when more cases were studied it became evident that the circulation in other territories could also be involved. Even ventral pontine disease has been observed (Hall and

Karp 1973). This disorder is the result of an isolated vascular accident within the spinal cord, but, at least in the case of narcotics abusers, it is not clear whether that accident is the result of thromboembolic phenomena, some sort of inflammatory vascular disease, or a toxic manifestation due to some contaminant injected along with the heroin. The most interesting new development in this regard is the recognition that heroin administration can increase or decrease blood flow to specific areas of the brain. Whether the decrease is ever large enough to produce neurologic symptoms remains to be determined (Fuller and Stein 1991).

5.11.6 PERIPHERAL NEUROPATHY

Peripheral nerve lesions occur in addicts for a number of reasons. Unsterile injections may lead to local infection with nerve involvement, as can the injection of toxic adulterants. Neuropathy associated with rhabdomyolysis is a well recognized entity. Nerve injury may be an indirect result of elevated compartment pressure, or a direct result of ischemia that can occur if compartment pressures rise high enough. Unperceived pressure or traction can also cause plexus or peripheral nerve injuries, even without muscle swelling (Kaku and Yuen 1990). There is evidence to suggest that all of these mechanisms come into play (Schreiber, Liebowitz et al. 1971) (Pearson, Challenor et al. 1972) (Penn, Rowland et al. 1972). In addition, HIV-positive patients are subject to peripheral and autonomic neuropathies, probably due to direct invasion by the virus, though it has also been suggested that an autoimmune etiology might be possible (Villa, Foresti et al. 1992).

Nerve injuries in narcotics addicts have been documented with electrophysiologic testing, but there have been no autopsy studies (Akmal and Massry 1983). The mechanism in these cases has never been elucidated, but toxic or allergic reactions seem likely candidates, because there have been cases of lumbar plexus involvement where pressure or traction are obviously not factors (Jacome 1982) (Challenor, Richter et al. 1973) (Greenwood 1974).

5.11.7 RHABDOMYOLYSIS

Heroin had been available for nearly 70 years before anyone ever observed that abusing it could cause acute myoglobinuria (Richter, Challenor et al. 1971) (Schreiber, Liebowitz et al. 1971) (Greenwood 1974) (D'Agostino and Annett 1979) (Jacome 1982) (DeGans, Stam et al. 1985) (Penn, Rowland et al. 1972) (Grossman, Hamilton et al. 1974) (Koffler, Freidler et al. 1976) (Nicholls, Niall et al. 1982) (Gibb 1985) (Hecker, Friedli 1988) (Strohmaier, Friedrich 1991). The incidence of rhabdomyolysis in heroin users is not known with any precision, but judging by the number of cases reported in the literature, rhabdomyolysis may be occurring more often than is generally appreciated. In some instances the cause of muscle injury is obvious: pressure necrosis from the weight of the patient's own body while the individual is lying comatose (Schreiber, Liebowitz et al. 1971). Many of the reported cases cannot be explained in this fashion (Chan, Wong et al. 1990). There are even cases with unequivocal evidence of concurrent cardiac necrosis, where the etiology could hardly have been pressure necrosis (Schwartz-farb, Singh et al. 1977). In such cases, a direct effect of heroin or of an adulterant seems to be responsible.

Patients usually complain of muscle weakness, pain, and swelling that begins several hours to several days after using heroin. The muscles of the lower limbs are involved more often than the upper limbs. Associated neurologic complaints and neuropathies of various sorts have been reported in conjunction with heroin-induced rhabdomy-olysis (DeGans, Stam et al. 1985). Diagnosis in these cases is usually suggested by the presence of muscle swelling and elevated creatinine phosphokinase levels. However, muscle swelling need not always be evident, and the presence of myoglobin in the serum is, at best, an unreliable indicator because myoglobin is rapidly cleared from the plasma. Early on, laboratory tests will disclose marked elevations of creatinine phosphokinase and aldolase. Some individuals may complain of dark urine, and about half will go on to develop full-blown renal failure, with typical laboratory findings.

5.11.8 STROKE

Occasional reports of stroke in heroin users have been published, but the incidence seems to be lower now than it was 20 years ago. In most cases the etiology is obscure. Twenty years ago it was thought that the re-exposure of addicts to heroin after a period of abstinence might lead to vascular hypersensitivity reactions, but the theory has never been substantiated (Rumbaugh, Begerson et al. 1971) (Ostor 1977) (Citron, Halpern et al. 1970) (Woods and Strewler 1972) (Caplan, Hier et al. 1982). Necrotizing angiitis (see below) can certainly cause cerebral infarction, but there is rarely evidence for this disorder, and the apparent decline in its incidence in general suggests that it may have been the result of some toxic contaminants mixed with the heroin (King, Richards et al. 1978) (Citron, Halpern et al. 1970). As often as not, angiographic studies will be normal (Herskowitz and Gross 1973) (Olson and Winther 1990). Table 5.11.8.1 lists additional mechanisms that can cause stroke in opiate abusers. The same mechanisms that cause stroke in stimulant abusers could also cause stroke in opiate abusers, but vasospasm seems unlikely in opiate users, since opiates share no common pharmacologic mechanisms with stimulants, and do not (except for pentazocine) cause elevations in circulating catecholamines .

TABLE 5.11.8.1
POSSIBLE ETIOLOGIES FOR STROKE IN OPIATE ABUSERS
Thromboembolism
Thrombocytopenia
Vasculitis
Septic emboli
Hypotension
        a.secondary to arrhythmia
        b.secondary to decreased cardiac output
        c.secondary to peripheral vasodilation
Positional vascular compression

A likely mechanism in many cases of stroke is positional vascular compression. The most recently published case involved a 35-year old addict with dense hemiparesis. Regional flow studies demonstrated severe hyperemia of the entire carotid territory on the affected side, but normal vessels on angiography. Such localized hyperemia is often seen following restoration of flow in stroke patients (Caplan, Hier et al. 1982), and after cerebral spasm (Voldby, Enevoldsen et al. 1985). Generalized hyperemia is more likely to be observed after global ischemia. Stroke in these patients may have been the result of an unfortunate set of circumstances. Large doses of narcotic lead to hypotension, decreased respiration, and generalized cerebral ischemia. If the carotid artery is then compressed, by lying in the wrong way, perfusion might be lowered beneath some critical level and stroke could occur in an already ischemic brain (Olson and Winther 1990). In the absence of experimental evidence such an explanation is speculative, but it could well account for an occasional infarct.

Hemorrhagic stroke in heroin abusers is the result of a deranged clotting mechanism, as might be encountered in cases of fulminant hepatitis or in individuals with AIDS-associated thrombocytopenia (Brust and Richter 1976). Rupture of a mycotic aneurysm, or underlying AV malformation is also possible, but extremely uncommon. This is in contrast to hemorrhagic stroke in cocaine users, where victims commonly bleed from a preexisting malformation or aneurysm.

5.11.9 NECROTIZING ANGIITIS

Reports of a polyarteritis-like disorder in intravenous drug abusers were first published in the late 1960s, and traditionally this disorder has been acknowledged to be a complication of intravenous heroin abuse (see section 5.11.5). Most of the patients described in the original report by Citron were intravenous amphetamine abusers, or polydrug abusers taking combinations of amphetamine and other drugs (Citron, Halpern et al. 1970). None of Citron's patients limiting themselves to heroin abuse had the syndrome, and only one other case of

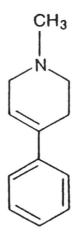

Figure 5.11.10 MPTP
1-Methyl-4-phenyl-1,2,3,6-tetrahydropyridine (MPTP) molecule.

arteritis in opiate abusers has been reported (King 1978).

5.11.10 PARKINSONISM

MPPP is a potent meperidine analog. When it is synthesized by clandestine chemists, inattention to detail occasionally results in the production of a neurotoxic byproduct, known as MPTP. Taken in sufficient quantity, MPTP can produce all the classic symptoms of parkinsonism, including resting tremor, rigidity, bradykinesia, and postural instability. At least three isolated outbreaks of recognized of MPTP toxicity have been reported.

The first reported case occurred in 1979 (Davis, Williams et al. 1979) and involved a graduate student who had been synthesizing and intravenously injecting MPPP for a period of six months. Just before he became symptomatic he had modified his synthetic methods, and later analysis by authorities disclosed that he had actually produced a mixture of MPPP and MPTP. His symptoms responded well to treatment, but he died of an unrelated drug overdose some two years later. Detailed neuropathologic examination of his brain disclosed degenerative changes within the substantia nigra that were confined to zona compacta. A marked astrocytic response and focal glial scarring was present, along with abundant collections of extraneuronal melanin pigment.

A second cluster of patients was reported in 1983. Four patients bought what they thought was "synthetic heroin" and, within a matter of days, developed striking features of parkinsonism. Analysis of material injected by these individuals showed they had been using mixtures of MPTP and MPPP (2.5 – 3.2% MPTP, 0.3 – 27% MPPP) (Langston, Ballard et al. 1983). Since that original report an additional 22 cases with less florid symptoms have been identified, all stemming from exposure to product from the same clandestine lab that had been operating in Northern California (Tetrud, Langston et al. 1989). The results of follow-up epidemiologic studies indicate that, during the three-year period from 1982 to 1985, over 500 individuals were exposed to MPTP, probably all from the same clandestine lab (Ruttenber 1991).

Additional cases stemming from exposure to products from other sources were reported in 1983 and 1984. The first case was in a non-drug abusing chemist exposed to MPTP at work. He developed classic symptoms of parkinsonism that responded to treatment. The last reported case was in a polydrug-abusing chemist who responded to initial treatment, but who died of unrelated causes 2 years later. This individual preferred to snort his drug, but his parkinsonian symptoms were no less severe than those of the intravenous users. When he accidentally drowned, examination of his brain was perfunctory, and the substantia nigra was never even examined (Wright, Wall et al. 1984).

Other than the fact that different age groups are involved (average age in the 30s vs. average age in the 60s), there is little to distinguish parkinsonism occurring after MPTP exposure from parkinsonism in the general population. Initial symptoms may be mild or quite severe, though there is some evidence to suggest that tremor is somewhat less common in the drug abusers.

It is an open question whether additional new cases are likely to be encountered. Only sporadic seizures of samples containing MPTP have been reported. The most recent of these were in 1985, the same year when production of MPTP was made illegal. A closely related analog of MPTP called PEPTP (1,2-phenylethyl-1,2,5,6-tetrahydropyridine) can be generated as a byproduct of PCP production, and may well possess the same neurotoxicity as MPTP, but no cases of parkinsonism attributable to PCP contamination have been reported to date.

References

Adams, J., J. Brierley, R. Connor et al. (1966). The effects of systemic hypotension upon the human brain: clinical and neuropathological observations in 11 cases. Brain. 89:235–268.

Adams, J., J. Corsellis and L. Duchen (1984). Greenfield's Neuropathology, 4th Edition, John Wiley & Sons, New York, 1126.

Adelman, L. and S. Aronson (1969). The neuropathologic complications of narcotics addiction. Bull New York Acad Med. 45(2):225–234.

Akmal, M. and S. Massry (1983). Peripheral nerve damage in patients with nontraumatic rhabdomyolysis. Arch Intern Med. 143:835.

Arlazoroff, A., C. Klein, N. Blumen and A. Ohry (1989). Acute transverse myelitis, a possible vascular etiology. Med Hypothesis. 30:27–30.

Brierley, J. (1972). The neuropathology of brain hypoxia. Scientific Foundations of Neurology. Critchley M. ed., Philadelphia, F.A. Davis Company.

Brust, J. and R. Richter (1976). Stroke associated with addiction to heroin. J Neurol Neurosurg Psychiatry. 39:194–199.

Budka, H. (1991). The definition of HIV-specific neuropathology. Acta Pathol Jpn. 41: 182–191.

Caplan, L., D. Hier and G. Banks (1982). Current concepts of cerebrovascular disease-stroke and drug abuse. Stroke. 13:869–872.

Challenor, Y., R. Richter, B. Bruun and Pearson (1973). Nontraumatic plexitis and heroin addiction. JAMA. 225:958–965.

Chan, Y., P. Wong and T. Chow (1990). Acute myoglobinuria as a fatal complication of heroin addiction. Am J Forensic Med & Pathol 11:160–164.

Chmel, H. and M. Grieco (1973). Cerebral mucormycosis and renal aspergillosis in heroin addicts without endocarditis. Am J Med Sci. 266:225–231.

Citron, B., M. Halpern, M. McCarron et al. (1970). Necrotizing angiitis associated with drug abuse. N Engl J Med. 283:1003–1011.

Creutzfeldt, H. (1926). Histologischer befund bei Morphinismus mit Morphium– und Veronalvergiftung. Ztsch f.d.g. Neurologie u Psychiatrie. 101:97–108.

D'Agostino, R. and E. Arnett (1979). Acute myoglobinuria and heroin snorting. JAMA. 241:277.

Davis, G., A. Williams, S. Markey et al. (1979). Chronic parkinsonism secondary to intravenous injection of meperidine analogues. Psychiatry Res. 1:249–254.

DeGans, J., J. Stam and R. Van Wijngaarden (1985). Rhabdomyolysis and concomitant neurological lesions after intravenous heroin abuse. J Neurol Neurosurg Psychiatr. 48:1057–1059.

Fuller, S. and E. Stein (1991). Effects of heroin and naloxone on cerebral blood flow in the conscious rat. Pharmacol Biochem Behav. 40(2):339–344.

Gibb, W., Shaw, I. (1985). Myoglobinuria due to heroin abuse. J Royal Soc Med. 78: 862–863.

Gill, P., A. Levine, P. Meyer et al. (1985). Primary central nervous system lymphoma in homosexual men: Clinical, immunologic, and pathologic features. Am J Med. 78:742–748.

Gray, G., Lescs, M., C. Keohane et al. (1992). Early brain changes in HIV infection: neuropathological study of 11 HIV seropositive, non-AIDS cases. J Neuropath and Exp Neurol, 51:177–185.

Greenwood, R. (1974). Lumbar plexitis and rhabdomyolysis following abuse of heroin. Postgrad Med J. 50:772–773.

Grindal, A., Cohen, R., Saul, R. et al. (1978). Cerebral infarction in young adults. Stroke, 9:39–42.

Grossman, R., R. Hamilton, B. Morse et al. (1974). Nontraumatic rhabdomyolysis and acute renal failure. N Engl J Med. 291:807–811.

Haan, J., E. Müller and L. Gerhard (1983). Spongiöseleukodystrophie nach drogenmisbrauch. Nervenartz. 54:489–490.

Hall, J. and H. Karp (1973). Acute progressive ventral pontine disease in heroin abuse. Neurology. 23:6–7.

Hameroff, S., J. Eckholdt and R. Lindenberg (1970). Cerebral phycomycosis in a heroin addict. Neurology. 20:261–265.

Hecker, E. and Friedli W. (1988). Plexusläsionen, Rhabdomyolyse und Heroin. Schweiz med Wschr, 118:1982–1988.

Herskowitz, A. and E. Gross (1973). Cerebral infarction associated with heroin sniffing. South Med J. 66:778–784.

Hugentobler, H. and Waespe, W. (1990). Leukoenzephalopathie nach inhalation von Heroin-Pyrolypsat. Schweiz Med Wochenschr, 120:1801–1905.

Jacome, D. (1982). Neurogenic bladder, lumbosacral plexus neuropathy, and drug-associated rhabdomyolysis. J Urol. 127:994.

Jensen, R. and Olsen, T. (1990). Severe non occlusive ischemic stroke in young heroin addicts. Acta Neurol Scand. 81:354–357.

Jervis, G. and F. Joyce (1948). Barbiturate-opiate intoxication with necrosis of the basal ganglia of the brain. Arch Pathol. 45:319–326.

Jones, H., Siekert, R., Geraci, J. (1969). Neurologic manifestations of bacterial endocarditis. Ann Intern Med, 71:21–28.

Kaku, D. and Y. So (1990). Acute femoral neuropathy and iliopsoas infarction in intravenous drug abusers. Neurology. 40(40):1317–1318.

Kasantikul, V., S. Shuangshoti and C. Taecholarn (1987). Primary phycomycosis of the brain in heroin addicts. Surg Neurol. 28:468–472.

King, J., M. Richards and B. Tress (1978). Cerebral arteritis associated with heroin abuse. Med J Aust. 2:444–445.

Koffler, A., R. Friedler and S. Massry (1976). Acute renal failure due to nontraumatic rhabdomyolysis. Ann Intern Med. 85:23–28.

Kreek, M.,Dodes L., S. Kane et al. (1972). Long-term methadone maintenance therapy: effects on liver function. Ann Intern Med,77:598–602.

Langston, J., P. Ballard, J. Tetrud and I. Irwin (1983). Chronic parkinsonism in humans due to a product of meperidine-analog synthesis. Science. 219: 979–980.

Levine, S. and E. Grimes (1973). Pulmonary edema and heroin overdose in Vietnam. Arch Pathol. 95(5):330–332.

McDonough, R., Madden, J., A. Falek et al. (1980). Alteration of T and null lymphocyte frequencies in the peripheral blood of human opiate addicts. *In vivo* evidence for opiate receptor sites on T lymphocytes. J Immunol, 125: 2539–2543.

Morgello, S., E. Cho, S. Nielsen et al. (1987). Cytomegalovirus encephalitis in patients with acquired immunodeficiency syndrome: An autopsy study of 30 cases and a review of the literature. Hum Pathol. 18:289–297.

Masucci, E., J. Fabara, N. Saini and J. Kurtzke (1982). Cerebral mucormycosis (phycomycosis) in a heroin addict. Arch Neurol. 39:304–306.

Micozzi, M. and C. Wetli (1985). Intravenous amphetamine abuse, primary cerebral mucormycosis and acquired immunodeficiency. J Forensic Sci. 30:504–510.

Navia, B., E. Cho, C. Petito and R. Price (1986). The AIDS dementia complex: II Neuropathology. Ann Neurol. 19:525–535.

Navia, B., C. Petito, J. Gold et al. (1986). Cerebral toxoplasmosis complicating the acquired immune deficiency syndrome: Clinical and neuropathological findings in 27 patients. Ann Neurol. 19:224–238.

Nicholls, K., J. Niall and J. Moran (1982). Rhabdomyolysis and renal failure. Med J Aust. 2:387–389.

Nissl, F. (1897). Die Hypothese der specifischen Nervenzellenfunction. Allg. Ztschr f Psychiatrie. 54:1–107.

Ostor, A. (1977). The medical complications of narcotic addiction. Med J Aust. 1: 497–499.

Pearson, J., Y. Challenor, M. Baden and R. Richter (1972). The neuropathology of heroin addiction. J Neuropath and Exp Neurol. 31(1):165–166.

Pearson, J. and R. Richter (1975). Neuropathological effects of opiate addiction. Medical aspects of drug abuse. New York, Evanston, San Francisco, London, Harper & Row.

Penn, A., L. Rowland and D. Fraser (1972). Drugs, coma, and myoglobinuria. Arch Neurol. 26:336–343.

Petito, C., E. Cho, W. Lemann et al. (1986). Neuropathology of acquired immunodeficiency syndrome (AIDS): An autopsy review. J Neuropathol Exp Neurol. 45: 635–646.

Petito, C., B. Navia, E. Cho et al. (1985). Vacuolar myelopathy pathologically resembling subacute combined degeneration in patients with the acquired immunodeficiency syndrome. N Engl J Med. 312:874–879.

Pierce, P., S. Solomon, L. Kaufman et al. (1982). Zygomycetes brain abscesses in narcotic addicts with serological diagnosis. JAMA. 248:2881–2882.

Richter, R., Y. Challenor, J. Pearson et al. (1971). Acute myoglobinuria associated with heroin addiction. JAMA. 216:1172–1176.

Richter, R. and R. Rosenberg (1968). Transverse myelitis associated with heroin addiction. JAMA. 206:1255–1257.

Ruttenber, A. (1991). Stalking the elusive designer drugs: techniques for monitoring new problems in drug abuse. J Addict Dis. 11(1):71–87.

Rodriguez, E., M. Smokvina, J. Sokolow and B. Grynbaum (1972). Encephalopathy and paraplegia occurring with use of heroin. NY State med J Med. 71: 2879–2880.

Roulet Perez, E., Maeder, P., Rivier, L., and Deonna, T. (1992). Toxic leucoencephalopathy after heroin ingestion in a 2½-year-old child. Lancet, 340:729.

Rumbaugh, C., T. Bergeron, H. Fang and R. McCormick (1971). Cerebral angiographic changes in the drug abuse patient. Radiology. 101:335–344.

Sapira, J. (1968). The narcotic addict as a medical patient. Am J Med 45:555–588.

Schein, P., L. Yessayan and C. Mayman (1971). Acute transverse myelitis associated with intravenous opium. Neurology. 21:101–102.

Schiffer, D., Brignolio, F., Giordana, M. et al. (1985). Spongiform encephalopathy in addicts inhaling pre-heated heroin. Clin Neuropathol, 4:174–180.

Schreiber, S., M. Liebowitz, L. Bernstein et al. (1971). Limb compression and renal impairment (crush syndrome) complicating narcotic overdose. N Engl J Med. 284:368–369.

Schawarz, J. (1982). Progress in pathology: the diagnosis of deep mycosis by morphologic methods. Hum Pathol. 13:519–533.

Schwartzfarb, L., G. Singh and D. Marcus (1977). Heroin-associated rhabdomyolysis with cardiac involvement. Arch Intern Med. 137:1255–1257.

Sempere, A., I. Posada, C. Ramo and A. Caabello (1991). Spongiform leukoencephalopathy after inhaling heroin. Lancet. 338:320.

Slayter, W. (1862). Poisoning by opium and gin: fatal result. Lancet,1:326.

So, Y., J. Beckstead and R. Davis (1986). Primary central nervous system lymphoma in acquired immune deficiency syndrome: A clinical and pathological study. Ann Neurol. 20:566–572.

Strassmann, G., W. Sturner and M. Halpern (1969). Gehirnschädigungen ins besondere linsenkernerweichungen bei Heroinsüchtigen nach Barbituratvergiftung, Spättod nach Erhängen und Herzstillstand in der Narkose Beitr Gerichtl Med. 25:236–242.

Strohmaier, A., and Friedrich, M. (1991). Rhabdomyolyse und plexusläsion nach Heroinintoxikation. Radiologe, 31:95–97.

Tetrud, J., J. Langston, P. Garbe and A. Ruttenber (1989). Mild parkinsonism in persons exposed to 1-methyl-4-phenyl-1,2,3,6- tetrahydropyridine (MPTP). Neurology. 39(11):1483–1487.

Thompson, W. and M. Waldman (1970). Cervical myelopathy following heroin administration. J Med Soc NJ. 67:223–224.

Villa, A., Foresti, V., and Confalonieri, F. (1992). Autonomic nervous system dysfunction associated with HIV infection in intravenous heroin users. AIDS, 6:85–89.

Voldby, B., E. Enevoldsen and F. Jensen (1985). Regional CBF, intraventricular pressure, and cerebral metabolism in patients with ruptured intracranial aneurysms. J Neurosurg. 62:48–58.

Wetli, C., S. Weiss, T. Cleary and F.Gyori (1984). Fungal cerebritis from intravenous drug abuse. J Forensic Sci. 29:260–268.

Wolters, E., G. Wijngaarden, F. Stam et al. (1982). Leukoencephalopathy after inhaling heroin pyrolysate. Lancet. ii:1233–1237.

Woods, B. and G. Strewler (1972). Hemiparesis occurring six hours after intravenous heroin injection. Neurology. 22:863–866.

Wright, J., R. Wall, T. Perry and D. Paty (1984). Chronic parkinsonism secondary to intranasal administration of a product of meperidine-analogue synthesis. N Engl J Med. 310:325.

Ziment, I. (1969). Nervous system complications in bacterial endocarditis. Am J Med, 47:593–607.

5.12 HORMONAL AND IMMUNE ALTERATIONS

Host resistance to most pathogens is reduced by opiate abuse. Even prior to the advent of HIV, heroin addicts were known to have higher rates of opportunistic infection and cancer than the population at large (Sapira 1968) (Harris and Garret 1972). Studies done in the early 1900s demonstrated the effects of morphine on lymphocytes (Atchard, Bernhard et al. 1909) (Terry and Pellens 1928). With the advent of intravenous narcotic abuse, sometime in the mid 1920's, other abnormalities of the immune system were observed. These included generalized lymphadenopathy (Halpern and Rho 1966), elevated serum immunoglobins (Kreek et al. 1972), lymphocytosis (Sapira 1968) and abnormal T-cell rosette formation (McDonough et al. 1980). Recently it has become apparent that opiates themselves, and not some associated life-style factor associated with drug abuse, are directly responsible for the immune alterations seen in addicts.

Morphine (but possibly not methadone) alters immune function via centrally mediated effects on neurons in the periacqueductal gray matter (Weber and Pert 1989). Opiates interact with receptors throughout the entire neuroimmune system. Opiate receptors are found on the surfaces of the two major classes of lymphocytes. Among the better known immunologic abnormalities in narcotic abusers are decreased cutaneous sensitivity, decreased mitogen responsiveness (Brown, Stimmel et al. 1974), and depressed levels of T cells as determined by the ability to form E type rosettes with sheep red blood cells (Wybran, Appelboom et al. 1979) (McDonough, Madden et al. 1980) (Donahue, Bueso-Ramos et al. 1987). The fact that this depression can be reversed with naloxone led to the discovery that opiate receptors were located on lymphocytes.

The ability of opiates to alter lymphocyte function is important because lymphocytes, in addition to compromising a major component of the immune system, also have a role in the regulation of macrophages, mast cells and granulocytes. Regulation is accomplished by the release of compounds such as prostaglandins, complement, cytokines and lymphokines. Release of these compounds is in turn modulated by the neuroendocrine axis. The resultant changes in immune response depend on whether or not opiate exposure is acute or chronic, since animals chronically exposed to opiates become tolerant to the initial immunologic effects (Donahoe 1990).

In addition to the indirect control of mast cell function by cytokine release, opiates can also bind directly to specific receptor sites on the mast cell membranes (Fjellner and Hagermark 1982). One result of such binding is histamine release that can lead to bronchospasm, hives, and flushing. Opiate-induced histamine release has occasionally been referred to as "pseudoallergy." IgG class antibodies to morphine and other opiates have been demonstrated in man, but it is not known if the presence of these antibodies has any clinical significance (Biagini, Bernstein et al. 1992) (Biagini, Klincewicz et al. 1990). IgE type opiate antibodies have not been identified, at least in humans. Most addicts have elevated serum immunoglobulins, especially IgM. The elevations are thought to be a consequence of repeatedly injecting antigenic material (Millian and Cherubin 1971). The changes revert when heroin use is discontinued (Cushman 1980).

Current research centers on the possible role of opiates as cofactors in HIV infection. Comparisons of HIV seronegative intravenous narcotic users with seronegative, rehabilitated methadone users and normals have shown that natural killer activity is significantly reduced in the heroin users when compared to activity measured in methadone maintenance patients and controls. Measurements made in these same individuals show higher absolute numbers of CD2, CD3, CD4, and CD8--positive cells (Novick et al. 1989). Similar changes have been observed in mice chronically treated with morphine. Mice treated with opiates have increased numbers of CD4 cells in the spleen and thymus (Arpra, Fride et al. 1990). Measurements in heroin users have confirmed the presence of increased numbers of CD4+/T cells. Since the CD4 antigen is the receptor the HIV virus uses to get into T cells, the presence of increased numbers of CD4 cells in narcotic abusers may favor HIV infection (Pillai, Nair et al. 1991). The observation is of clinical significance, since it has also been shown that long-term methadone maintenance normalizes lymphocyte function (Novick, Ochshorn et al. 1989).

TABLE 5.12
IMMUNE ABNORMALITIES IN OPIATE ABUSERS
Depressed E-rosette formation (in vitro)
Depressed cutaneous sensitivity
Depressed mitogenic response
Elevated CD4 cells
Elevated CD4/CD8 ratio
Elevated levels of CD4 receptor
Elevated neopterin levels
Elevated soluble interleukin 2 receptors
Elevated gamma interferon levels

Adapted from Pillai et al., 1991.

References

Arora, L., E. Fride, J. Petitto et al. (1990). Morphine induced immune alterations in vivo. Cell Immunol. 126:343–353.

Achard, C., H. Bernard and C. Gagneux (1909). Action de la morphine sur les propriétés leucocytaires: leuco-diagnostic du morphinisme. Bull et Mem Soc Med Hosp Paris. 28:958–966.

Biagini, R., S. Klincewicz, G. Henningsen et al. (1990). Antibodies to morphine in workers occupationally exposed to opiates at a narcotics-manufacturing facility and evidence for similar antibodies in heroin abusers. Life Sci 47:897–908.

Biagini, R., D. Bernstein, S. Klincewicz et al. (1992). Evaluation of cutaneous responses and lung function from exposure to opiate compounds among ethical narcotics-manufacturing workers. J Allerg Clin Immunol. 89(1):108–118.

Brown, S., B. Stimmel, R. Taub et al. (1974). Immunologic dysfunction in heroin addicts. Arch Int Med. 134:1001–1006.

Cushman, P. (1980). The major medical sequelae of opioid addiction. Drug Alcohol Depend. 5:239–254.

Donohoe, R. (1991). Immune effects of opiates in test tubes and monkeys. Problems of Drug Dependence, 1990: Proceedings of the 52nd Annual Scientific Meeting of the Committee on Problems of Drug Dependence. Rockville, MD, NIDA Research Monograph Series,105:103–108.

Donohoe, R., C. Bueso-Ramos, F. Donahoe et al. (1987). Mechanistic implications of the findings that opiates and other drugs of abuse moderate T cell surface receptors and antigenic markers. Ann NY Acad Sci. 496:711–721.

Fjellner, B. and Ö. Hägermark (1982). Potentiation of histamine-induced itch and flare responses in human skin by the enkephalin analogue FK-33-824, beta-endorphin, and morphine. Arch Derm Res. 274:29–37.

Harris, P. and R. Garret (1972). Susceptibility of addicts to infection and neoplasia. N Engl J Med. 287:310.

Helpern, M. and Y. Rho (1966). Deaths from narcotism in New York City. N.Y. State Med J. 66:2391–2408.

McDonough, R., J. Madden, A. Falek et al. (1980). Alteration of T and null lymphocyte frequencies in the peripheral blood of human opiate addicts: in vivo evidence for opiate receptor sites on T lymphocytes. J Immunol. 125:2539–2543.

Millian, S. and C. Cherubin (1971). Serologic investigations in narcotic addicts. Am J Clin Pathol. 56:693–698.

Novick, D., M. Ochshorn, V. Ghali et al. (1989). Natural killer cell activity and lymphocyte subsets in parenteral heroin abusers and long-term methadone maintenance patients. J Pharm and Exp Ther. 250(2): 606–610.

Pillai, R., B. Nair and R. Watson (1991). Aids, drugs of abuse and the immune system: a complex immunotoxicological network. Arch Toxicol. 65:609–617.

Sapira, J. (1968). The narcotic addict as a medical patient. Am J Med. 45:555–588.

Terry, C. and M. Pellens (1928). The opium problem. New York, Committee on Drug Addictions in collaboration with the Bureau of Social Hygiene, Inc.

Weber, R. and A. Pert (1989). The periaqueductal gray matter mediates opiate-induced immunosuppression. Science. 245:188–190.

Wybran, J., T. Appelboom, J. Famaey and A. Govaerts (1979). Suggestive evidence for receptors for morphine and methionine-enkephalin on normal human blood lymphocyter. J Immunol, 123:1068–1070.

5.13 BONE AND SOFT TISSUE DISORDERS

5.13.1 INTRODUCTION

Except for the fibrous myopathy associated with chronic pentazocine abuse, virtually all of the bone and soft tissue disorders seen in opiate abusers are infectious in origin. Infectious complications are, in fact, the main reason that drug abusers are hospitalized (White 1973) (Cherubin 1967). Directly or indirectly, especially if HIV infection is included, infectious complications also account for the majority of deaths. In the past such exotic infections as malaria and tetanus were common. These disorders have been replaced by endocarditis, hepatitis, and HIV infection, but much more mundane conditions such as cellulitis, soft tissue abscess, and septic thrombophlebitis are the conditions which most often bring the abuser to medical attention.

5.13.2 BONE AND JOINT INFECTION

In most instances, the source of bone and soft tissue infections is either the solution used to dissolve the drug or the abuser's own skin flora (Tuazon, Hill et al. 1974). Once introduced into the body, the infection may spread locally or hematogenously. The pattern of sites most frequently infected, and the organism responsible for the infection, appears to be changing. In the past, the skeletal sites most frequently infected were the vertebral column and sternoarticular joints (Waldvogel and Vasey 1980). In more recent studies the extremities, especially the left knee (Chandrasekar and Narula 1986), were found to be involved much more than the sternoarticular joint. The shift seems to be due to the fact that more addicts are injecting themselves in the groin, and the fact that infection is most likely to occur in the structures closest to the injection site. Since most individuals are right handed, the left side is most frequently injected.

In early studies *P aeruginosa* was responsible for most (more than 80%) of the joint and bone infections in intravenous drug abusers (Waldvogel and Vasey 1980) (McHenry, Alfidi et al. 1975). The results of studies published in the mid 1980's indicate that a shift to gram positive organism has occurred (Chandrasekar and Narula 1986) (Ang-Fonte, Rozboril et al. 1985) (Dreyfuss, Djedaini et al. 1992). Infections with *candida* are increasingly frequent, but it is not obvious that the increase has anything to do with HIV infection.

Except in addicts, infections of the cervical spine are rare in adults. While rare in the past, infection of the upper spine is becoming more common, and the infectious agent is, more often than not, *staphylococcus*. Just as addicts are using the large vessels in the groin, they are also injecting into the great veins of the neck, introducing *staphylococcus* from their skin (Endress, Guyot et al. 1990). In life, CT scanning will show an inflammatory reaction about the carotid sheath with prevertebral soft-tissue masses adjacent to the areas of bone destruction.

Candida bone infections, on the other hand, almost never involve the cervical spine. They occur with increased frequency in intravenous abusers and in patients with indwelling venous catheters, and the route of *candida* infection is hematogenous. Just why the blood supply should favor the lower lumbar spine is not obvious, but almost all cases of *Candida* osteomyelitis have involved the lower lumbar area. Infection spreads into the endplate of the vertebral body, which is supplied by ventral branches of the spinal arteries. *C. albicans* is the responsible agent in two thirds of the cases (Almekinders and Greene 1991).

Tuberculosis is occurring with increased frequency in addicts, especially those that are HIV seropositive. Extrapulmonary involvement, with or without obvious lung lesions, is seen in 15% of cases (Alvarez 1984), and in many of these the extrapulmonary site involved is osteoarticular, usually the vertebral bodies and their intervertebral discs. Involvement of the bony arch usually produces a compression syndrome. Fortunately, involvement of the arch is rare, but it has been reported in intravenous heroin users (Mallolas, 1988).

5.13.3 SOFT TISSUE INFECTIONS

Though skin and soft tissue infections are common among intravenous abusers, there is nothing to distinguish their appearance from similar lesions in non-drug users. The bacteriology of these infections is somewhat controversial, with conflicting results being reported from different centers. In one series, most infections were polymicrobial, and only 19% had isolates of *S. aureus*, the remainder being anaerobes, including clostridia and *Bacteroides spp* (Webb and Thadepalli 1979). Other series have also described polymicrobial infections, with *S. aureus* present in almost every case, along with enteric gram negative aerobes and oropharyngeal organisms (Orangio, Pitalick et al. 1984). *E. corrodens*, a gram negative anaerobe, part of the normal flora in the mouth, is occasionally seen when addicts use their saliva to dilute or dissolve their drug for injection (Brooks, O'Donoghue et al. 1979)

5.13.4 FIBROUS MYOPATHY OF PENTAZOCINE ABUSE

Woody infiltration, cutaneous ulcers and abnormal pigmentation can be seen surrounding areas of repeated pentazocine injection. Clinically the syndrome is marked by limitation of motion, neuropathic symptoms, and even muscle and joint contractures (Oh 1975). The contractures and neuropathic symptoms are secondary to nerve damage and reflex sympathetic dystrophy (Roberson 1983) (Hertzman 1986).

The syndrome may be the result of a foreign body reaction, with crystallization of the drug within the muscle (Levin 1973) (Oh 1975). This possibility is suggested by the fact that birefringent crystals have been demonstrated in the areas of most intense induration (Adams 1983). Myocytes are destroyed and replaced with dense, fibrotic tissue. Inflammatory infiltrates may or may not be present. Dystrophic calcification may be so marked that it sometimes can be detected by CT scanning or sonography.

References

Adams, E., Horowitz, H., and W. Sundstrom (1983). Fibrous myopathy in association with pentazocine. Arch Intern Med, 143:2203–2204.

Almekinders, L. C. and W. B. Greene (1991). Vertebral candida infections - a case report and review of the literature. Clin Orthop. (267):174–178.

Alvarez, S., McCabe, W. (1984). Extrapulmonary tuberculosis revisited: a review of experience at Boston City and other hospitals. Medicine, 63:25–55.

Ang-Fonte, G., M. Rozboril and G. Thompson (1985). Changes in nongonococcal septic arthritis: drug abuse and methicillin-resistant *Staphylococcus aureus*. Arthritis Rheum. 28:210–213.

Brooks, G., J. O'Donoghue, J. Rissing et al. (1979). *Eikenella Corrodens* A recently recognized pathogen: infections in medical-surgical patients in association with methylphenidate abuse. Medicine. 53(5):325–42.

Chandrasekar, P. and A. Narula (1986). Bone and joint infections in intravenous drug abusers. Rev Infect Dis. 8(6):904–911.

Cherubin, C. (1967). The medical sequelae of narcotic addiction. Ann Intern Med. 67: 23–33.

Dreyfuss, D., Djedaini, K, Bidault-Lapomme, C. et al. (1992). Nontraumatic acute anterior mediastinitis in two HIV-positive heroin addicts. Chest, 101:583–585.

Endress, C., D. Guyot, J. Fata and G. Salciccioli (1990). Cervical osteomyelitis due to IV heroin use: radiologic findings in 14 patients. Am J Radiol.155:333–335.

Hertzman, A., Toone, E. and C. Resnik (1986). Pentazocine induced myocutaneous sclerosis. J Rheumatol, 13:210–214.

McHenry, M, R. Alfidi, A. Wilde and W. Hawk (1975). Hematogenous osteomyelitis: a changing disease. Clevel Clin Q. 42:125–153.

Mollalas, J., Gatell, J., M. Rovira et al. (1988). Vertebral arch tuberculosis in two human immunodeficiency virus-seropositive heroin addicts. Arch Intern Med, 148:1125–1127.

Oh, S., Rollins, J. and I. Lewis (1975). Pentazocine-induced fibrous myopathy. JAMA, 231:271–273.

Orangio, G., S. Pitlick, P. Latta et al. (1984). Soft tissue infections in parenteral drug abusers. Ann Surg. 199:97–100.

Roberson, J., and J. Dimon (1983). Myofibrosis and joint contractures caused by injections of pentazocine. J Bone Joint Surg, 65A:1007–1009.

Tuazon, C., R. Hill and J. Sheagren (1974). Microbiologic study of street heroin and injection paraphernalia. J Infect Dis. 129:327–329.

Waldvogel, F. and H. Vasey (1980). Osteomyelitis: the past decade. N Engl J Med. 303:360–370.

Webb, D. and H. Thadepalli (1979). Skin and soft tissue polymicrobial infections from intravenous abuse of drugs. West J Med. 130:200–204.

White, A. (1973). Medical disorders in drug addicts: 200 consecutive admissions. JAMA 223:1469–1471.

6 Anabolic Steroids

6.1 INTRODUCTION

Anabolic steroids are synthetic compounds that are structurally related to testosterone, the male sex hormone. Testosterone has two different effects on the body: it promotes the development of secondary male sexual characteristics (androgenic effects), and it accelerates muscle growth (anabolic effects). The hormonal basis for male sexual characteristics was discovered by Berthold in 1849. He observed that the male characteristics of roosters disappeared when they were castrated, and reappeared when the testes were implanted in the abdomen. Berthold correctly deduced that the testes were secreting something into the blood that controlled the development of male traits. In 1930, another scientist from the same medical school in Gottingen, where Berthold had made his original discovery, succeeded in isolating 15 mg of a compound with anabolic activity, from 25,000 liters of policemen's urine. The compound was named androsterone because it was virilizing (andro from the Greek for male), because the nucleus of its molecule was like that of cholesterol's ("ster" for sterol), and because it contained a ketone group ("one"). A few years later testosterone was crystallized from bull testes (testo = testis) and its chemical structure characterized (Kochakian 1990).

When experimenters in the 1940's were finally able to synthesize testosterone, they were disappointed to find that it had minimal effect when given orally. Subsequent research demonstrated that testosterone's positive effects on nitrogen balance and muscle growth could, at least partially, be separated from its androgenic effects. In the process of trying to separate the androgenic from the anabolic effects, it was observed that substitutions at the 17-position produced orally absorbed compounds that had anabolic effects with only a fraction of testosterone's androgenic effects. Further manipulations of the testosterone molecule at the 17-position have led to the production of a series of "anabolic" steroids that are active when taken orally.

No agent is purely anabolic. All so-called "anabolic steroids" exert androgenic effects, and the only difference between agents is the proportion of anabolic to androgenic effects that are produced. When commercially prepared anabolic steroids became available, just before

aging without wasting...

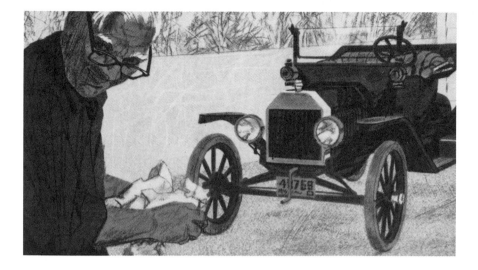

supportive oral anabolic therapy • potent • well-tolerated

With advancing age, weakness and weight loss may indicate a "wasting" of dietary protein due to poor protein metabolism. A potent, well-tolerated anabolic agent plus a diet high in protein can make a remarkable difference. Patients show a notable increase in strength, vigor and sense of well-being. There is marked improvement in appetite, measurable weight gain. The natural anabolic processes are helped in the utilization of dietary protein for tissue building and other vital functions.

WINSTROL® brand of STANOZOLOL

...a new oral anabolic agent, combines high anabolic activity with outstanding tolerance. Although its androgenic influence is extremely low*, women and children should be observed for signs of slight virilization (hirsutism, acne or voice change), and young women may experience milder or shorter menstrual periods. These effects are reversible when dosage is decreased or therapy discontinued. Patients with impaired cardiac or renal function should be observed because of the possibility of sodium and water retention. Liver function tests may reveal an increase in BSP retention, particularly in elderly patients, in which case therapy should be discontinued. Although it has been used in patients with cancer of the prostate, its mild androgenic activity is considered by some investigators to be a contraindication.

Dosage in adults, *usually 1 tablet t.i.d.; young women, 1 tablet b.i.d.; children (school age), up to 1 tablet t.i.d.; children (pre-school age), ½ tablet b.i.d. Shows best results when administered with a high protein diet. Available as scored tablets of 2 mg. in bottles of 100.*

The therapeutic value of anabolic agents depends on the ratio of anabolic potency to androgenic effect. This anabolic androgenic ratio of Winstrol is especially great because it combines high potency with low androgenic activity.

Winthrop Laboratories, New York, N. Y.

Figure 6.1 Anabolic steroids
When these agents first became available, they were often used for indications that are no longer considered acceptable today. This advertisement is from a 1961 issue of JAMA.

World War II, they were used to promote healing, and speed recovery. It quickly became apparent that these drugs also had the ability to alter mood, and they were even used to treat depression (Bahrke, Yesalis et al. 1990). It is alleged that steroids were given to German storm troopers to increase both strength and hostility. The notion that steroids might improve physical performance is attributed to Boje, who published his ideas in 1939 (Boje 1939). Table 6.2.1.1 lists the anabolic steroids most commonly abused today. There is a thriving black market for these drugs, and much clandestine production and importation. Analysis of confiscated samples has shown wide variation in steroid content. Many products are falsely labeled.

Athletes use steroids because the believe that by taking them they will improve their performance. Specifically, it has been claimed that steroid use (1) increases lean body mass, (2) increases strength, (3) increases aggressiveness, and (4) leads to a shorter recovery time between workouts. There is some evidence to support all of these claims, particularly the increases in strength (Plymate & Friedl, 1992), but rigidly controlled studies have never been done, nor are they likely to be. Athletes use doses of steroids that most physicians consider dangerous, and ethical considerations prevent physicians from participating in "megadose" steroid studies. Anecdotal reports suggest that East German scientists have done many of the requisite studies, but their results have never been published.

The steroid-abusing subculture recognizes three patterns of steroid use. These are referred to as stacking, cycling, and pyramiding. "Stacking" refers to the practice of using several different steroid preparations at once. The hope is that maximal anabolic effects will be achieved while, at the same time, the androgenic effects are minimized. "Cycling" describes a pattern of usage where combinations of drugs are taken in alternating six to twelve week cycles. The rationale here is that the practice will prevent tolerance from occurring. "Pyramiders" start with low doses of the drug and gradually increase the amount of drug taken over several weeks, tapering off entirely before a competition. Not uncommonly, serious steroid abusers combine all three approaches.

The real incidence of steroid abuse in general, and as a cause of medical problems in particular, is hard to evaluate. The DAWN report for 1990 contains no mention of steroid-related deaths or emergency room visits (National Institute on Drug Abuse 1990). Single case reports of steroid related deaths and vascular disease have increased, but are still uncommon. Multiple surveys have confirmed steroid abuse in at least 7% of high-school aged males and 1% of females. When an announced drug testing program was initiated by the National Collegiate Athletic Association, steroid use was detected in fewer than 1% of the athletes, but when the International Olympic committee performed surprise, nonpunitive, testing in 1984-1985, approximately 50% of those tested were positive for steroids (Yesalis, Anderson et al. 1990)!

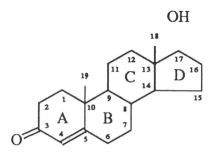

Testosterone

Figure 6.2.1 Testosterone
Testosterone is rapidly degraded by the liver when it is given orally. Modifications at the 17 position, such as esterification of the β hydroxyl group, prevent
hepatic breakdown and allow the drug to be given orally.

6.2 PHARMACOLOGY

6.2.1 SYNTHESIS AND METABOLISM

Testosterone is synthesized in the testes and adrenal glands, but
only about 5% originates in the adrenals. It is a 19-carbon molecule
synthesized from cholesterol. Cholesterol is produced from acetate
stored in the testes, not from circulating cholesterol bound to low-
density lipoprotein. Conversion from cholesterol to pregnenolone occurs
in the mitochondria. From there the pregnenolone is transported to the
endoplasmic reticulum, where a three-step synthesis converts it to testosterone. Once it is produced, testosterone is immediately released into
the circulation. It has been estimated that a normal adult male produces
6 mg of testosterone per day.

Once it is released into the blood stream, approximately 50% of
the testosterone circulates tightly bound to sex-hormone-binding
globulin (SHBG). The latter is a glycoprotein produced in the liver.
Much smaller amounts circulate loosely bound to albumin. The bond
between albumin and testosterone is so weak that for practical purposes
it can be considered unbound. Free testosterone seems to enter cells by
simple diffusion. Once it does, it or a metabolite binds to a steroid
receptor in the cytosol that is transported to the nucleus where it
initiates DNA transcription. Because the testosterone bound to SHBG is
so tightly bound, it probably never enters cells. For that reason, changes
in the concentration of SHBG must be considered when measuring total
testosterone blood levels, since they may drastically affect the observed

half-life of the drug. Half-life values reported in the literature have ranged anywhere from 10 to 100 minutes.

When testosterone is given orally, nearly half will be metabolized on the first pass through the liver, so very large oral doses are required to produce any therapeutic effect. Agents such as methyltestosterone are not as extensively metabolized by the liver, which is why they can be used orally. There are two pathways in the liver by which testosterone is broken down into a series of 17 ketosteroids. The latter are excreted in the urine, along with much larger amounts of 17 keto steroids that are produced in the adrenal cortex. About 90% of a dose of testosterone is excreted in the urine either as the glucuronic or sulfuric acid conjugates. Approximately 6% is excreted unconjugated in the feces, and small amounts of glucuronide may appear in the bile. Less than 250 μg per day of testosterone appears unchanged in the urine. For testing purposes, most programs monitor the ratio of testosterone to epitestosterone that is excreted in the urine. In healthy young men this ratio is known to be less than 1.2, but the International Olympic Committee accepts as normal any value of less than 1.6.

TABLE 6.2.1.1
COMMERCIALLY AVAILABLE STEROID PREPARATIONS

Injectable agents:
  Deca-Durbolin (Nandrolone decanoate)
  Depo-Testosterone (Testosterone cypionate)
  Delatestryl (Testosterone enanthate)
  Durabolin (Nandrolone phenpropionate)
  Oreton (Testosterone propionate)
  Primobolan (Methenolone enanthate)

Oral agents:
  Anadrol-50 (Oxymetholone)
  Anavar (Oxandrolone)
  Dianabol (Methandrostenolone)
  Halotestin (Fluoxymesterone)
  Maxibolin (Ethylestrenol)
  Metandren (Methyltestosterone)
  Nibal (Methenolone acetate)
  Nilevar (Norethandrolone)
  Winstrol (Stanozolol)

6.3 LEGITIMATE CLINICAL INDICATIONS

In males the only legitimate indication for androgen is replacement therapy when, for whatever reason (trauma, congenital), there is testicular failure. Androgens are occasionally used to treat women who have metastatic breast cancer with bone involvement. Steroids classified as anabolic agents, such as stanozolol (Winstrol™) are indicated only for use in the treatment of hereditary angioedema. Compounds with both androgenic and anabolic effects are also indicated for the treatment of deficient red cell production, as occurs in acquired aplastic anemia and myelofibrosis. Methyltestosterone is occasionally sold in combination with estrogens (Premarin™) for the relief of symptoms associated with menopause.

6.4 STEROID RELATED DISORDERS

6.4.1 LIVER DISEASE

Elevated liver enzymes have been observed in steroid-abusing athletes, but since exercise itself can be associated with some enzyme changes (depending on when the sample is drawn in relation to exercise), it is hard to be sure that any connection exists at all (Graham and Kennedy 1990). The connections between peliosis hepatis and steroid use is much firmer, and the evidence that anabolic steroid use can cause hepatic adenomas is convincing, but evidence for hepatoma and other malignancies is not so strong (especially given the enormous number of people taking these drugs).

6.4.1.1 Peliosis hepatis

This obscure disorder has been recognized for well over 100 years. Histologically its appearance is characterized by the presence of scattered, small, cystic, blood-filled lakes scattered throughout the liver. Some of the cysts may be lined with epithelium while others are not (Kalra, Mangla et al. 1976). These collections of blood often abut on zones of hepatocellular necrosis. The lungs may also be involved in the same process, as may the entire reticuloendothelial system. Lesions have been described in the spleen, lymph nodes, and bone marrow (Kent and Thompson 1961) (Taxy 1978).

Peliosis was first described in tuberculosis patients (Zak 1950), but over the years reports have been published linking peliosis to many other conditions. The connection between anabolic steroids and peliosis was first noted in 1952 (Burger and Marcuse 1952), and since then has been reconfirmed on many occasions. In one series of 38 patients with peliosis, 27 had hematologic disorders and all 27 had been treated with 17 alpha-alkyl substituted steroids (Boyer 1978). In an autopsy study of patients with aplastic anemia, one third of the patients treated with steroids had peliosis. Only 3 percent of the patients who had not been so treated had peliosis (Wakabayashi, Onda et al. 1984). Other studies have confirmed the steroid connection (Friedl 1990). Testosterone and the testosterone esters have not been implicated. In all of the steroid/peliosis case reports, 17-alkylated androgens have been the responsible agents.

Peliosis is not easily diagnosed in life. If studied, patients with peliosis will have abnormal liver scans (Lowdell and Murray-Lyon 1985), but since they are mostly asymptomatic, the probability that they will be scanned is small. Patients with peliosis occasionally bleed to death from these lesions (Bagheri and Boyer 1974b) (Nadell and Kosek 1977) (Taxy 1978), or die of hepatic coma, but since most of them were gravely ill with other disorders, it is hard to tell what prompted the fatal event. Recently peliosis has been described in AIDS patients, where the lesions may be confused with Kaposi's sarcoma (Czapar, Weldon-Linne et al. 1986).

At first it was thought that peliosis was congenital (Zak 1950), however that explanation seems unlikely, especially since cows with peliosis (referred to as St. George's disease) have been cured simply by change of pasture (Graham and Kennedy 1990). Another explanation was suggested by Paradinas et al. who, after analyzing biopsy material from individuals with peliosis, suggested that the 17-alkylated androgens induce hepatocyte hyperplasia. If the hyperplasia is marked, then the hepatocytes can obstruct venous drainage, and maybe even the bile canaliculi (Paradinas, Bull et al. 1977). The problem with this theory is that it doesn't explain how some of the cysts come to have an endothelial lining. The results of the most recent study on the subject suggest that peliosis may be the result of an infectious process related to, or possibly the same as, bacillary angiomatosis, a lesion usually found only in individuals with HIV infection (Leong, Cazen, Yu et al. 1992). The bacilli responsible for bacillary angiomatosis have staining and histologic similarities with the bacilli known to cause cat scratch disease, but whether infection with this agent is responsible for all cases of peliosis remains to be seen.

6.4.1.2 Cholestasis

The 17 alpha-alkyl substituted steroids can cause cholestatic jaundice. Bile accumulates in the canaliculi, but without evidence of inflammation or necrosis (Foss and Simpson 1959). There are many cases in the literature and the connection with steroid abuse seems clear (Foss and Simpson 1959) (Lucey and Moseley 1987). However, the frequency with which cholestasis occurs is not clear. Different estimates have placed the incidence of cholestasis at anywhere from less than 1% to at least 17% (Friedl 1990). Several deaths from cholestatic jaundice have been attributed to steroids, but they occurred in elderly, debilitated patients, and the evidence of causality is far from convincing (Friedl 1990). Based on animal studies, the mechanism for bile accumulation appears to involve a disruption of the microfilaments within the hepatocytes that reduces the ability of the cells to transport bile (Phillips, Oda et al. 1978).

6.4.1.3 Hepatic Tumors

A clear association exists between use of C-17 alkylated androgens and hepatic tumors. Hepatocellular adenomas, similar in many ways to the adenomas that arise in the livers of women taking birth control pills, are not uncommon, even in non-steroid using men. Judging from the number of reports, the incidence is 1 to 3 per cent among the 17 alkylated androgen users (Friedl 1990). The difficulty of assessing the frequency of the lesion is the fact that, like peliosis, it is usually silent, only coming to medical attention when adenomas are found incidentally at autopsy, or when they rupture and cause hemoperitoneum (Bruguera 1975) (Lesna, Spencer et al. 1976) (Paradinas, Bull et al. 1977) (Boyd and Mark 1977) (Hermandez-Nieto, Bruguera et al. 1977) (Bird, Vowles et al. 1979) (Westaby, Portmann et al. 1983) (Creagh, Rubin et al. 1988).

Adenomas have the same appearance in both androgen and birth-control users. They are comprised of sheets of cells that look like normal hepatocytes. There are, however, some differences. For one thing, androgen-related adenomas tend to be bigger. Adenomas in steroid users range in size from a few millimeters to several centimeters across. Androgen-related adenomas often form bile-containing acini, and absent a history of androgen abuse, acini formation is usually considered to be histologic evidence of malignancy. Adenomas in steroid users may also display other features which are suspect for malignancy, such as bizarre nuclei and even rare mitoses (Creagh, Rubin et al. 1988). The benign nature of most such lesions is confirmed by their sharply demarcated margins, their failure to metastasize, the absence of demonstrable alpha feto protein, and the absence of associated cirrhosis (which is the setting where hepatocellular carcinoma is most often found). The fact that adenomas regress when androgens are discontinued also argues against their malignant nature (Friedl 1990). Nonetheless, hepatocellular carcinoma has been reported in C-17 substituted androgen users (Overly, Dankoff et al. 1984), so the possibility for conversion from adenoma to carcinoma cannot be ruled out (Boyd and Mark 1977).

Like peliosis, hepatic adenomas can be difficult to diagnose in life. Liver function tests may well be normal (Westaby, Portmann et al. 1983), and the distribution of these lesions can be patchy (Bagheri and Boyer 1974a) (Westaby, Ogle et al. 1977), so that percutaneous biopsy may well miss the lesions. There are proven instances where nodular hyperplasia resulted in portal hypertension, even in the face of a normal biopsy (Stromeyer and Ishak 1981). This possibility is confirmed by one report of bleeding varices in a steroid abuser, where biopsy was negative and there were no other risk factors or findings to account for the bleeding (Winwood, Robertson et al. 1990).

6.4.2 CARDIOVASCULAR DISEASE

Myocardial infarction, sudden arrhythmic death, and stroke have all been described in young steroid abusers. There are many good reasons why that should be, including the fact that highly conditioned athletes, the individuals most likely to abuse steroids, do not have anatomically normal hearts to begin with (Huston, Puffer et al. 1985), and the fact that anabolic androgens have direct effects on cardiac growth and metabolism (Kinson, Layberry & Hébert 1991). Relevant animal studies are almost entirely lacking and so few cases reports have been published that generalization is impossible.

The first documented steroid-related infarct was reported in 1988. Angiography showed no lesions, but the patient was hyperlipidemic and had evidence of increased platelet aggregation (McNutt, Ferenchick et al. 1988). Another case associated with hyperlipidemia was reported in 1989 (Graham and Kennedy 1990), and a third case with thrombotic occlusion of both the left main and left anterior descending coronary arteries was briefly described in 1991 (Ferenchick 1991). Infarction has even been reported in a weight lifter who was abusing aspirin and testosterone simultaneously (Ferenchick and Adelman, 1992). Arterial thrombosis manifested as saddle pulmonary embolus in a steroid-abusing weight lifter has been described (Montine and Gaede 1992), and another paper recounts the clinical history a of 32-year old with "cardiomyopathy" and stroke (Mochizuki and Richter 1988). Since this last patient did not undergo angiography or biopsy, the diagnosis of cardiomyopathy remains in question, but the autopsy findings in another recent case of sudden arrhythmic death did, in fact, demonstrate prominent myocardial fibrosis (Luke, Farb et al. 1991), not unlike the changes that have been described in stimulant abusers' hearts (Karch and Billingham 1988).

If, in fact, steroid abusers are more prone to thrombosis and infarction than the rest of the population, it might be explained by the 50% decrease in high-density lipoprotein levels that has been documented in some steroid-abusing athletes. At the same time, low-density lipoprotein levels increase by more than 36% (Glazer 1991). Hyperlipidemia, in turn, initiates a train of events, all of which have unfavorable effects on the vascular system. There is even evidence that hypercholesteremia potentiates coronary-artery response to epinephrine (Rosendorff, Hoffman et al. 1981). Hyperlipidemia leads to hyperinsulinemia (Friedl, Jones et al. 1989), and hyperinsulinemia is known to be associated with accelerated atherogenesis (Ducimetriere, Eschwere et al. 1980). Hyperlipidemia also favors increased platelet aggregation (Sano, Motomiya et al. 1983). The problem with implicating lipids as the cause of thrombosis in the steroid abusing subpopulation is that different steroids have different effects on the lipid profile (Thompson, Cullinane et al. 1989). In some instances the effects may even be beneficial (Maciejko, Holmes et al.

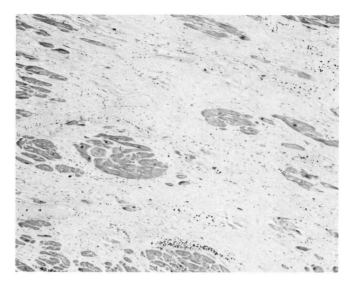

Figure 6.4.2 Myocardial fibrosis
Section of an interventricular septum taken from a steroid-abusing weight lifter
who died of an arrythmia. There is no extensive myocardial fibrosis which
probably accounts for the occurrence of the arrythmia. Original magnification
60x. Courtesy of Dr. Renu Virmani, Chairman, Department of Cardiovascular
Pathology, Armed Forces Institute of Pathology.

1983), but since the steroid abusers themselves rarely know what drug
they are really taking, determining cause-and-effect relationships is
nearly impossible.

Even though only one case of "cardiomyopathy" has been described, the argument for steroid-induced alterations in the myocardium is
strong and could conceivably account for some cases of sudden death
in athletes. In experimental studies, guinea pigs and rats treated with
methandrostenolone predictably develop myocyte necrosis, cellular
edema, and mitochondrial swelling (Behrendt and Boffin 1977) (Appell,
Heller-Umpfenbach et al. 1983). Clinical echocardiographic studies have
yielded conflicting results as to whether anabolic steroids counteract the
improvement of cardiac performance that results from endurance training (Takala, Ramo et al. 1991), but there is no question that animals
given steroids have morphologic alterations in their hearts, and that
these alterations are different from those produced by exercise alone
(Appell, Heller-Umpfenbach et al. 1983). In beagles, anabolic steroids
modulate the increased collagen production normally seen in the hearts
of animals that have undergone endurance training (Takala, Ramo et al.
1991). In murine peripheral muscle, anabolic steroid administration
results in mitochondrial disruption and, most importantly, a decrease in
myocyte capillary supply. Decreases also occur in the total number of

mitochondria present when compared to muscle fibers from animals not treated with steroids (Tesch 1987) (Soares and Duarte 1991).

If similar subcellular changes occur in human hearts, it could explain the histologic picture recently seen in a case of sudden death reported by Luke et al (Luke, Farb et al. 1991). They described the findings in a 21-year-old, previously healthy, steroid abusing (nandrolone and testosterone) weight lifter who died of cardiac arrest. In addition to renal hypertrophy and hepatosplenomegally, there was biventricular hypertrophy with chamber dilatation. The heart weighed 530 grams, but the valves and coronary arteries were entirely normal. Sectioned myocardium showed extensive fibrosis, especially in the subendocardium and the central parts of the left ventricle and intraventricular septum. One area of fibrosis measured more than 8 cm across. Microscopic sections disclosed small foci of necrosis with sparse neutrophilic and round cell infiltrates. In some of these small foci of necrosis, myocytes with contraction band necrosis were evident. While there is no way to rule out occult myocarditis in this particular individual, the similarities to catechol toxicity are quite striking (Reichenbach and Benditt 1970).

Several mechanisms could explain fibrosis in these cases. If muscle fiber hypertrophy is not accompanied by proportionate increases in blood supply, small areas of infarction may result. When these areas of infarction heal, they are replaced by fibrosis. Alternatively, it has been known for many years that steroids can also cause contraction band necrosis (Karch and Billingham, 1986). It is even conceivable that steroid use might in some way produce catechol elevation, but studies are lacking. Whatever the cause, fibrotic material has conduction properties quite unlike those of normal muscle, and areas of fibrosis may later provide the anatomic substrate for lethal reentrant arrhythmias. However, until more autopsy material becomes available, the mechanism for sudden death in these individuals remains speculative.

6.4.3 NEUROLOGIC DISORDERS

Cases of cerebral thrombosis have been reported (Mochizuki and Richter 1988) (Frankle, Eichberg et al. 1988), but they are decidedly rare events. Psychiatric disturbances are, on the other hand, relatively common, and steroid-related psychosis has been used as a defense in several murder trials. One study of 41 self-admitted steroid abusers found that 22% of those interviewed had affective disorders and that 12% had episodes of frank psychosis (Pope and Katz 1988). Another study described three men, none with previous psychiatric histories, who committed violent crimes, including murder, while they were taking steroids. In each instance, anabolic steroids were thought to have played a role, and in all three cases the men returned to their normal premorbid personalities when the steroids were withdrawn (Pope and Katz 1990).

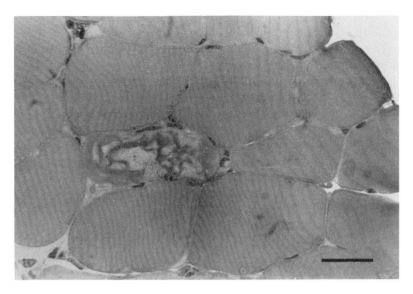

Figure 6.4.3.1 Degenerating muscle in steroid treated rat
The peripheral muscle of rat treated with nandrolone decanoate and forced to exercise. Microscopic analysis discloses focal necrosis; degenerating fibers intermingled with normal appearing fibers (scale bar = 50 μm). Morphometric analysis of these same fibers show decreased numbers of capillaries when compared to controls. Courtesy of Dr. J. M. Soares, Faculty of Sport Sciences, University of Porto, Porto, Portugal.

As yet, no jury has been willing to accept a "steroid defense" (Moss 1988), but the role of steroid abuse in the case of individual violent crimes is well worth considering. There is a firm physiologic basis for arguing that psychiatric disturbances can result from steroid abuse. Along with PCP and cocaine, steroids bind with the sigma receptor (Su 1991). This receptor is located in nonsynaptic regions of plasma membranes in the central nervous system, and peripherally in endocrine and immune tissues. Binding to the sigma receptor is thought to be the explanation for cocaine's dysphoric effects (Sharkey, Glen et al. 1988), and possibly for progesterone-related mood disturbances seen during the menstrual cycle (Backstrom, Baird et al. 1983). Since PCP also binds at the sigma receptor site, it should hardly be surprising that steroids binding to these same receptors should cause behavior changes.

6.4.4 MUSCULOSKELETAL DISEASE

Mice chronically treated with anabolic steroids have abnormal tendons. The collagen fibrils, which under normal circumstances are neatly aligned and symmetric, become crimped, fragmented, and frayed (Mincha 1986b) (Mincha 1986a). Stress testing shows that the tensile

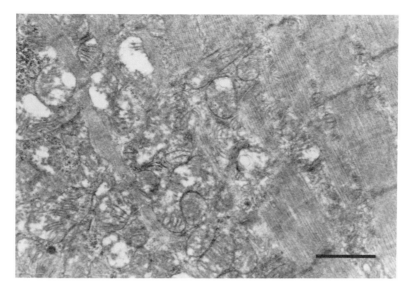

Figure 6.4.3.2 Steroid induced mitochondrial damage in rat
Electron micrographs of rats chronically treated with nandrolone show mitochondrial swelling and disruption very similar to what is seen in the hearts of animals exposed to high levels of catecholamines (Scale bar = 2 μm). Courtesy of Dr. J. M. Soares, Faculty of Sport Sciences, University of Porto, Porto, Portugal.

strength of the fibers is reduced. Light microscopic examination of tendons from these experimental animals shows no evident abnormalities, although electron microscopy will disclose alterations in the size of the collagen fibrils (Miles, Grana et al. 1992). These alterations may explain the occasional report of steroid-related tendon rupture (Hill, Suker et al. 1983) (Kramhoft and Solgaard 1986) (Laseter and Russell 1991). Avascular necrosis of the femoral heads, similar to that seen with long-term glucocorticoid therapy, has also been reported, but it is not clear that the phenomenon is due to anabolic steroid abuse. It could just as easily be an idiosyncratic reaction (Pettine 1991). Exercise-conditioned animals given anabolic steroids have reduced numbers of capillaries per muscle fiber, while at the same time the amount of fatty and connective tissue in their muscles increases (Soares and Duarte 1991). The relative decrease in the number of capillaries per fiber means that there is inefficient exchange of respiratory gases and substrates in the hypertrophied muscles. The typical histologic picture in these animals is patchy fiber necrosis. Degenerating fibers are surrounded by fibers which have normal morphology. Similar control studies in humans are lacking.

TABLE 6.4
PROFILE OF A STEROID ABUSER

Social
> Recent changes in friends, acquaintances
> Obsession with health, exercise, weight lifting
> Spends most of time in gyms or health clubs
> Takes large amounts of vitamins and food supplements
> Very high calorie intake
> Does not abuse other drugs because of concern with leading a "healthy life style"

Physical
> Rapid weight gain and muscle development
> Increased body hair, deepening of voice
> Acne (both sexes)
> Hair loss (both sexes)
> Breast enlargement (males)
> Testicular atrophy
> Difficulty urinating
> Elevated blood pressure
> Complaints of stomach upset
> Jaundice
> Edema of extremities

Mental Changes
> Increased aggression
> Hyperactivity, irritability
> Auditory hallucinations
> Paranoid delusions
> Manic episodes
> Depression and anxiety
> Panic disorders
> Suicidal thoughts

Laboratory Findings
> Decreased HDL cholesterol
> Decreased luteinizing hormone
> Decreased follicle stimulating hormone
> Decreased thyroid stimulating hormone
> Decreased thyroid hormone (T3 & T4)
> Increased liver enzymes (LDH, SGPT)
> Increased hematocrit (number of red cells)
> Increased LDL cholesterol
> Increased triglycerides
> Increased glucose

Adapted from Narducci et al: Anabolic steroids, a review of the clinical toxicology and diagnostic screening. Clinical Toxicology, 28(3):287–310.

6.4.5 DETECTING STEROID ABUSE

Medical review officers must correlate laboratory with physical findings in the diagnosis of narcotic abuse, and the situation is not dissimilar in cases of steroid abuse. A clinical profile of typical steroid abusers can be drawn, and reference to it is often helpful when the history is unclear. Typical findings are shown in Table 6.4. Testosterone blood levels remain poorly characterized. A recent study measured mean testosterone levels in conditioned athletes both before and after exercising. Resting levels were 16–17 nmol/dL. After an intense period of strength training, levels increased by 27%. Testosterone levels increased even more after endurance training (37%), but after both types of training levels returned to normal within a few hours (Jensen, Oftebro et al. 1991). At least for the time being, testosterone blood levels remain too poorly characterized to be of any use in abuse detection. Because blood testing is not yet reliable, and because it is so invasive, steroid detection programs rely entirely on the results of urine testing. Competitive athletes, who know they are subject to testing, rarely use oral anabolic agents, because it is widely known that such agents can be detected for weeks after their last use. Largely for that reason the use of injectable testosterone is becoming more and more popular. The only practical way to detect testosterone abuse is to measure the ratio of testosterone to epitestosterone in the urine. The latter is a natural breakdown product of testosterone, and the normal T/E ratio is known for the population at large. In normal young men that ratio is less than 1:3 and is probably closer to 1:1. However the International Olympic Committee, and other official sports bodies, accept any ratio of less than 1:6 as normal. In practice that means that an athlete who wants to take steroids can do so with impunity, because modest doses of testosterone will not alter the ratio sufficiently to lead to disqualification. There are even reports of testosterone abusers who titrate their dose. One week after an injection they have their T/E ratio measured. If the ratio is still low enough, they can even increase their dosage. In 1992 there was a report of college football player who vehemently denied testosterone abuse, but who nonetheless was found to have persistent ratios as high as 1:10 (Baylis, Chan et al. 1992).

Because such large sums of money are involved, considerable effort is expended on finding new ways to beat steroid testing programs. One of the newest approaches is to inject epitestosterone along with testosterone, thereby keeping the ratio of the two compounds within accepted limits. The only problem with this approach is that the absolute amount of epitestosterone in the urine will be abnormally high. As a result the International Olympic Committee (IOC) has recently banned epitestosterone use and ruled that any specimen found to contain more than 150 ng/mL of epitestosterone is suspect. The IOC is also experimenting with other ways of detecting testosterone abuse, such as measuring the ratio of testosterone to 17 alpha-hydroxyprogesterone (Carlström, Palonek, Garle et al. 1992) (Catlin, Cowan 1992).

References

Appell, H., B. Heller-Umpfenbach, M. Feraudi and H. Weicker (1983). Ultrastructural and morphometric investigations on the effects of training and administration of anabolic steroids on the myocardium of guinea pigs. Int J Sports Med. 4: 268–274.

Bäckström, T., Sanders, D., Leask, R. et al. (1989). Mood, sexuality, hormones, and the menstrual cycle II. Hormone levels and their relationship to the premenstrual syndrome. Psychosom Med 45(6):503–507.

Bagheri, S. and J. Boyer (1974). Peliosis hepatis associated with androgenic-anabolic steroid therapy. Ann Intern Med. 81:610–618.

Bahrke, M., C. Yesalis and J. Wright (1990). Psychological and behavioral effects of endogenous testosterone levels and anabolic-androgenic steroids among males. Sports Med. 10(5):303–337.

Baylis, B., S. Chan and P. Przybylski (1992). A case of naturally high urinary ratio of testosterone to epitestosterone. 44th Annual Meeting of the American Academy of Forensic Sciences.

Behrendt, H. and H. Boffin (1977). Myocardial cell lesions caused by an anabolic hormone. Cell Tissue Res. 181:423–426.

Bird, D., K. Vowles and P. Anthony (1979). Spontaneous rupture of a liver cell adenoma after long term methyl testosterone: report of a case successfully treated by emergency right hepatic lobectomy. Br J Surg. 66:212–213.

Boje, O. (1939). Doping. Bull Hlth Org League Nations 8:439–469.

Boyd, P. and G. Mark (1977). Multiple hepatic adenomas and a hepatocellular carcinoma in a man on oral methyl testosterone for 11 years. Cancer. 40: 1765–770.

Boyer, J. (1978). Androgenic-anabolic steroid associated peliosis hepatis in man - a review of 38 reported cases. Advances in pharmacology and therapeutics. Volume 8. Drug-action modifications, comparative pharmacology. Oxford, Pergamon Press.

Bruguera, M. (1975). Hepatoma associated with androgenic steroids. Lancet. i:1295.

Burger, R. and P. Marcuse (1952). Peliosis hepatis: report of a case. Am J Clin Pathol. 22:569–573.

Carlström, K., Palonek, E., Garle, M. et al. (1992). Detection of testosterone administration by increased ratio between serum concentrations of testosterone and 17 alpha-hydroxyprogesterone. Clin Chem, 38:1770–1784.

Catlin, D., Cowan, D. (1992). Detecting testosterone administration. Clin Chem, 38: 1685–1686.

Creagh, T., A. Rubin and D. Evans (1988). Hepatic tumors induced by anabolic steroids in an athlete. J Clin Pathol. 41:441–443.

Czapar, C., M. Weldon-Linne, D. Mooor and D. Rhone (1986). Peliosis hepatis in the acquired immunodeficiency syndrome. Arch Pathol Lab Med. 110:611–613.

Ducimetriere, P., E. Eschwere, L. Papoz et al. (1980). Relationship of plasma insulin levels to the incidence of myocardial infarction and coronary heart disease mortality in a middle-aged population. Diabetologia. 19:205–210.

Ferenchick, G. (1991). Anabolic/androgenic steroid abuse and thrombosis - is there a connection. Med Hypotheses. 35(1):27–31.

Ferenchick, G., and Adelman, S. (1992). Myocardial infarction associated with anabolic steroid use in a previously healthy 37-year-old weight lifter. Am Heart J, 124: 507–508.

Foss, G. and S. Simpson (1959). Oral methyltestosterone and jaundice. Br Med J. 1:259–263.

Frankle, M., R. Eichberg and S. Zachariah (1988). Anabolic androgenic steroids and a stroke in an athlete: case report. Arch Phys Med Rehabil. 69(8):632–633.

Friedl, K. (1990). Reappraisal of the health risks associated with the use of high doses of oral and injectable androgenic steroids. Anabolic Steroid Abuse. Rockville, MD, National Institute on Drug Abuse.

Friedl, K., R. Jones, C. Hannan and S. Plymate (1989). The administration of pharmacological doses of testosterone or 19-nortestosterone to normal men is not associated with increased insulin secretion or impaired glucose tolerance. J Clin Endocrinol Metab. 68:971–975.

Glazer, G. (1991). Atherogenic effects of anabolic steroids on serum lipid levels. A literature review. Arch Intern Med. 151(10):1925–1923.

Graham, S. and M. Kennedy (1990). Recent developments in the toxicology of anabolic steroids. Drug Safety. 5(6):458–476.

Hermandez-Nieto, L., M. Bruguera, S. Bombi et al. (1977). Benign liver cell adenoma associated with long term administration of an androgenic - anabolic steroid (methandienone). Cancer. 40:1761–1764.

Hill, J., J. Suker, K. Sachs and C. Brigham (1983). The athletic polydrug abuse phenomenon. A case report. Am J Sports Med. 11:269–271.

Huston, T., J. Puffer and W. Rodney (1985). The athletic heart syndrome. N Engl J Med. 313(1):24–31.

Jensen, J., H. Oftebro, B. Breigan et al. (1991). Comparison of changes in testosterone concentrations after strength and endurance exercise in well-trained men. Eur J Appl Physiol. 63(6):467–471.

Kalra, T., J. Mangla and E. DePapp (1976). Benign hepatic tumors and oral contraceptive pills. Am J Med. 61:871–877.

Karch, S. and M. Billingham (1988). The pathology and etiology of cocaine - induced heart disease. Arch Pathol Lab Med. 112:225–230.

Karch, S. and M. Billingham (1986). Myocardial contraction bands revisited. Hum Pathol. 17:9–13.

Kent, G. and J. Thompson (1961). Peliosis hepatis: involvement of reticuloen-dothelial system. Arch Pathol Lab Med. 72:658–664.

Kinson, G., Lyberry, R. & Hebert, B. (1991). Influences of anabolic androgens on cardiac growth and metabolism in the rat. Can J Physiol Pharmacol 69: 1698–1704.

Kochakian, C. (1990). History of anabolic-androgenic steroids. Anabolic Steroid Abuse. Rockville, MD, National Institute on Drug Abuse.

Kramhoft, M. and S. Solgaard (1986). Spontaneous rupture of the extensor pollicis longus tendon after anabolic steroids. J Hand Surg. 11B:87.

Laseter, J. and J. Russell (1991). Anabolic steroid-induced tendon pathology - a review of the literature. Med Sci Sports Exerc. 23(1):1–3.

Leong, S., Cazen, R., Yu, G., et al. (1992). Abdominal visceral peliosis associated with bacillary angiomatosis. Ultrastructural evidence for endothelial destruction by bacilli. Arch Pathol Lab Med, 116:866–871.

Lesna, M., I. Spencer and W. Walker (1976). Liver nodules and androgens. Lancet. i: 1124.

Lowdell, C. and I. Murray-Lyon (1985). Reversal of liver damage due to long term methyltestosterone and safety of non-17a-alkylated androgens. Br Med J. 291: 636.

Lucey, M. and R. Moseley (1987). Severe cholestasis associated with methyltestosterone: a case report. Am J Gastroenterol. 82:461–462.

Luke, J., A. Farb, R. Virmani and R. Sample (1991). Sudden cardiac death during exercise in a weight lifter using anabolic androgenic steroids: pathological and toxicological findings. J. Forensic Sci. 35(6):1441–1447.

Maciejko, J., D. Holmes, B. Kottke et al. (1983). Apolipoprotein A-I as a marker of angiographically assessed coronary-artery disease. N Engl J Med. 309:385–389.

McNutt, R., G. Ferenchick, P. Kirlin and N. Hamlin (1988). Acute myocardial infarction in a 22-year old world class weight lifter using anabolic steroids. Am J Cardiol. 62(1):164.

Miles, J., W. Grana, D. Egle, K. Min and J. Chitwood (1992). The effect of anabolic steroids on the biomechanical and histological properties of rat tendon. J Bone Joint Surg [Am]. 74A(3):411–422.

Mincha, H. (1986a). Organisation of collagen fibrils in tendon: changes induced by anabolic steroid. I. A morphometric and sterologic analysis. Virchows Arch (B). 52:87–89.

Mincha, H. (1986b). Organisation of collagen fibrils in tendon: changes induced by anabolic steroid. I. Functional and ultrastructural studies. Virchows Arch (B). 52:75–86.

Mochizuki, R. and K. Richter (1988). Cardiomyopathy and cerebrovascular accident associated with anabolic-androgenic steroid use. Physician Sportsmed. 16: 109–114.

Montine, T. and J. Gaede (1992). Massive pulmonary embolus and anabolic steroid abuse. JAMA. 267(17):2328–2329.

Moss, D. (1988). And now the steroid defense? Am Bar Assn J.(October 1):22.

Nadell, J. and J. Kosek (1977). Pelosis hepatis: 12 cases associated with oral androgen therapy. Arch Pathol Lab Med. 101:405–410.

National Institute on Drug Abuse (1990). Annual Medical Examiner Data. Data from the Drug Abuse Warning Network. Statistical Series, Number 10-B. Rockville, Maryland, U.S. Department of Health and Human Services.

Overly, W., J. Dankoff, B. Wang and U. Singh (1984). Androgens and hepatocellular carcinoma in an athlete. Ann Intern Med. 100(1):158–159.

Paradinas, F., T. Bull, D. Westaby and I. Murray-Lyon (1977). Hyperplasia and prolapse of hepatocytes into hepatic veins during long term methyltestosterone therapy: possible relationships of these changes to the development of peliosis hepatis and liver tumors. Histopathology. 1:225–226.

Pettine, K. (1991). Association of an anabolic steroids and avascular necrosis of femoral heads. Am J Sports Med. 19(1):96–98.

Phillips, M., M. Oda and K. Funatsu (1978). Evidence for microfilament involvement in norethandrolone-induced intrahepatic cholestasis. Am J Pathol. 93:729–744.

Pope, H. and D. Katz (1988). Affective and psychotic symptoms associated with anabolic steroid use. Am J Psychiatry. 145(4):487–490.

Pope, H. and D. Katz (1990). Homicide and near homicide by anabolic steroid users. J Clin Psych. 51:28–31.

Plymate, S., and Friedl, K. (1992). Anabolic steroids and muscle strength. Ann Intern Med, 116(3):270.

Reichenbach, D. and E. Benditt (1970). Catecholamines and cardiomyopathy. Hum Pathol. 1(1):125–150.

Rosendorff, C., J. Hoffman, E. Verner et al. (1981). Cholesterol potentiates the coronary artery response to norepinephrine in anesthetized and conscious dogs. Circ Res. 48(3):320–329.

Sano, T., T. Motomiya and H. Yamazaki (1983). Influence of lipids on platelet activation in vivo. Thromb Res. 31:675–684.

Sharkey, J., K. Glen, S. Wolfe and M. Kuhar (1988). Cocaine binding at sigma receptors. Euro J Pharmacol. 149:171–174.

Soares, J. and J. Duarte (1991). Effects of training and an anabolic steroid on murine red skeletal muscle - a stereological analysis. Acta Anat. 142(2):183–187.

Stromeyer, F. and K. Ishak (1981). Nodular transformation of the liver: a clinicopathologic study of 30 cases. Hum Pathol. 12:60–71.

Su, T.-P. (1991). Review: Sigma receptors. Putative links between nervous, endocrine and immune systems. Euro J Biochem. 200:633–642.

Takala, T., P. Ramo, K. Kiviluoma et al. (1991). Effects of training and anabolic steroids on collagen synthesis in dog heart. Eur J Appl Physiol. 62(1):1–6.

Taxy, J. (1978). Peliosis: a morphologic curiosity becomes an iatrogenic problem. Hum Pathol. 9:331–340.

Tesch, P. (1987). Acute and long-term metabolic changes consequent to heavy-resistance exercise. Med Sport Sci. 26:67–89.

Thompson, P., Cullinane, E, Sady,S. et al. (1989). Contrasting effects of testosterone and stanozolol on serum lipoprotein levels. JAMA. 261:1165–1168.

Wakabayashi, T., H. Onda, T. Tada et al. (1984). High incidence of peliosis hepatis in autopsy cases of aplastic anemia with special reference to anabolic steroid therapy. Acta Pathol Jpn. 34:1079–1086.

Westaby, D., S. Ogle, F. Paradinas et al. (1977). Liver damage from long-term methyl-testosterone. Lancet. ii:261–263.

Westaby, D., B. Portmann and R. Williams (1983). Androgen related primary hepatic tumors in non-Fanconi patients. Cancer. 51:1947–1952.

Winwood, P., D. Robertson and R. Wright (1990). Bleeding oesophageal varices associated with anabolic steroid use in an athlete. Postgrad Med J. 66:864–865.

Yesalis, C., W. Anderson, W. Buckley and J. Wright (1990). Incidence of the nonmedical use of anabolic-androgenic steroids. Anabolic Steroid Abuse. Rockville, MD, National Institute on Drug Abuse.

Zak, F. (1950). Peliosis hepatis. Am J Pathol. 26:1–15.

Index